D0743591

ORGAN PHYSIOLOGY

STRUCTURE AND FUNCTION OF THE NERVOUS SYSTEM

Second Edition

ARTHUR C. GUYTON, M.D.

*Professor and Chairman of the Department of Physiology
and Biophysics, University of Mississippi School of Medicine*

1976

W. B. SAUNDERS COMPANY · PHILADELPHIA · LONDON · TORONTO

W. B. Saunders Company: West Washington Square
Philadelphia, PA 19105

12 Dyott Street
London, WC1A 1DB

833 Oxford Street
Toronto, Ontario M8Z 5T9, Canada

ORGAN PHYSIOLOGY—Structure and Function of the Nervous System   ISBN 0-7216-4366-3

Last digit is the print number: 9   8   7   6   5   4   3   2   1

PREFACE

This text, which is derived almost entirely from my Textbook of Medical Physiology, 5th Edition, is intended for those persons—medical students, paramedical students, students of psychology, students of basic physiology, and others—who wish to study the general organization and function of the nervous system without the detail often associated with a research-oriented text. Also, neuroanatomy is presented only to the extent that it is important to understanding how the nervous system performs its many tasks; this means mainly emphasis on nerve tracts and on function of the nerve signals when they reach their destination.

I have tried above all to present the beauty and logic intrinsic in the design of the nervous system—the automaticity of such feats as walking, sleeping, waking, and even search for food; the inbred pace-setting effects of emotions; and the almost magic processes for channeling, storing, and deciphering information. The nervous system is an overall controller of our bodily function. It is a computer with capabilities that have never yet been duplicated by the most massive electronic computer. And it is that quality of our being that makes life meaningful, thoughtful, exciting.

At many points in the text, one will find discussion of neurological illnesses as examples of abnormal function of the nervous system. These are presented not with the view that this book is dedicated only to medical students but, instead, because of the enlightening experience that a student can achieve when he correlates basic conceptual knowledge with happenings in the world about him. Indeed, in many instances, understanding the neurological abnormality adds immeasurably to one's understanding of basic neurophysiological concepts. Therefore, even for the non-medically oriented student, the discussions of abnormal function in the nervous system are meant to give values that are difficult to establish in other ways.

I wish to thank many others who have made this text possible, particularly Mrs. Billie Howard for her excellent secretarial service, Mrs. Carolyn Hull and Miss Tomiko Mita for preparing the figures, and the staff of the W. B. Saunders Company for its continued excellence in editing and preparing the text for publication.

ARTHUR C. GUYTON

CONTENTS

PART I   NERVE AND MUSCLE

CHAPTER 1

PART II   THE NERVOUS SYSTEM

CHAPTER 5

TRANSMISSION AND PROCESSING OF INFORMATION IN THE NERVOUS SYSTEM

CHAPTER 6

SENSORY RECEPTORS AND THEIR BASIC MECHANISMS OF ACTION

CHAPTER 9

MOTOR FUNCTIONS OF THE SPINAL CORD AND THE CORD REFLEXES

CHAPTER 10

MOTOR FUNCTIONS OF THE BRAIN STEM AND BASAL GANGLIA—RETICULAR FORMATION, VESTIBULAR APPARATUS, EQUILIBRIUM, AND BRAIN STEM REFLEXES

CHAPTER 13

THE CEREBRAL CORTEX AND INTELLECTUAL FUNCTIONS OF THE BRAIN

CHAPTER 14

BEHAVIORAL FUNCTIONS OF THE BRAIN: THE LIMBIC SYSTEM, ROLE OF THE HYPOTHALAMUS, AND CONTROL OF VEGETATIVE FUNCTIONS OF THE BODY

PART III   THE SPECIAL SENSES

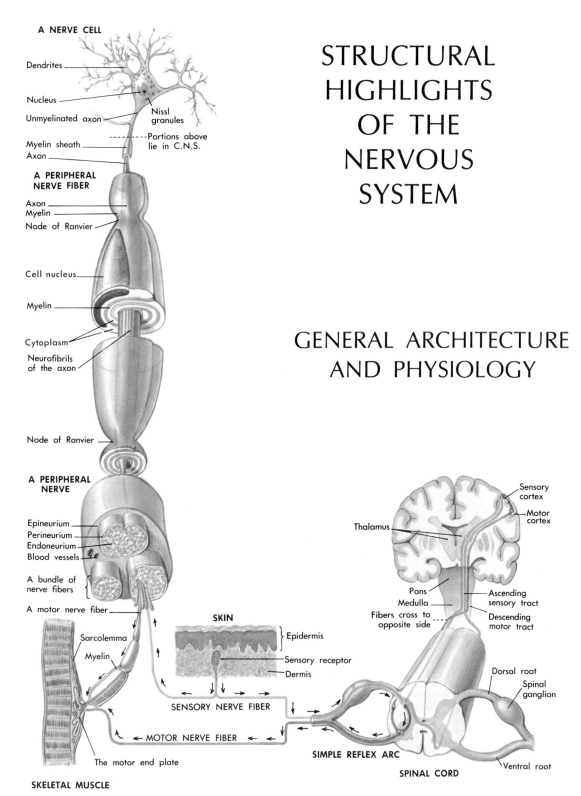

A NERVE CELL

Dendrites

Nucleus

Unmyelinated axon

Nissl granules

Myelin sheath

Portions above lie in C.N.S.

Axon

A PERIPHERAL NERVE FIBER

Axon

Myelin

Node of Ranvier

Cell nucleus

Myelin

Cytoplasm

Neurofibrils of the axon

Node of Ranvier

A PERIPHERAL NERVE

Epineurium

Perineurium

Endoneurium

Blood vessels

A bundle of nerve fibers

A motor nerve fiber

Sarcolemma

Myelin

The motor end plate

SKELETAL MUSCLE

SKIN

Epidermis

Sensory receptor

Dermis

SENSORY NERVE FIBER

← MOTOR NERVE FIBER ←

SIMPLE REFLEX ARC

STRUCTURAL HIGHLIGHTS OF THE NERVOUS SYSTEM

GENERAL ARCHITECTURE AND PHYSIOLOGY

Sensory cortex

Motor cortex

Thalamus

Pons

Medulla

Fibers cross to opposite side

Ascending sensory tract

Descending motor tract

Dorsal root

Spinal ganglion

Ventral root

SPINAL CORD

Plate 1

BRAIN AND SPINAL NERVES

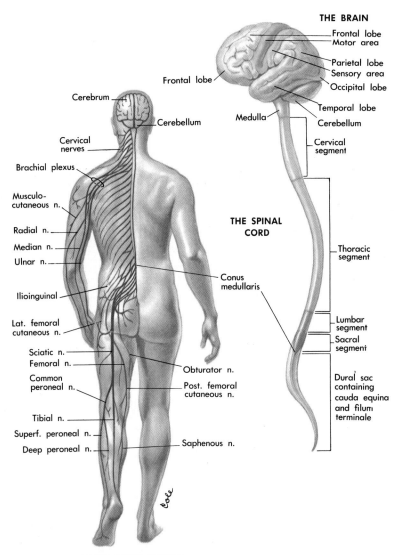

THE BRAIN

Frontal lobe
Motor area
Parietal lobe
Sensory area
Occipital lobe
Temporal lobe
Cerebellum

Frontal lobe

Medulla

Cervical
segment

Cerebrum

Cerebellum

Cervical
nerves

Brachial plexus

Musculo-
cutaneous n.

**THE SPINAL
CORD**

Radial n.

Median n.

Ulnar n.

Thoracic
segment

Ilioinguinal

Conus
medullaris

Lat. femoral
cutaneous n.

Sciatic n.

Femoral n.

Obturator n.

Common
peroneal n.

Post. femoral
cutaneous n.

Lumbar
segment

Sacral
segment

Dural sac
containing
cauda equina
and filum
terminale

Tibial n.

Superf. peroneal n.

Deep peroneal n.

Saphenous n.

THE MAJOR SPINAL NERVES

Plate 2

AUTONOMIC NERVES

Brain

Ciliary ganglion

Lacrimal gland

Eye

Sphenopalatine ganglion

Oculomotor nerve III

Facial nerve VII

Glossopharyngeal nerve IX

Sup. cervical ganglion

Parotid gland

Otic ganglion

Sublingual and submandibular glands

Submandibular ganglion

Vagus nerve X

Trachea

T1
2
3
4
5
6
7
8
9
10
11
12
L1
2
3

Lung

Heart

Greater splanchnic nerve

Lesser splanchnic nerve

Liver
Gallbladder

Least splanchnic nerve

Suprarenal gland

Renal plexus

Kidney

Stomach

Celiac plexus

Aortic plexus

Colon

Sup. mesenteric plexus

Small intestine

Inf. mesenteric plexus

Hypogastric plexus

S2

S3

S4

Spinal cord

Vertebral ganglia (sympathetic trunk)

Ovary

Uterus

Testis

Bladder

Pelvic nerves

Pelvic plexus

Urethra

SYMPATHETIC
Thoracolumbar outflow

Preganglionic sympathetic fibers
Postganglionic sympathetic fibers
Preganglionic parasympathetic fibers
Postganglionic parasympathetic fibers

PARASYMPATHETIC
Craniosacral outflow

Plate 3

ORGANS OF SPECIAL SENSE

Middle ear bones:

Malleus
Incus
Stapes

Epitympanic recess
in temporal bone

External ear

External ear canal

Inner ear:

Semicircular canals

Cochlea

Eardrum
Tympanic cavity
Eustachian tube

THE ORGAN OF HEARING

Lacrimal sac
Lacrimal ducts

Lacrimal glands

Excretory ducts

Conjunctiva

Pupil

Iris

Nasolacrimal
duct

THE LACRIMAL APPARATUS AND THE EYE

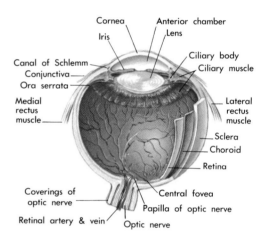

HORIZONTAL SECTION OF THE EYE

Cornea
Iris

Anterior chamber
Lens

Ciliary body
Ciliary muscle

Canal of Schlemm
Conjunctiva
Ora serrata

Medial
rectus
muscle

Lateral
rectus
muscle

Sclera
Choroid

Retina

Coverings of
optic nerve

Retinal artery & vein

Central fovea

Papilla of optic nerve

Optic nerve

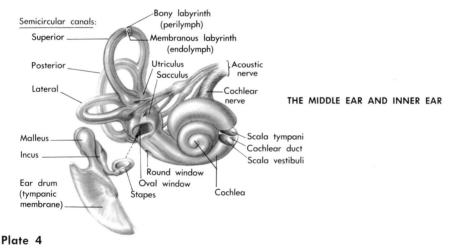

Semicircular canals:

Superior

Posterior

Lateral

Malleus

Incus

Ear drum
(tympanic
membrane)

Bony labyrinth
(perilymph)

Membranous labyrinth
(endolymph)

Utriculus
Sacculus

Acoustic
nerve

Cochlear
nerve

Round window
Oval window
Stapes

Scala tympani
Cochlear duct
Scala vestibuli

Cochlea

THE MIDDLE EAR AND INNER EAR

Plate 4

PART I
NERVE AND MUSCLE

1

Membrane Potentials, Action Potentials, Excitation, and Rhythmicity

Electrical potentials exist across the membranes of essentially all cells of the body, and some cells, such as nerve and muscle cells, are "excitable"—that is, capable of transmitting electrochemical impulses along their membranes. And in still other types of cells, such as glandular cells, macrophages, and ciliated cells, changes in membrane potentials probably play significant roles in controlling many of the cell's functions. However, the present discussion is concerned with membrane potentials generated both at rest and during action by nerve and muscle cells.

BASIC PHYSICS OF MEMBRANE POTENTIALS

Before beginning this discussion, let us first recall that the fluids both inside and outside the cells are electrolytic solutions containing approximately 155 mEq./liter of anions and the same concentration of cations. Generally, a very minute excess of negative ions (anions) accumulates immediately inside the cell membrane along its inner surface, and an equal number of positive ions (cations) accumulates immediately outside the membrane. The effect of this is the development of a *membrane potential*.

The two basic means by which membrane potentials can develop are: (1) active transport of ions through the membrane, thus creating an imbalance of negative and positive charges on the two sides of the membrane, and (2) diffusion of ions through the membrane as a result of a concentration difference between the two sides of the membrane, this also creating an imbalance of charges.

MEMBRANE POTENTIALS CAUSED BY ACTIVE TRANSPORT—THE "ELECTROGENIC PUMP"

Figure 1–1A illustrates how the process of active transport can create a membrane potential. In this figure equal concentrations of anions, which are *negatively charged,* are present both inside and outside the nerve fiber. However, in the membrane is a chemical system called the "sodium pump." This actively transports *positively charged* sodium ions to the exterior of the fiber. Thus, more negatively charged anions than positively charged sodium ions remain inside the nerve fiber, causing negativity on the inside. On the other hand, outside the fiber there are more positively charged sodium ions than negatively charged anions, thus causing positivity outside the fiber. A pump such as this, which causes the development of a membrane potential, is called an *electrogenic pump*.

In most nerve and muscle cells potassium is pumped into the cell at the same time that sodium is pumped out; usually, however, two to five times as much sodium as potassium is pumped. Because of this imbalance of pumping, the pump is still considered electrogenic.

The Cell Membrane as a Capacitor. Note in Figure 1–1A that the negative and positive ionic charges are shown lined up against the membrane. This occurs because the negative charges inside the membrane and the positive charges on the outside pull each other together at the membrane barrier, thus creating an abrupt change in electrical potential across the cell membrane.

This alignment of electrical charges on the two sides of the membrane is exactly the same process that takes place when an electrical capacitor becomes charged with electricity. In the cell membrane, the lipid matrix of the cell is the *dielectric*, much as mica is frequently used as a dielectric in an electrical capacitor. It will be recalled that a capacitor's capacity for holding electrical charges is inversely proportional to the thickness of the membrane. Because of the extreme thinness of the cell membrane (70 to 100 Ångstroms), the capacitance of the cell membrane is tremendous for its area—about 1 microfarad per square centimeter.

Though the figures of this chapter will show large numbers of negative or positive ions (or charges) lined up against the nerve membrane, in actuality, very few positive or negative ions actually need to line up on the two sides of the membrane to create the usual membrane potential of nerves. In the case of the usual nerve fiber, only about 1/50,000 to 1/500,00 of the positive charges inside the nerve fiber need to be transferred to the outside of the fiber to create the normal nerve potential of −85 millivolts inside the fiber.

MEMBRANE POTENTIALS CAUSED BY DIFFUSION

Figure 1–1B illustrates the nerve fiber under another condition in which the permeability of the membrane to sodium has increased so much that diffusion of sodium through the membrane is now great in comparison with the transport of sodium by active transport. Since the sodium and anion concentrations are great outside the cell and slight inside, the positively charged sodium ions now move rapidly to the inside of the membrane, leaving an excess of negative charges outside, but creating an excess of positive charges inside.

Relationship of the Diffusion Potential to the Concentration Difference—The Nernst Equation. When a concentration difference of ions across a membrane causes diffusion of ions through the membrane, thus creating a membrane potential, the magnitude of the potential is determined by the ratio of tendency for the ions to diffuse in one direction versus the other direction, which is determined by the following formula (at body temperature, 38°C.):

$$\text{EMF (in millivolts)} = 61 \log \frac{\text{Conc. inside}}{\text{Conc. outside}} \quad (1)$$

Thus, when the concentration of ions on one side of a membrane is 10 times that on the other, the log of 10 is 1, and the potential difference calculates to be 61 millivolts. This equation is called the *Nernst Equation*.

However, two conditions are necessary for a membrane potential to develop as a result of diffusion: (1) The membrane must be semipermeable, allowing ions of one charge to diffuse through the pores more readily than ions of the opposite charge. (2) The concentration of the diffusible ions must be greater on one side of the membrane than on the other side.

Calculation of the Membrane Potential when the Membrane is Permeable to Several Different Ions. When a membrane is permeable to several different ions, the diffusion potential that will develop depends on three factors: (1) the polarity of the electrical charge of each ion, (2) the permeability of the membrane (P) to each ion, and (3) the concentration of the respective ions on the two sides of the membrane. Thus, the following formula, called the *Goldman equation*, gives the calculated membrane potential when two univalent cations (C) and two univalent anions (A) are involved.

Figure 1–1. (A) Establishment of a membrane potential as a result of active transport of sodium ions. (B) Establishment of a membrane potential of opposite polarity caused by rapid diffusion of sodium ions from an area of high concentration to an area of low concentration.

$$\text{EMF(in millivolts)} =$$

$$-61 \log \frac{C_{1_i}P_1 + C_{2_i}P_2 + A_{3_o}P_3 + A_{4_o}P_4}{C_{1_o}P_1 + C_{2_o}P_2 + A_{3_i}P_3 + A_{4_i}P_4} \quad (2)$$

Note that a cation gradient from the inside (*i*) to the outside (*o*) of a membrane causes electronegativity inside the membrane, while an anion gradient in *exactly the opposite direction* also causes electronegativity on the inside.

ORIGIN OF THE CELL MEMBRANE POTENTIAL

Role of Sodium and Potassium Pumps and of Nondiffusible Anions in the Origin of the Cell Membrane Potential. Before attempting to explain the origin of the cell membrane potential, several basic facts need to be understood as follows:

1. The nerve membrane is endowed with a sodium and a potassium pump, sodium being pumped to the exterior and potassium to the interior. These pumps were discussed in Chapter 4.

2. The resting nerve membrane is normally 50 to 100 times as permeable to potassium as to sodium. Therefore, potassium diffuses with relative ease through the resting membrane, whereas sodium diffuses only with difficulty.

3. Inside the nerve fiber are large numbers of anions (negatively charged) that cannot diffuse through the nerve membrane at all or that diffuse very poorly. These anions include especially organic phosphate ions, sulfate ions, and protein ions.

Now, let us put the above facts together to see how the resting nerve membrane potential comes about. First, sodium is pumped to the outside of the fiber, while potassium is pumped to the inside. However, because two to five sodium ions are pumped out of the fiber for every potassium ion that is pumped in, more positive ions are continually being pumped out of the fiber than into it. Since most of the anions inside the nerve fiber are nondiffusible, the negative charges remain inside the nerve fiber so that the inside of the fiber becomes electronegative, while the outside becomes electropositive, as illustrated in Figure 1–2.

Equilibration of Sodium Ion Transfer in the Two Directions Across the Membrane—Maximum Potential Caused by the Electrogenic Sodium Pump. As progressively more sodium ions are pumped out of the nerve

Figure 1–2. Establishment of a membrane potential of −85 millivolts in the normal resting nerve fiber, and development of concentration differences of sodium and potassium ions between the two sides of the membrane. The dashed arrows represent diffusion and the solid arrows represent active transport (pumps).

fiber, they begin to diffuse back into the nerve fiber for two reasons: (1) a sodium concentration gradient develops from the outside of the fiber toward the inside, and (2) a negative membrane potential develops inside the fiber and attracts the positively charged sodium ions inward. Eventually, there comes a point at which the inward diffusion equals the outward pumping by the sodium pump. When this occurs, the pump has reached its maximum capability to cause net transfer of sodium ions to the outside. This occurs when the sodium ion concentration inside the nerve fiber falls to about 10 mEg./liter (in contrast to 142 mEg./liter in the extracellular fluids) and when the membrane potential inside the fiber falls to approximately −85 millivolts. Therefore, this −85 millivolts is also the *resting potential* of the nerve membrane.

Equilibration of Potassium Ion Transfer Across the Membrane. At the same time that the sodium pump pumps sodium ions to the exterior, a coupled potassium pump pumps about one third as many potassium ions to the interior. However, the resting membrane is 50 to 100 times as permeable to potassium ions as to sodium ions, which means that each time potassium ions are pumped in they tend to diffuse back out of the fiber almost immediately. Therefore, because the potassium pump is considerably weaker than the sodium pump and because the back leakage of potassium ions is very great, the potassium pump by itself can build up only a slight excess of potassium ions inside the nerve fiber.

Yet, it is known that potassium ions do build up to a high concentration inside the nerve fiber. How could this be, if it is not caused by the potassium pump? The answer is that there is a high degree of negativity created inside the fiber by the sodium pump. The −85 millivolts inside the fiber attracts the positive potassium ions from the exterior to the inside, and this attraction accounts for most of the buildup of potassium ions inside the fiber, while the potassium pump accounts for only a small proportion of the buildup.

Thus, from a quantitative point of view, once the membrane has reached a steady state condition, there are three factors that affect the equilibration of potassium ions on the two sides of the membrane: (1) the potassium pump pumping potassium ions *inward,* (2) the electrical gradient causing *inward* diffusion of potassium ions, and (3) the concentration gradient caused by the buildup of potassium ions inside the fiber causing diffusion of potassium ions *outward.* In the steady state condition, the above three factors all come to exact quantitative equilibrium; that is, the two factors causing inward movement of potassium become exactly equal to the single factor causing outward movement.

Application of the Nernst Equation to the Dynamics of Potassium Transfer Equilibration Across the Nerve Fiber Membrane. Since the resting membrane is quite permeable to potassium ions and since the pump is a very weak one, the factors that dominate the distribution of potassium ions across the membrane are the two factors that cause potassium ion diffusion, that is, (1) the concentration gradient that causes potassium ion diffusion out of the fiber and (2) the voltage gradient that causes potassium ion diffusion inward. If the pump were entirely inactive, the rates of diffusion of potassium ions in opposite directions caused by these two factors would be

exactly equal, and under these conditions the Nernst equation would give the exact relationship between the concentrations on the two sides of the membrane and the equilibrium membrane potential. Therefore, let us assume that the negative voltage of −85 millivolts has already been created by the sodium pump and that the extracellular fluid potassium ion concentration is 5 mEq./liter. Substituting these values in the Nernst equation, we obtain the following:

$$-85 = -61 \log \frac{K^+ \text{ Conc. (inside)}}{5}$$

Now, solving this equation for the concentration of potassium ions inside the nerve fiber, we find that the equilibrium level of potassium ions inside would be about 125 mEq./liter. Thus, of the 140 mEq./liter of potassium inside the nerve fiber, 125 of these are caused simply by diffusion into the nerve fiber resulting from the −85 millivolts that had previously been created by the sodium pump. The remaining 15 mEq./liter of potassium ions results from the action of the potassium pump.

We can also use the Nernst equation in still another way to test the degree of diffusional equilibration of potassium ions across the membrane. Given a concentration of potassium ions inside the fiber of 140 mEq./liter and a concentration outside of 5 mEq./liter what membrane potential would be required to establish diffusional equilibrium at the membrane, assuming that there were no potassium pump? Substituting these values in the Nernst equation and solving gives a membrane potential of −88.3 millivolts. This is only 3.3 millivolts more negative than the usual resting membrane potential of the nerve fiber. Therefore, under most conditions, the distribution of potassium ions between the inside of the fiber and the outside can be considered to be very nearly that required to satisfy the Nernst equation.

The Nernst Potential for Sodium Distribution. Now, let us calculate the Nernst potential for sodium as follows:

$$\text{Nernst potential} \atop (Na^+) = -61 \log \frac{Na^+ \text{ (inside)}}{Na^+ \text{ (outside)}}$$

$$= -61 \log \frac{10}{142}$$

$$= +70 \text{ millivolts}$$

Thus, it is clear that the −85 millivolts of the

resting nerve is actually opposite to the +70 millivolts predicted by the Nernst equation. The reason for this is that the sodium pump completely dominates the picture in the resting state, and the diffusional factors (which cause development of the Nernst potential) are of very little significance. We shall see, however, that when a nerve impulse is being conducted, this is not true. During conduction of an impulse the membrane permeability to sodium increases several thousand-fold, sodium diffusion becomes very great, and the membrane potential inside the fiber then rises abruptly from -85 millivolts to about $+45$ millivolts, approaching the Nernst potential for sodium.

Role of Chloride and Other Ions. Chloride ions are not pumped through the nerve membrane in either direction. However, they readily diffuse through the membrane. Because there is no pump to force buildup of a concentration difference of chloride ions across the membrane, the distribution of chloride ions on the two sides of the membrane is determined entirely by electrical potential. That is, the negativity that develops inside the membrane repels chloride ions from inside the fiber and causes the chloride concentration to fall to a very low value, about 4 mEq./liter in comparison with an extracellular fluid concentration of about 103 mEq./liter. Because there is no chloride pump, the Nernst equation can be used to calculate the exact concentration ratio of chloride ions on the two sides of the membrane when the membrane potential is known and when the membrane is in an equilibrium state. Thus, chloride ions play only a passive role. Later in the chapter we will discuss instantaneous changes in membrane potential caused by the so-called action potential. Under these conditions, chloride ions move rapidly through the membrane and affect the duration and the magnitude of the action potential, but again their role is a passive one.

Essentially the same principles as those for sodium, potassium, and chloride distribution across the membrane also apply to other ions. Magnesium ions are affected in much the same way as potassium, and calcium ions in much the same manner as sodium ions. However, the concentrations and permeabilities of magnesium and calcium ions are small enough that the total number of electrical charges actually involved is also small. Yet both of these ions affect membrane potentials in another way, by altering the permeability of the membrane to other ions, a subject that is discussed at greater length later in the chapter.

Membrane Potentials Measured in Nerve and Muscle Fibers. Figure 1–3 illustrates a method that has been used for measuring the resting membrane potential. A micropipet is made from a minute capillary glass tube so that the tip of the pipet has a diameter of only 0.25 to

Figure 1–3. Measurement of the membrane potential of the nerve fiber using a microelectrode.

2 microns. Inside the pipet is a solution of potassium chloride, which acts as an electrical conductor. The fiber whose membrane is to be measured is pierced with the pipet and electrical connections are made from the pipet to an appropriate meter, as illustrated in the figure. The resting membrane potential measured in many different nerve and skeletal muscle fibers of mammals has usually ranged between -75 and -95 millivolts, with -85 millivolts as a reasonable average of the different measurements.

THE ACTION POTENTIAL

So long as the membrane of the nerve fiber remains completely undisturbed, the membrane potential remains approximately -85 millivolts, which is called the *resting potential*. However, any factor that suddenly increases the permeability of the membrane to sodium is likely to elicit a *sequence of rapid changes* in membrane potential lasting a minute fraction of a second, followed immediately thereafter by return of the membrane potential to its resting value. This sequence of potential changes is called the *action potential*.

Some of the factors that can elicit an action potential are *electrical stimulation* of the membrane, *application of chemicals* to the membrane to cause increased permeability to sodium, *mechanical damage* to the membrane, *heat, cold,* or almost any other factor that momentarily disturbs the normal resting state of the membrane.

Depolarization and Repolarization. The action potential occurs in two separate stages called depolarization and repolarization, which may be explained by referring to Figure 1–4. Figure 1–4A illustrates the resting state of the membrane, with negativity inside and positivity outside. When the permeability of the mem-

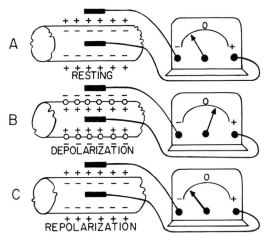

Figure 1–4. Sequential events during the action potential, showing: (A) the normal resting potential, (B) development of a reversal potential during depolarization, and (C) re-establishment of the normal resting potential during repolarization.

brane pores to sodium ions suddenly increases, many of the sodium ions rush to the inside of the fiber, carrying enough positive charges to the inside to cause complete disappearance of the normal resting potential and usually enough charges actually to develop a positive state inside the fiber instead of the normal negative state, as illustrated in Figure 1–4B. This positive state inside the fiber is called the *reversal potential.*

Almost immediately after depolarization takes place, the pores of the membrane again become almost totally impermeable to sodium ions. Because of this, the positive reversal potential inside the fiber disappears, and the normal resting membrane potential returns. This is called *repolarization* (Fig. 1–4C).

Now, let us explain in more detail *how* this sequence of events occurs.

MEMBRANE PERMEABILITY CHANGES FOR SODIUM AND POTASSIUM DURING THE ACTION POTENTIAL

The action potential is caused by a sequence of changes in the membrane permeability for sodium and potassium.

The *first event* is a tremendous *increase in sodium permeability*—as much as a 5000-fold increase. Because of the very high concentration of sodium outside the fiber, sodium ions now diffuse rapidly to the inside, carrying positive charges and changing the inside electrical potential from negativity to positivity.

The *second event* is an *increase in potassium permeability* coupled with a simultaneous *decrease of the sodium permeability* back to normal. This allows large quantities of positively charged potassium ions to diffuse out of the fiber, a diffusion which returns the inside membrane potential back to its negative resting level.

The *third event* is a *decrease of the potassium permeability* back to normal.

The *fourth event* is *active transport of sodium back out of the nerve fiber* and, concurrently, both active transport and diffusion of potassium ions back into the nerve fiber, thus re-establishing the original state of the fiber.

Sodium "Channels" and Potassium "Channels."   The sodium and potassium ions are believed to diffuse through pores in the membrane. However, the sodium ions are thought to move through one set of pores called *sodium channels* whereas the potassium ions move through another set of pores called *potassium channels.* The actual anatomical structures of these channels are not known, but some physiologists believe that they are actual physical pores. Other physiologists believe that they are openings within the latticeworks of complex protein molecules that penetrate all the way through the membrane; still others have differing concepts of the "pores." Yet, regardless of what these structures are, they have physiological properties *as if* the sodium channels were actual oval pores with dimensions of about 3 by 5 Ångstroms and the potassium channels were round pores with dimensions of about 3 by 3 Ångstroms.

Each channel is believed to be guarded by a "gate" that can open and close the channel. Under resting conditions both the sodium and potassium channels are almost completely closed; therefore, relatively few sodium and potassium ions can diffuse through the two respective channels (though the potassium channels are some 50 to 100 times as permeable as the sodium channels, which allows far more potassium diffusion than sodium, as already explained). Yet, when the gates open, the permeability of the sodium channels can increase as much as 5000-fold and the permeability of the potassium channels as much as 50-fold.

Opening the Gates—the Gating Potential.   The gates themselves are believed to be positive charges that are fixed inside the channels, at their openings, or in the lipid matrix adjacent to the channels. These positive charges create a positive electric field that protrudes far into the channels and, therefore, blocks positive ion permeability. Alternatively, the field can be pulled back from the channel and thereby increase the channel permeability. It is believed that this closing and opening of the gates is caused by electrical potentials called *gating potentials* that occur in the lipid matrix of the cell membrane adjacent to the channels. That is, an appropriate electrical potential appearing in the lipid matrix near a pore can either close or open the gate, depending on the polarity of the potential.

With this background we can now discuss more intelligently the mechanisms for the changes in sodium and potassium permeabilities during the action potential.

Sudden Increase in Sodium Permeability at the Onset of the Action Potential—"Activation" of the Membrane. In the resting state the gate of the sodium channel is closed. However, any sudden change in electrical potential across the membrane that causes the potential inside the fiber to become suddenly less negative will also cause a simultaneous change in the gating potential of the sodium channel and increase the channel's permeability; that is, the gate will begin to open. Once the gate has begun this opening, the process becomes a *regenerative* vicious cycle: sodium ions diffuse to the interior; the internal negativity becomes still less; the gate opens even more widely; and the process continues until the gate is wide open. Therefore, the permeability of the sodium gate increases rapidly and drastically. This is illustrated by the lowermost curve of Figure 1–5, which shows that at the onset of the action potential the permeability of the membrane for sodium (measured as sodium "conductance") increases several thousand-fold in only a small fraction of a millisecond. This tremendous increase in sodium permeability is called *activation of the membrane.*

Closure of the Sodium Gates and Decrease in Sodium Permeability—Membrane Inactivation. Immediately after the sodium gates have opened widely, for reasons not now known, these gates immediately begin to close again. This is illustrated by the rapid decrease in sodium conductance in Figure 1–5. This closure of the sodium gates is called *membrane inactivation.*

Thus, at the onset of an action potential, the sodium channels open widely for a fraction of a millisecond and then they close almost equally as rapidly. Yet, during this short period of time, large quantities of sodium ions diffuse to the

interior of the fiber, thereby increasing the membrane potential from its normal negative value of −85 millivolts up to a positive value of approximately +45 millivolts.

Closure of the sodium channels—that is, inactivation of the membrane—does not in itself return the potential back to the negative value because once the sodium ions have moved to the interior, the inside of the fiber has become charged to a positive voltage, and will remain at this voltage until some other movement of ions through the membrane changes the voltage again. But, within a fraction of a millisecond potassium ions diffuse to the exterior, as described below, to return the membrane potential back to its resting value.

Possible Role of Calcium Ions in Closing the Sodium Gates. When calcium ions are deficient

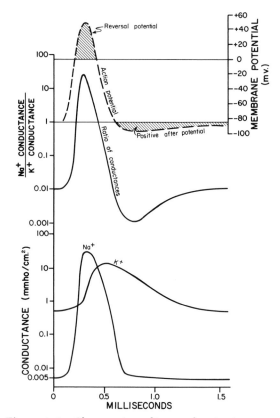

Figure 1–5. Changes in sodium and potassium conductances during the course of the action potential. Note that sodium conductance increases several thousand-fold during the early stages of the action potential, while potassium conductance increases only about 30-fold during the latter stages of the action potential and for a short period thereafter. (Curves constructed from data in Hodgkin and Huxley papers but transposed from squid axon to apply to the membrane potentials of large mammalian nerve fibers.)

in the extracellular fluids, the sodium gates will not close fully between action potentials, and the membrane remains very leaky to sodium ions—sometimes so much so that the membrane remains depolarized continuously or fires repetitively. Because of this effect, it is believed that calcium ions in some way play a significant role in the closure of the sodium gates. One theory is that the calcium ions bind with the outside of the cell membrane at or near the openings to the sodium channels. The presence of the electropositive charge created by the calcium ions then creates a positive field near the channels and blocks entry of sodium ions. At the onset of the next action potential, the first event is theoretically to remove these calcium ions, an occurrence which supposedly increases the permeability of the sodium channels to sodium ions.

Delayed Increase, and Subsequent Decrease, in Potassium Permeability During the Action Potential. Referring again to Figure 1–5, we see that the potassium permeability (as measured by conductance) does not change significantly during the first half of the action potential. Yet, toward the end of the action potential, the potassium permeability now increases about fifty-fold. This allows very rapid movement of potassium ions out of the fiber to the exterior. Because the sodium gates have already closed by this time, this loss of positive charges from the interior of the fiber causes rapid return of the membrane potential back to its normal resting value of −85 millivolts.

Figure 1–5 also shows that the potassium permeability remains elevated for a short period even after the major portion of the action potential is over, but within a millisecond or so it returns to normal. By this time the membrane potential has returned almost exactly to its original resting negative level.

Unfortunately, the factors that cause opening and closing of these potassium channels are even less well understood than those for the sodium channels. However, the potassium ion permeability does seem to be determined mainly by the electrical potential that exists at any given time across the membrane. When the potential becomes positive on the inside, the potassium ion permeability increases; when negative, it decreases. Therefore, when the action potential becomes positive, after a fraction of a millisecond lag time, potassium permeability automatically increases, and then when the action potential becomes negative again, after another millisecond or so lag, the potassium

permeability decreases back to its original level.

Therefore, for the time being, without knowing the reasons why, we are forced simply to accept the major changes in sodium and potassium permeabilities during the course of the action potential. A simple way to remember these is that the sodium channels open widely for a fraction of a millisecond at the onset of the action potential, and at this time the inward flux of sodium ions increases the inside potential from negativity to positivity. Then, within another fraction of a millisecond the sodium channels close while the potassium channels open for about a millisecond; the resulting efflux of potassium ions returns the membrane potential back approximately to its resting negative level.

SUMMARY OF THE EVENTS OF THE ACTION POTENTIAL

We can now summarize the action potential by referring specifically to the action potential shown at the top of Figure 1–5 and to the conductance changes for sodium and potassium at the bottom of this figure. When the sodium channels open and sodium ions pour to the inside of the membrane, the positive charges of the sodium ions not only neutralize the normal electronegativity inside the fiber but also create an excess of positive charges, thereby making the membrane potential inside the fiber positive. This is called the *reversal potential,* and for large myelinated nerve fibers it is normally about +45 millivolts.

Then, after a fraction of a millisecond, the sodium conductance decreases to its normal level. At the same time the potassium conductance *increases* and allows rapid flow of potassium ions outward through the membrane. This now transfers large numbers of positive charges to the outside, once again creating negativity inside the membrane and returning the membrane potential approximately to its original −85 millivolts.

Quantity of Ions Lost from the Nerve Fiber During the Action Potential. The actual quantity of ions that must pass through the nerve membrane to cause the action potential—that is, to cause a 135 millivolt increase in the membrane potential and then to return this potential back to its normal resting level—is extremely slight. For large myelinated nerve fibers only about 1/100,000 to 1/500,000 of the ions normally inside the fiber are exchanged during this process. Nevertheless, this does cause a very slight increase of sodium ions inside the fiber and a corresponding very slight decrease in potassium ions. As we shall see later in the chapter, the active transport processes restore these ions within a few milliseconds or seconds.

SOME EXPERIMENTAL METHODS THAT HAVE BEEN USED TO STUDY THE ACTION POTENTIAL

The events of the action potential, as discussed in the preceding few pages, have been studied most widely in the *squid axon,* a nerve fiber that is sometimes as large as 1 mm. in diameter. This fiber is large enough that potentials are easily measured on its inside, and it is even possible to remove the axoplasm from inside the fiber and to replace this with artificial solution. Also, electrodes can be placed inside the fiber to excite it or to "clamp" the voltage across the membrane—that is, to fix the voltage across the membrane at a constant level by running current through the electrodes. Use of this clamping process has made it possible to study the effect of voltage changes on sodium and potassium fluxes and also on sodium and potassium permeabilities.

Two drugs have proved to be invaluable in the study of the sodium and potassium channels. One drug, *tetrodotoxin,* will block the sodium channels. However, it will block these channels only when applied to the outside of the nerve fiber. Nevertheless, when the sodium channels are blocked it is then possible to study the permeability of the potassium channels independently of the sodium channels. In a similar manner, application of *tetraethylammonium ion* to the inside of the fiber membrane blocks the potassium channels. In this state, the sodium channels can be studied independently of the potassium channels. Thus, by a painstaking process of elimination, the separate effects on the two types of channels are gradually being elucidated.

PROPAGATION OF THE ACTION POTENTIAL

In the preceding paragraphs we have discussed the action potential as it occurs at one spot on the membrane. However, an action potential elicited at any one point on an excitable membrane usually excites adjacent portions of the membrane, resulting in propagation of the action potential. The mechanism of this is illustrated in Figure 1–6. Figure 1–6A shows a normal resting nerve fiber, and Figure 1–6B shows a nerve fiber that has been excited in its midportion—that is, the midportion has suddenly developed increased permeability to

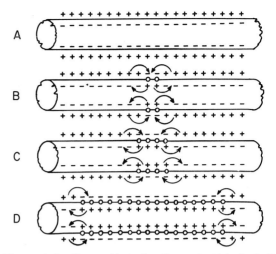

Figure 1–6. Propagation of action potentials in both directions along a conductive fiber.

sodium. The arrows illustrate a *local circuit* of current flow between the depolarized and the resting membrane areas; current flows inward through the depolarized membrane and outward through the resting membrane, thus completing a circuit. In some way not understood, *the outward current flow through the resting membrane now increases the membrane's permeability to sodium,* which immediately allows sodium ions to diffuse inward through the membrane, thus setting up the vicious cycle of membrane activation discussed earlier in the chapter. As a result, depolarization occurs at this area of the membrane as well. Therefore, as illustrated in Figure 1–6C and D, successive portions of the membrane become depolarized. And these newly depolarized areas cause local circuits of current flow still farther along the membrane, causing progressively more and more depolarization. Thus, the depolarization process travels in both directions along the entire extent of the fiber. The transmission of the depolarization process along a nerve or muscle fiber is called a *nerve* or *muscle impulse.*

Direction of Propagation. It is now obvious that an excitable membrane has no single direction of propagation, but that the impulse can travel in both directions away from the stimulus—and even along all branches of a nerve fiber—until the entire membrane has become depolarized.

The All-or-Nothing Principle. It is equally obvious that, once an action potential has been elicited at any point on the membrane of a normal fiber, the depolarization process will travel over the entire membrane. This is called the all-or-nothing principle, and it applies to all normal excitable tissues. Occasionally, though, when the fiber is in an abnormal state the impulse will reach a point on the membrane at which the action potential does not generate sufficient voltage to stimulate the adjacent area of the membrane. When this occurs the spread of depolarization will stop. Therefore, for normal propagation of an impulse to occur, the ratio of action potential to threshold for excitation, called the *safety factor,* must at all times be greater than unity.

Propagation of Repolarization. The action potential normally lasts almost the same length of time at each point along a fiber. Therefore, repolarization normally occurs first at the point of original stimulus and then spreads progressively along the membrane, moving in the same direction that depolarization had previously spread. Figure 1–7 illustrates the same nerve fiber as that in Figure 1–6, showing that the polarization process is propagated in the same direction as the depolarization process but a few ten-thousandths of a second later.

"RECHARGING" THE FIBER MEMBRANE—IMPORTANCE OF ENERGY METABOLISM

Since transmission of large numbers of impulses along the nerve fiber reduces the ionic concentration gradients, these gradients must be re-established. This is achieved by the action of the sodium and potassium pump in exactly the same way as that described in the first part of the chapter for establishment of the original resting potential. That is, the sodium ions that, during the action potentials, have diffused to the interior of the cell and the potassium ions that have diffused to the exterior are returned to their original state by the sodium and potassium pump. Since this pump requires energy for operation, this process of "recharging" the nerve fiber is an active metabolic one, utilizing energy derived from the adenosine triphosphate energy

Figure 1–7. Propagaton of repolarization in both directions along a conductive fiber.

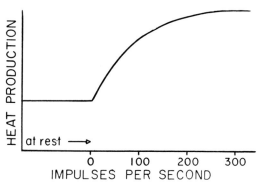

Figure 1–8. Heat production in a nerve fiber at rest and at progressively increasing rates of stimulation.

"currency" system of the cell.

Heat Production by the Nerve Fiber. Figure 1–8 illustrates the relationship of heat production in a nerve fiber to the number of impulses transmitted by the fiber each second. The rate of heat production is a measure of the rate of metabolism in the nerve, because heat is always liberated as a product of the chemical reactions of energy metabolism. Note that the heat production increases markedly as the number of impulses per second increases. It is this increased energy that causes the "recharging" process.

Unimportance of Energy Metabolism During Actual Transmission of the Action Potential. The role of the sodium and potassium pump to recharge the nerve fiber is to maintain adequate concentration differences of sodium and potassium across the nerve membrane. However, if metabolism in the nerve fiber suddenly ceased and the sodium and potassium ions that move through the membrane with each action potential were not returned to their original sides of the membrane, the nerve fiber would still be able to transmit perhaps fifty thousand to a million nerve impulses before it would be necessary to recharge the fiber again. The reason for this is that the quantities of sodium and potassium ions that diffuse through the nerve membrane with each action potential are extremely minute, allowing tremendous numbers of action potentials to occur before the recharging process is necessary.

Thus, the action potential itself is a passive process in contrast to the charging and recharging processes, which are active metabolic processes requiring the utilization of ATP as an energy source.

THE SPIKE POTENTIAL AND THE AFTER-POTENTIALS

Figure 1–9 illustrates an action potential recorded with a much slower time scale than that illustrated in

Figure 1–5; many milliseconds of recording are shown in comparison with only the first 1.5 milliseconds of the action potential in Figure 1–5.

The Spike Potential. The initial very large change in membrane potential shown in Figure 1–9 is called the spike potential. In large type A myelinated nerve fibers it lasts for about 0.4 millisecond. The spike potential is analogous to the action potential that has been discussed in the preceding paragraphs, and it is the spike potential that is also called the *nerve impulse.*

The Negative After-Potential. At the termination of the spike potential, the membrane potential fails to return all the way to its resting level for another few milliseconds, as shown in Figure 1–9. This is called the *negative after-potential.* It is believed to result from a buildup of potassium ions immediately outside the membrane; this causes the concentration ratio of potassium across the membrane to be temporarily less than normal and therefore prevents full return of the normal resting membrane potential for a few additional milliseconds.

The Positive After-Potential. Once the membrane potential has returned to its resting value, it becomes a little more negative than its normal resting value; this excess negativity is called the *positive after-potential.* It is a fraction of a millivolt to, at most, a few millivolts more negative than the normal resting membrane potential, but it lasts from 50 milliseconds to as long as many seconds.

This positive after-potential is caused principally by the electrogenic pumping of sodium outward through the nerve fiber membrane, which is the recharging process that was discussed previously. If the active transport processes are poisoned, the positive after-potential is lost, though both the action potential and the negative after-potential continue to occur.

(The student might wonder why greater negativity in the resting membrane potential is called a positive rather than a negative after-potential, and likewise,

Figure 1–10. An action potential from a Purkinje fiber of the heart, showing a "plateau."

why the so-called negative after-potential is not named positive. The reason for this is that these potentials were first measured *outside* the nerve fibers rather than inside, and all potential changes on the outside are of exactly opposite polarity, whereas modern terminology expresses membrane potentials in terms of the inside potential rather than the outside potential.)

PLATEAU IN THE ACTION POTENTIAL

In some instances the excitable membrane does not repolarize immediately after depolarization, but, instead, the potential remains on a plateau near the peak of the spike sometimes for many milliseconds before repolarization begins. Such a plateau is illustrated in Figure 1–10, from which one can readily see that the plateau greatly prolongs the period of depolarization. It is this type of action potential that occurs in the heart, where the plateau lasts for as long as two- to three-tenths second and causes contraction of the heart muscle during this entire period of time.

The cause of the action potential plateau is probably a combination of several different factors. First, there is delay in inactivation of the sodium channels, which allows sodium ions to continue flowing into the fiber for a long time after the onset of the action potential. Second, there is a small amount of calcium current flowing into the fiber at the same time, and these two currents together maintain the positive state inside the membrane that causes the plateau. However, probably equally as important is the fact that the permeability of the potassium channels decreases about five-fold at the onset of the action potential in excitable membranes that exhibit plateaus, and this prevents rapid outflow of potassium ions to the

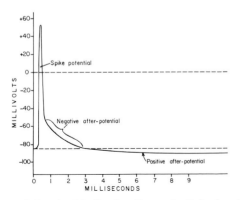

Figure 1–9. An idealized action potential, showing: the initial spike followed by a negative after-potential and a positive after-potential.

outside of the fiber and, therefore, delays the repolarization process.

Yet, when inactivation of the sodium channels does begin, the inactivation process proceeds unabated; simultaneously, the potassium permeability of the membrane increases a hundred-fold or more. Therefore, sodium and calcium ions stop diffusing to the interior of the fiber, while potassium ions diffuse outward extremely rapidly. Consequently, the membrane potential returns quickly to its normal negative level, as llustrated in Figure 1–10, by the rapid decline of the potential at the end of the plateau.

RHYTHMICITY OF CERTAIN EXCITABLE TISSUES—REPETITIVE DISCHARGE

All excitable tissues can discharge repetitively if the threshold for stimulation is reduced low enough. For instance, even nerve fibers and skeletal muscle fibers, which normally are highly stable, discharge repetitively when they are veratrinized or when the calcium ion concentration falls below a critical value. Repetitive discharges, or rhythmicity, occur normally in the heart, in most smooth muscle, and probably also in some of the neurons of the central nervous system.

The Re-excitation Process Necessary for Rhythmicity. For rhythmicity to occur, the membrane, even in its natural state, must be already permeable enough to sodium ions to allow automatic membrane activation and consequent depolarization. That is, (a) sodium ions flow inward, (b) this further increases the membrane permeability, (c) still more sodium ions flow inward, (d) the permeability increases more, and so forth, thus eliciting the regenerative process of membrane activation until an action potential is generated. Then, at the end of the action potential the membrane returns to its normal resting potential. Shortly thereafter, the activation process begins again and a new action potential occurs spontaneously—this cycle continuing again and again and causing self-induced rhythmic excitation of the excitable tissues.

Yet why does the membrane not remain depolarized all the time instead of re-establishing a membrane potential, only to beome depolarized again shortly thereafter? The answer to this can be found by referring back to Figure 1–5, which shows that toward the end of the action potential, and continuing for a short period thereafter, the membrane becomes ex-cessively permeable to potassium. The excessive outflow of potassium carries tremendous numbers of positive charges to the outside of the membrane, creating inside the fiber considerably more negativity than would otherwise occur for a short period after the preceding action potential is over. This is a state called *hyperpolarization*. As long as this state exists, re-excitation will not occur; but gradually the excess potassium conductance (and the state of hyperpolarization) disappears, thereby allowing the onset of a new action potential.

Figure 1–11 illustrates this relationship between repetitive action potentials and potassium conductance. The state of hyperpolarization is established immediately after each preceding action potential; but it gradually recedes, and the membrane potential correspondingly increases until it reaches the *threshold* for excitation; then suddenly a new action potential results, the process occurring again and again.

SPECIAL ASPECTS OF IMPULSE TRANSMISSION IN NERVES

"Myelinated" and Unmyelinated Nerve Fibers. Figure 1–12 illustrates a cross-section of a typical small nerve trunk, showing a few very large nerve fibers that comprise most of the cross-sectional area and many more small fibers lying between the large ones. The large fibers are *myelinated* and the small ones are *unmyelinated*. The average nerve trunk contains about twice as many unmyelinated fibers as myelinated fibers.

Figure 1–13 illustrates a typical myelinated fiber. The central core of the fiber is the *axon,* and the membrane of the axon is the actual *conductive membrane.* The axon is filled in its center with *axoplasm,* which is a viscid intracellular fluid. Surrounding the axon is a *myelin*

Figure 1–11. Rhythmic action potentials, and their relationship to potassium conductance and to the state of hyperpolarization.

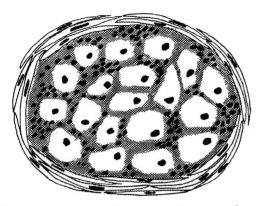

Figure 1–12. Cross section of a small nerve trunk containing myelinated and unmyelinated fibers.

sheath that is approximately as thick as the axon itself, and about once every millimeter along the extent of the axon the myelin sheath is interrupted by a *node of Ranvier.*

The myelin sheath is deposited around the axon by Schwann cells in the following manner: The membrane of a Schwann cell first envelops the axon. Then the cell rotates around the axon several times, laying down multiple layers of cellular membrane containing the lipid substance *sphingomyelin.* This substance is an excellent insulator that prevents almost all flow of ions. However, at the juncture between each two successive Schwann cells along the axon, a small uninsulated area remains where ions can

flow with ease between the extracellular fluid and the axon. This area is the node of Ranvier.

Saltatory Conduction in Myelinated Fibers. Even though ions cannot flow to a significant extent through the thick myelin sheaths of myelinated nerves, they can flow with considerable ease through the nodes of Ranvier. Indeed, the membrane at this point is 500 times as permeable as the membranes of some unmyelinated fibers. Impulses are conducted from node to node by the myelinated nerve rather than continuously along the entire fiber as occurs in the unmyelinated fiber. This process, illustrated in Figure 1–14, is called *saltatory conduction.* That is, electrical current flows through the surrounding extracellular fluids and also through the axoplasm from node to node, exciting successive nodes one after another. Thus, the impulse jumps down the fiber, which is the origin of the term "saltatory."

Saltatory conduction is of value for two reasons: First, by causing the depolarization process to jump long intervals along the axis of the nerve fiber, this mechanism greatly increases the velocity of nerve transmission in myelinated fibers. Second, saltatory conduction conserves energy for the axon, for only the nodes depolarize, allowing several hundred times less loss of ions than would otherwise be necessary and therefore requiring little extra metabolism for retransporting the ions across the membrane.

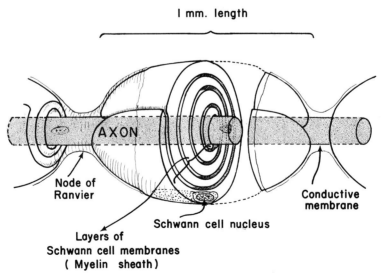

Figure 1–13. The myelin sheath and its formation by Schwann cells. (Modified from Elias and Pauley: Human Microanatomy, Davis Co., 1966.)

Figure 1–14.   Saltatory conduction along a myelinated axon.

VELOCITY OF CONDUCTION IN NERVE FIBERS

The velocity of conduction in nerve fibers varies from as little as 0.5 meter per second in very small unmyelinated fibers up to as high as 130 meters per second (the length of a football field) in very large myelinated fibers. The velocity increases approximately with the fiber diameter in myelinated nerve fibers and approximately with the square root of fiber diameter in unmyelinated fibers.

EXCITATION—THE PROCESS OF ELICITING THE ACTION POTENTIAL

Chemical Stimulation.   Basically, any factor that causes sodium ions to begin to diffuse inward through the membrane in sufficient numbers will set off the automatic, regenerative "activation" mechanism, noted earlier in the chapter, that eventuates in the action potential. Thus, certain chemicals can stimulate a nerve fiber by increasing the membrane permeability. Such chemicals include acids, bases, almost any salt solution of very strong concentration, and, most importantly, the substance *acetylcholine.* Many nerve fibers, when stimulated, secrete acetylcholine at their endings where they synapse with other neurons or where they end on muscle fibers. The acetylcholine in turn stimulates the successive neuron or muscle fiber. This is discussed in much greater detail in Chapter 3, and it is one of the most important means by which nerve and muscle fibers are stimulated. Likewise, *norepinephrine* secreted by sympathetic nerve endings can stimulate cardiac muscle fibers and some smooth muscle fibers, and still other hormonal substances can stimulate successive neurons in the central nervous system.

Mechanical Stimulation.   Crushing, pinching, or pricking a nerve fiber can cause a sudden surge of sodium influx and, for obvious reasons, can elicit an action potential. Even slight pressure on some specialized nerve endings can stimulate these; this will be discussed in Chapter 6 in relation to sensory perception.

Electrical Stimulation.   Electrical stimulation also can initiate an action potential. An electrical charge artificially induced across the membrane causes excess flow of ions through the membrane; this in turn can initiate an action potential. However, not all methods of applying electrical stimuli result in excitation, and, since this is the usual means by which nerve fibers are excited when they are studied in the laboratory, the process of electrical excitation deserves more detailed comment.

Cathodal versus Anodal Currents.   Figure 1–15 illustrates a battery connected to two electrodes on the surface of a nerve fiber. At the cathode, or negative electrode, the potential outside the membrane is negative with respect to that on the inside, and the current that flows outward through the membrane at this point is called *cathodal current.* At the anode, the electrode is positive with respect to the potential immediately inside the membrane, and the inward current flow at this point is called *anodal current.*

A cathodal current excites the fiber whereas an anodal current actually makes the fiber more resistant to excitation than normal. Though the cause of this difference between the two types of current cannot be explained completely, it is known that the normal impermeability of the membrane to sodium results partially from the high resting membrane potential across the membrane, and any condition that lessens this potential causes the membrane to become progressively more permeable to sodium. Obviously, at the cathode the applied voltage is opposite to the resting potential of the membrane, and this reduces the net potential. As a result, the membrane becomes far more permeable than usual to sodium followed by subsequent development of an action potential.

On the other hand, at the anode, the applied potential actually enhances the membrane potential. This makes the membrane less permeable to sodium than ever, resulting in increased resistance of the membrane to stimulation by other means.

Threshold for Excitation and "Acute Subthreshold Potential."   A very weak cathodal potential cannot excite the fiber. But, when this potential is progressively increased, there comes a point at which excitation takes place. Figure 1–16 illustrates the effects of successively applied cathodal stimuli of progressing strength. A very weak stimulus at point A causes the membrane potential to change from -85 to -80 millivolts, but this is not a sufficient change for the automatic regenerative processes of the action potential to develop. At point B the stimulus is greater, but, here again, the intensity still is not enough to set off the automatic action potential. Nevertheless, the membrane voltage is disturbed for

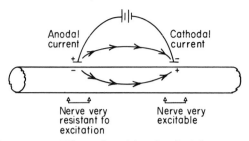

Figure 1–15. Effects of anodal and cathodal currents on excitability of the nerve membrane.

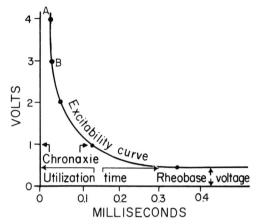

Figure 1–17. Excitability of a large myelinated nerve fiber.

as long as a millisecond or more after both of the weak stimuli; the potential changes during these small intervals of time are called *acute subthreshold potentials,* as illustrated in the figure.

At point C in Figure 1–16 the stimulus elicits an acute membrane potential that is not subthreshold but slightly more than the threshold value, and, after a short "latent period," it initiates an action potential. At point D the stimulus is still stronger, and the acute membrane potential initiates the action potential even sooner. Thus, this figure shows that even a very weak stimulus always causes a local potential change at the membrane, but that the intensity of the *local potential* must rise to a *threshold value* before the automatic action potential will be set off.

"Accommodation" to Stimuli. When a cathodal potential applied to a nerve fiber is made to increase very slowly, rather than rapidly, the threshold voltage required to cause firing is considerably increased. This phenomenon is called *accommodation;* in other words, the excitable membrane is said to "accommodate" itself to slowly increasing potentials rather than firing. It is probable that a slowly increasing stimulatory current allows time for ions to build up (or become depleted) in the areas immediately adjacent to the fibers, these changes in ion concentrations partially opposing the stimulus.

Excitability Curve of Nerve Fibers. A so-called "excitability curve" of a nerve fiber is shown in Figure 1–17. To obtain this curve a high voltage

stimulus (4 volts, in this instance) is first applied to the fiber, and the minimum duration of stimulus required to excite the fiber is found. The voltage and minimal time are plotted as point A. Then a stimulus voltage of 3 volts is applied, and the minimal time required is again determined; the results are plotted as point B. The same is repeated at 2 volts, 1 volt, 0.5 volt, and so forth, until the least voltage possible at which the membrane is stimulated has been reached. On connection of these points, the excitability curve is determined.

The excitability curve of Figure 1–17 is that of a large myelinated nerve fiber. The least possible voltage at which it will fire is called the *rheobase,* and the time required for this least voltage to stimulate the fiber is called the *utilization time.* Then, if the voltage is increased to twice the rheobase voltage, the time required to stimulate the fiber is called the *chronaxie;* this is often used as a means of expressing relative excitabilities of different excitable tissues. For instance, the chronaxie of a large type A fiber is about 0.0001 to 0.0002 second; of smaller myelinated nerve fibers, approximately 0.0003 second; of unmyelinated fibers, 0.0005 second; of skeletal muscle fibers, 0.00025 to 0.001 second; and of heart muscle, 0.001 to 0.003 second.

The Refractory Period. A second action potential cannot occur in an excitable fiber as long as the membrane is still depolarized from the preceding action potential. Therefore, even an electrical stimulus of maximum strength applied before the first spike potential is almost over will not elicit a second one. This interval of inexcitability is called the *absolute refractory period.* The absolute refractory period of large myelinated nerve fibers is about $1/2500$ second. Therefore, one can readily calculate that such a fiber can carry a maximum of about 2500 impulses per second. Following the absolute refractory period is a *relative refractory period* lasting about one quarter as long. During this period, stronger than normal stimuli are required to excite the fiber. In some types of

Figure 1–16. Effect of stimuli on the potential of the excitable membrane, showing the development of "acute subthreshold potentials" when the stimuli are below the threshold value required for eliciting an action potential.

fibers, a short period of supernormal excitability follows the relative refractory period.

FACTORS THAT INCREASE MEMBRANE EXCITABILITY

Any condition that increases the natural permeability of the membrane usually causes it to become more excitable than usual. For instance, the drug *veratrine* has a direct action on the membrane to increase its permeability to sodium, and, as a consequence, the strength of stimulus needed to elicit an impulse is greatly reduced; or, on occasion, the fiber becomes so excitable that spontaneous impulses are generated without any extraneous excitation.

Low Calcium Tetany. An extremely important potentiator of excitability is low concentration of calcium ions in the extracellular fluids. Calcium ions normally decrease the permeability of the membrane to sodium. If sufficient calcium ions are not available, however, the permeability becomes increased, and, as a result, the membrane excitability greatly increases—sometimes so greatly that many spontaneous impulses result and cause muscular spasm. This condition is known as low calcium tetany. It often occurs in patients who have lost their parathyroid glands and who therefore cannot maintain normal calcium ion concentrations.

INHIBITION OF EXCITABILITY— "STABILIZERS" AND LOCAL ANESTHETICS

Contrary to the factors that increase excitability, still others called *membrane stabilizing factors* can decrease excitability. For instance, a *high calcium ion concentration* decreases the membrane permeability and simultaneously reduces its excitability. Therefore, calcium ions are said to be a "stabilizer." Also, *low potassium ion concentration* in the extracellular fluids, because it increases the negativity of the resting membrane potential (a process called "hyperpolarization"), likewise acts as a stabilizer and reduces membrane excitability. Indeed, in a hereditary disease known as *familial periodic paralysis*, the extracellular potassium ion concentration is often so greatly reduced that the person actually becomes paralyzed, but he reverts to normalcy instantly after intravenous administration of potassium.

Local Anesthetics and the "Safety Factor." Among the most important stabilizers are the many substances used clinically as local anesthetics, including *cocaine, procaine, tetracaine,* and many other drugs. These act directly on the membrane, decreasing its permeability to sodium and, therefore, also reducing membrane excitability. When the excitability has been reduced so low that the ratio of *action potential strength to excitability threshold* (called the "safety factor") is reduced below unity, a nerve impulse fails to pass through the anesthetized area.

RECORDING MEMBRANE POTENTIALS AND ACTION POTENTIALS

The Cathode Ray Oscilloscope. Earlier in this chapter we have noted that the membrane potential changes very rapidly throughout the course of an action potential. Indeed, most of the action potential complex of large nerve fibers takes place in less than $1/1000$ second. In some figures of this chapter a meter has been shown recording these potential changes. However, it must be understood that any meter capable of recording them must be capable of responding extremely rapidly. For practical purposes the only type of meter that is capable of responding accurately to the very rapid membrane potential changes of most excitable fibers is the cathode ray oscilloscope.

Figure 1–18 illustrates the basic components of a cathode ray oscilloscope. The cathode ray tube itself is composed basically of an *electron gun* and a *fluorescent surface* against which electrons are fired. Where the electrons hit the surface, the fluorescent material glows. If the electron beam is moved across the surface, the spot of glowing light also moves and draws a fluorescent line on the screen.

In addition to the electron gun and fluorescent surface, the cathode ray tube is provided with two sets of plates: one set, called the *horizontal deflection plates,* positioned on either side of the electron beam, and the other set, called the *vertical deflection plates,* positioned above and below the beam. If a negative charge is applied to the left-hand plate and a positive charge to the right-hand plate, the electron beam will be repelled away from the left plate and attracted toward the right plate, thus bending the beam toward the right, and this will cause the spot of light on the fluorescent surface of the cathode ray

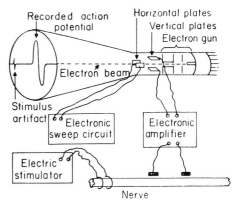

Figure 1–18. The cathode ray oscilloscope for recording transient action potentials.

screen to move to the right. Likewise, positive and negative charges can be applied to the vertical deflection plates to move the beam up or down.

Since electrons travel at extremely rapid velocity and since the plates of the cathode ray tube can be alternately charged positively or negatively within less than a millionth of a second, it is obvious that the spot of light on the face of the tube can also be moved to almost any position in less than a millionth of a second. For this reason, the cathode ray tube oscilloscope can be considered to be an inertialess meter capable of recording with extreme fidelity almost any change in membrane potential.

To use the cathode ray tube for recording action potentials, two electrical circuits must be employed. These are (1) an *electronic sweep circuit* that controls the voltages on the horizontal deflection plates and (2) an *electronic amplifier* that controls the voltages on the vertical deflection plates. The sweep circuit automatically causes the spot of light to begin at the left-hand side and move slowly toward the right. When the spot reaches the right side it jumps back immediately to the left-hand side and starts a new trace.

The electronic amplifier amplifies signals that come from the nerve. If a change in membrane potential occurs while the spot of light is moving across the screen, this change in potential will be amplified and will cause the spot to rise above or fall below the mean level of the trace, as illustrated in the figure. In other words, the sweep circuit provides the lateral movement of the electron beam while the amplifier provides the vertical movement in direct proportion to the changes in membrane potentials picked up by appropriate electrodes.

Figure 1–18 also shows an electric stimulator used to stimulate the nerve. When the nerve is stimulated, a small *stimulus artifact* usually appears on the oscilloscope screen prior to the action potential.

Recording the Monophasic Action Potential. Throughout this chapter monophasic action potentials have been shown in the different diagrams. To record these, an electrode such as that illustrated earlier in the chapter in Figure 1–3 must be inserted into the interior of the fiber. Then, as the action potential spreads down the fiber, the changes in the potential inside the fiber are recorded as illustrated earlier in the chapter in Figures 1–5, 1–9, and 1–10.

Recording a Biphasic Action Potential. When one wishes to record impulses from a whole nerve trunk, it is not feasible to place electrodes inside the nerve fibers. Therefore, the usual method of recording is to place two electrodes on the outside of fibers. However, the record that is obtained is then biphasic for the following reasons: When an action potential moving down the nerve fiber reaches the first electrode, it becomes charged negatively while the second electrode is still unaffected. This causes the oscilloscope to record in the negative direction. Then as the action potential passes beyond the first electrode and reaches the second electrode, the mem-

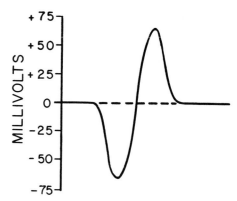

Figure 1–19. Recording of a biphasic action potential.

brane beneath the first electrode becomes repolarized while the second electrode is still negative, and the oscilloscope records in the opposite direction. When these changes are recorded continuously by the oscilloscope, a graphic record such as that illustrated in Figure 1–19 is recorded, showing a potential change first in one direction and then in the opposite direction.

REFERENCES

Abbott, B. C., and Howarth, J. V.: Heat studies in excitable tissues. *Physiol. Rev.*, 53:120, 1973.

Agin, D.: Negative conductance and electrodiffusion in excitable membrane systems. *Membranes*, 1:249, 1972.

Baker, P. F., Hodgkin, A. L., and Shaw, T. I.: Replacement of the axoplasm of giant nerve fibers with artificial solutions. *J. Physiol. (Lond.)*, 164:330, 1962.

Baker, P. F., Hodgkin, A. L., and Shaw, T. I.: The effects of changes in internal ionic concentrations on the electrical properties of perfused giant axons. *J. Physiol. (Lond.)*, 164:355, 1962.

Caldwell, P. C.: Factors governing movement and distribution of inorganic ions in nerve and muscle. *Physiol. Rev.*, 48:1, 1968.

Cohen, L. B.: Changes in neuron structure during action potential propagation and synaptic transmission. *Physiol. Rev.*, 53:373, 1973.

Cole, K. S.: Electrodiffusion models for the membrane of squid giant axon. *Physiol. Rev.*, 45:340, 1965.

De Weer, P.: Aspects of the recovery process in nerve. *In* Guyton, A. C. (ed.): MTP International Review of Science: Physiology. Baltimore, University Park Press, 1975, Vol. 3, p. 231.

Ehrenstein, G., and Lecar, H.: The mechanism of signal transmission in nerve axons. *Ann. Rev. Biophys. Bioeng.*, 1:347, 1972.

Evans, M. H.: Tetrodotoxin, saxitoxin, and related substances: their applications in neurobiology. *Int. Rev. Neurobiol.*, 15:83, 1972.

Glynn, I. M., and Karlish, S. J. D.: The sodium pump. *Ann. Rev. Physiol.*, 37:13, 1975.

Hodgkin, A. L.: The Conduction of the Nervous Impulse. Springfield, Ill., Charles C Thomas, Publisher, 1963.

Hodgkin, A. L., and Horowicz, P.: The effect of sudden changes in ionic concentrations on the membrane potential of single muscle fibres. *J. Physiol. (Lond.)*, 153:370, 1960.

Hodgkin, A. L., and Huxley, A. F.: Movement of sodium and potassium ions during nervous activity. *Cold Spr. Harb. Symp. Quant. Biol.*, 17:43, 1952.

Hodgkin, A. L., and Huxley, A. F.: Quantitative description of membrane current and its application to conduction and excitation in nerve. *J. Physiol. (Lond.)*, 117:500, 1952.

Hubbard, J. I. (ed.): The Peripheral Nervous System. New York, Plenum Publishing Corp., 1974.

Jack, J. J. B., Noble, D., and Tsien, R. W.: Electric Current Flow in Excitable Cells. New York, Oxford University Press, 1975.

Kater, S. B., Heyer, C. B., and Kaneko, C. R. S.: Invertebrate behavior and identifiable neurons. In Guyton, A. C. (ed.): MTP International Review of Science: Physiology. Baltimore, University Park Press, 1975, Vol. 3, p. 1.

Katz, B.: Nerve, Muscle, and Synapse. New York, McGraw-Hill Book Company, 1968.

Koketsu, K.: Calcium and the excitable cell membrane. Neurosci. Res., 2:1, 1969.

Landowne, D., Potter, L. T., and Terrar, D. A.: Structure-function relationships in excitable membranes. Ann. Rev. Physiol., 37:485, 1975.

Läuger, P., and Neumcke, B.: Theoretical analysis of ion conductance in lipid bilayer membranes. Membranes, 2:1, 1973.

Lerman, L., Watanabe, A., and Tasaki, I.: Intracellular perfusion of squid giant axons: recent findings and interpretations. Neurosci. Res., 2:71, 1969.

Lieberstein, H. M.: Mathematical Physiology, Blood Flow, and Electrically Active Cells. New York, American Elsevier Publishing Co., Inc., 1973.

Martin, A. R., and Veale, J. L.: The nervous system at the cellular level. Ann. Rev. Physiol., 29:401, 1967.

Mystrom, R. A.: Membrane Physiology. Englewood Cliffs, N.J., Prentice-Hall, Inc., 1973.

Nachmansohn, D.: Chemical and Molecular Basis of Nerve Activity. New York, Academic Press, Inc., 1975.

Narahashi, T.: Chemicals as tools in the study of excitable membranes. Physiol. Rev., 54:813, 1974.

Nelson, P. G.: Nerve and muscle cells in culture. Physiol. Rev., 55:1, 1975.

Noble, D.: Applications of Hodgkin-Huxley equations to excitable tissues. Physiol. Rev., 46:1, 1966.

Noble, D.: Conductance mechanisms in excitable cells. Biomembranes, 3:427, 1972.

Peskoff, A., and Eisenberg, R. S.: Interpretation of some microelectrode measurements of electrical properties of cells. Ann. Rev. Biophys. Bioeng., 4:65, 1973.

Reuter, H.: Divalent cations as charge carriers in excitable membranes. Prog. Biophys. Mol. Biol., 26:1, 1973.

Ritchie, J. M.: Energetic aspects of nerve conduction: The relationships between heat production, electrical activity, and metabolism. Prog. Biophys. Mol. Biol., 26:147, 1973.

Roche e Silva, M., and Suarez-Kurtz, G. (eds.): Concepts of Membranes in Regulation and Excitation. New York, Raven Press, 1975.

Schultz, S. G.: Principles of electrophysiology and their application to epithelial tissues. In Guyton, A. C. (ed.): MTP International Review of Science: Physiology. Baltimore, University Park Press, 1974, Vol. 4, p. 69.

Shanes, A. M.: Electrochemical aspects of physiological and pharmacological action in excitable cells. Pharmacol. Rev., 10:59, 1958; 10:165, 1958.

Somjen, G. G.: Electrogenesis of sustained potentials. Prog. Neurobiol., 1:201, 1973.

Spurway, N. C.: Mechanisms of anion permeation. A review of available data, principally on muscle cells, with the fixed charge concept in mind. Biomembranes, 3:363, 1972.

Tasaki, I., and Hallett, M.: Bioenergetics of nerve excitation. J. Bioenerg., 3:65, 1972.

Thomas, R. C.: Electrogenic sodium pump in nerve and muscle cells. Physiol. Rev., 52:563, 1972.

Thompson, R. F., and Patterson, M. M. (eds.): Bioelectric Recording Techniques, Part A, Cellular Processes and Brain Potentials. New York, Academic Press, Inc., 1973.

Trautwein, W.: Membrane currents in cardiac muscle fibers. Physiol. Rev., 53:793, 1973.

Zachar, J.: Electrogenesis and Contractility in Skeletal Muscle Cells. Baltimore, University Park Press, 1973.

2

Contraction of Skeletal Muscle

Approximately 40 per cent of the body is skeletal muscle and another 5 to 10 per cent is smooth or cardiac muscle. Many of the same principles of contraction apply to all these different types of muscle, but in the present chapter the function of skeletal muscle is considered mainly, while the specialized functions of smooth muscle will be discussed in the following chapter.

PHYSIOLOGIC ANATOMY OF SKELETAL MUSCLE

THE SKELETAL MUSCLE FIBER

All skeletal muscles of the body are made up of numerous muscle fibers ranging between 10 and 80 microns in diameter. In most muscles the fibers extend the entire length of the muscle, and except for about 2 per cent of the fibers, each of these is innervated by only one nerve ending located near the middle of the fiber.

The Sarcolemma. The sarcolemma is the cell membrane of the muscle fiber. However, the sarcolemma consists of a true cell membrane, called the *plasma membrane,* and a thin layer of polysaccharide material similar to that of the basement membrane surrounding blood capillaries; thin collagen fibrillae are also present in the outer layer of the sarcolemma. At the ends of the muscle fibers, these surface layers of the sarcolemma fuse with tendon fibers, which in turn collect into bundles to form the muscle tendons, and thence insert into the bones.

Myofibrils; Actin and Myosin Filaments. Each muscle fiber contains several hundred to several thousand myofibrils, which are illustrated by the small dots in the cross-sectional view of Figure 2–1. Each myofibril in turn has, lying side-by-side, about 1500 *myosin filaments* and two times this many *actin filaments,* which are large polymerized protein molecules that are responsible for muscle contraction. These can be seen in longitudinal view in the electron micrograph of Figure 2–2, and are represented diagrammatically in Figure 2–3. The thick filaments are *myosin* and the thin filaments are *actin.* Note that the myosin and actin filaments partially interdigitate and thus cause the myofibrils to have alternate light and dark bands. The light bands, which contain only actin filaments, are called *I bands* because they are mainly *isotropic* to polarized light. The dark bands, which contain the myosin filaments as well as the ends of the actin filaments where

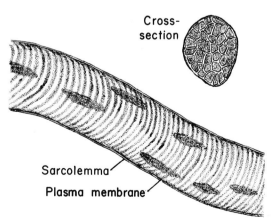

Figure 2–1. Side and cross-sectional views of a skeletal muscle fiber.

Figure 2–2. Electron micrograph of muscle myofibrils, showing the detailed organization of actin and myosin filaments in the fibril. Note the mitochondria lying between the myofibrils. (From Fawcett: The Cell, 1966).

they overlap the myosin, are called *A bands* because they are *anisotropic* to polarized light. Note also the small projections from the sides of the myosin filaments. These are called *cross-bridges*. They protrude from the surfaces of the myosin filaments along the entire extent of the filament, except in the very center. It is interaction between these cross-bridges and the actin filaments that causes contraction.

Figure 2–3. Arrangement of the myosin and actin filaments in the sarcomeres.

Figure 2–3 also shows that the actin filaments are attached to the so-called *Z membrane* or *Z line,* and the filaments extend on either side of the Z membrane to interdigitate with the myosin filaments. The Z membrane also passes from myofibril to myofibril, attaching the myofibrils to each other all the way across the muscle fiber. Therefore, the entire muscle fiber has light and dark bands, as is also true of the individual myofibrils. It is these bands that give skeletal and cardiac muscle their striated appearance.

The portion of a myofibril (or of the whole muscle fiber) that lies between two successive Z membranes is called a *sarcomere.* When the muscle fiber is at its normal fully stretched resting length, the length of the sarcomere is about 2.0 microns. At this length, the actin filaments completely overlap the myosin filaments and are just beginning to overlap each other. We shall see later that it is at this length that the sarcomere also is capable of generating its greatest force of contraction.

When a muscle fiber is stretched beyond its

resting length, the ends of the actin filaments pull apart, leaving a light area in the center of the A band. This light area, called the *H zone,* is illustrated in Figure 2–3. Such an H zone rarely occurs in the normally functioning muscle because normal sarcomere contraction occurs when the resting length of the sarcomere is from 2.0 microns to 1.6 microns. In this range the ends of the actin filaments not only overlap the myosin filaments but also overlap each other.

The Sarcoplasm. The myofibrils are suspended inside the muscle fiber in a matrix called *sarcoplasm,* which is composed of usual intracellular constituents. The fluid of the sarcoplasm contains large quantities of potassium, magnesium, phosphate, and protein enzymes. Also present are tremendous numbers of *mitochondria* that lie between and parallel to the myofibrils, a condition which is indicative of the great need of the contracting myofibrils for large amounts of ATP formed by the mitochondria.

The Sarcoplasmic Reticulum. Also in the sarcoplasm is an extensive endoplasmic reticulum, which in the muscle fiber is called the *sarcoplasmic reticulum.* This reticulum has a special organization that is extremely important in the control of muscle contraction, which will be discussed later in the chapter. The electron-micrograph of Figure 2–4 illustrates the arrangement of this sarcoplasmic reticulum and shows how extensive it can be. The more rapidly contracting types of muscle have especially extensive sarcoplasmic reticulums, indicating that this structure is important in causing rapid muscle contraction, as will also be discussed later.

One can see from the figure that the sarcoplasmic reticulum is composed of *longitudinal tubules* that lie parallel to the myofibrils. The reader can also note that the two ends of each longitudinal tubule terminate in *cisternae* that are bulbous structures quite different from the main body of the tubules. We shall see later that the two respective portions of the sarcoplasmic reticulum play specific roles in muscle contraction.

The Transverse Tubule System—T Tubules. In addition to the sarcoplasmic reticulum, each muscle fiber also has another extensive tubular system called the *transverse tubules* or *T tubules*. These tubules run *perpendicular* to the myofibrils, in contrast to the sarcoplasmic reticulum that runs parallel. They are illustrated in Figure 2–4, which shows the T tubules cut in cross-sections (see arrows). Note that each T tubule is very small and lies between the ends of two successive longitudinal tubules with the cisternae of the longitudinal tubules abutting the T tubule. This area of contact between the sarcoplasmic reticulum and a T tubule is called a *triad* because it is composed of a central small tubule and, on its sides, two bulbous cisternae of the sarcoplasmic reticulum. In skeletal muscle, a triad occurs adjacent to each area where the actin and myosin filaments overlap, and since this occurs at each

Figure 2–4. Sarcoplasmic reticulum surrounding the myofibril, showing the longitudinal system paralleling the myofibrils. Also shown in cross-section are the T tubules that lead to the exterior of the fiber membrane and that contain extracellular fluid (arrows). (From Fawcett: The Cell, 1966).

end of each myosin filament, there are two triads per sarcomere. (However, in heart muscle there is only one triad per sarcomere, located adjacent to the Z membrane.)

Another important characteristic of the T tubules is that they pass all the way through the fiber from one side of the membrane to the other; they open to the exterior rather than to the interior of the cell and contain *extracellular fluid* that is continuous with the fluid outside the cell rather than intracellular fluid. When an action potential spreads over the muscle fiber membrane, electrical currents, probably in the form of an action potential, are transmitted to the interior of the muscle fiber by way of the T tubule system, and it is these currents that cause the muscle to contract, as we shall discuss shortly.

MOLECULAR MECHANISM OF MUSCLE CONTRACTION

Sliding Mechanism of Contraction. Figure 2–5 illustrates the basic mechanism of muscle contraction. It shows the relaxed state of a sarcomere (above) and the contracted state (below). In the relaxed state, the ends of the actin filaments derived from two successive Z membranes barely overlap each other while at the same time completely overlapping the myosin filaments. On the other hand, in the contracted state these actin filaments have been pulled inward among the myosin filaments so that they now overlap each other to a major extent. Also, the Z membranes have been pulled by the actin filaments up to the ends of the myosin filaments. Indeed, the actin filaments can be pulled together so tightly that the ends of the myosin

RELAXED

CONTRACTED

Figure 2–5. The relaxed and contracted states of a myofibril, showing sliding of the actin filaments into the channels between the myosin filaments.

filaments actually buckle during very intense contraction. Thus, muscle contraction occurs by a *sliding filament mechanism.*

But what causes the actin filaments to slide inward among the myosin filaments? Unfortunately, we do not completely know the answer to this question. Yet we do know that it is caused by attractive forces that develop between the actin and myosin filaments. Almost certainly, these attractive forces are the result of mechanical, chemical, or electrostatic forces generated by the interaction of the cross-bridges of the myosin filaments with the actin filaments.

Under resting conditions, the attractive forces between the actin and myosin filaments are inhibited, but when an action potential travels over the muscle fiber membrane, this causes the release of large quantities of calcium ions into the sarcoplasm surrounding the myofibrils. These calcium ions activate the attractive forces between the filaments and contraction begins. But energy is also needed for the contractile process to proceed. This energy is derived from the high energy bonds of adenosine triphosphate (ATP), which is degraded to adenosine diphosphate (ADP) to give the energy required.

In the next few sections we will describe what is known about the details of the molecular processes of contraction. To begin this discussion, however, we must first characterize in detail the myosin and actin filaments.

MOLECULAR CHARACTERISTICS OF THE CONTRACTILE FILAMENTS

The Myosin Filament. The myosin filament is composed of approximately 200 myosin molecules, each having a molecular weight of 450,000. Figure 2–6, section A illustrates an individual molecule; section B illustrates the organization of the molecules to form a myosin filament as well as its interaction with two actin filaments.

The myosin molecule is composed of two parts; one part called *light meromyosin* and the other part called *heavy meromyosin.* The light meromyosin consists of two peptide strands wound around each other in a helix. The heavy meromyosin in turn consists of two parts: first, a double helix similar to that of the light meromyosin; second, a head attached to the end of the double helix. The head itself is a composite of two globular protein masses.

It is believed that the myosin molecule is

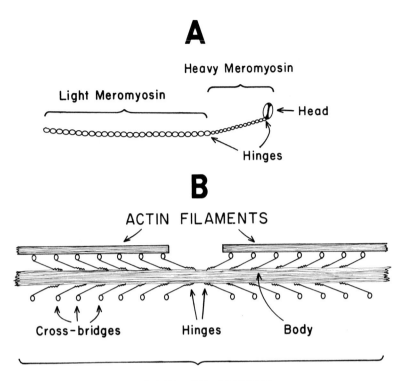

Figure 2–6. (A) the myosin molecule. (B) Combination of many myosin molecules to form a myosin filament. Also shown are the cross-bridges and the interaction between the heads of the cross-bridges with adjacent actin filaments.

especially flexible at two points—the juncture between the light meromyosin and the heavy meromysin and between the body of the heavy meromyosin and the head. These two areas are called hinges.

In section B of Figure 2–6 the central portion of a myosin filament is illustrated. The body of this filament is composed of parallel strands of light meromyosin from multiple myosin molecules. In fact, whenever myosin molecules are precipitated from solution, it is found that the light meromyosin portions of the myosin molecules have a natural tendency to aggregate together to form filaments almost precisely like those of the myosin filaments found in muscle. On the other hand, the heavy meromyosin portions of myosin molecules protrude from all sides of the myosin filament, as illustrated in the figure. These protrusions constitute the *cross-bridges*. The heads of the cross-bridges lie in apposition to the actin filaments, whereas the rod portions of the cross-bridges act as hinged arms that allow the heads to extend either far outward from the body of the myosin filament or to lie close to the body. The length of the head is 120 Ångstroms while the length of the hinged arm is 400 Ångstroms. Therefore, the combination of the

arm and the head allows the cross-bridges to extend far laterally. This is very important because during contraction of the muscle the actin and myosin filaments are spread progressively apart from each other by the engorgement of fluid in the shortened myofibrils.

Note also that the arms of the cross-bridges extend toward the two ends of the filament and away from the center of the filament. Therefore, in the very center of the myosin filament, for a length of about 0.2 micron, there are no cross-bridge heads.

The total length of the myosin filament is 160 Ångstroms, and the 200 myosin molecules allow the formation of 100 pairs of cross-bridges—50 pairs on each end of the myosin filament.

Now, to complete the picture, the myosin filament is twisted so that it makes one complete revolution for each three pairs of cross-bridges. Each twist has a length of 429 Ångstroms, and each pair of cross-bridges lies 143 Ångstroms from the next pair and is axially displaced from the previous pair by 120°.

The Actin Filament. The actin filament is also complex. It is composed of three different components; *actin, tropomyosin,* and *troponin.*

The backbone of the actin filament is a

double-stranded F-actin protein molecule, illustrated in Figure 2–7. The two strands are wound in a helix, making a complete 360° revolution approximately every 700 Ångstroms.

Each strand of the double F-actin helix is composed of polymerized G-actin molecules, each having a molecular weight of 47,000 and a length of 54 Ångstroms. There are approximately 13 of these molecules in each revolution of each strand of helix. And attached to each one of the G-actin molecules is one molecule of ADP. It is believed that these ADP molecules are the active sites on the actin filaments with which the cross-bridges of the myosin filaments interact to cause muscle contraction. The active sites on the two F-actin strands of the double helix are staggered, giving one active site on the overall actin filament approximately every 27 Ångstroms.

The Troponin-Tropomyosin Complex. The actin filament also contains two additional protein strands that are polymers of tropomyosin molecules, each molecule having a molecular weight of 70,000. It is believed that these protein strands lie in the two grooves formed by the two F-actin strands of the actin helix. Each tropomyosin molecule in the tropomyosin strand extends for a length of 400 Ångstroms, and attached to each tropomyosin molecule is a molecule of still another protein, *troponin.* Troponin has a very high affinity for calcium ions. It is believed that the combination of calcium ions with troponin is the trigger that initiates muscle contraction, as will be discussed in the following section.

INTERACTION OF MYOSIN AND ACTIN FILAMENTS TO CAUSE CONTRACTION

Inhibition of the Actin Filament by the Troponin-Tropomyosin Complex; Activation

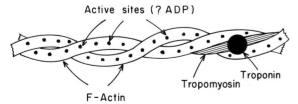

Figure 2–7. The actin filament, composed of two helical strands of F-actin. Also shown is a small portion of one of the two tropomyosin strands that lie in the grooves between the actin strands. On the surface of the tropomyosin one large molecule of troponin is shown schematically.

by Calcium Ions. A pure actin filament without the presence of the troponin-tropomyosin complex binds strongly with myosin molecules in the presence of magnesium ions and ATP, both of which are normally abundant in the myofibril. But, if the troponin-tropomyosin complex is added to the actin filament, this binding does not take place. Therefore, it is believed that the normal active sites on the normal actin filament of the relaxed muscle are inhibited (or perhaps physically covered) by the troponin-tropomyosin complex. Consequently, they cannot interact with the myosin filaments to cause contraction. Before contraction can take place the inhibitory effect of the troponin-tropomyosin complex must itself be inhibited.

Now, let us discuss the role of the calcium ions. In the presence of large amounts of calcium ions the inhibitory effect of the troponin-tropomyosin on the actin filaments is itself inhibited. The mechanism of this is not known, but one suggestion is the following: When calcium ions combine with troponin, which has an extremely high affinity for calcium ions even when they are present in minute quantities, the troponin molecule supposedly undergoes a conformational change that in some way tugs on the tropomyosin protein strand. This in turn supposedly moves the tropomyosin strand deeper into the groove between the two actin strands and thereby "uncovers" the active sites of the actin, thus allowing contraction to proceed. Though this is a hypothetical mechanism, nevertheless it does emphasize that the normal relationship between the tropomyosin-troponin complex and actin is altered by calcium ions—a condition which leads to contraction.

Interaction Between the "Activated" Actin Filament and the Myosin Molecule—The Ratchet Theory of Contraction. As soon as the actin filament becomes activated by the calcium ions, it is believed that the heads of the cross-bridges from the myosin filaments immediately become attracted to the active sites of the actin filament, and this in some way causes contraction to occur. Though the precise manner by which this interaction betwen the cross-bridges and the actin causes contraction is still unknown, a suggested hypothesis for which considerable circumstantial evidence exists is the so-called *ratchet theory of contraction.*

Figure 2–8 illustrates the postulated ratchet mechanism for contraction. This figure shows the heads of two cross-bridges attaching to and disengaging from the active sites of an actin

Figure 2–8. The ratchet mechanism for contraction of the muscle.

filament. It is postulated that when the head attaches to an active site this attachment alters the bonding forces between the head and its arm, thus causing the head to tilt toward the center of the myosin filament, and to drag the actin filament along with it. This tilt of the head of the cross-bridge is called the *power stroke*. Then, immediately after tilting, the head automatically splits away from the active site and returns to its normal perpendicular direction. In this position it combines with an active site further down along the actin filament; then, a similar tilt takes place again to cause a new power stroke, and the actin filament moves another step. Thus, the heads of the cross-bridges bend back and forth and step by step pull the actin filament toward the center of the myosin filament. Thus, the movements of the cross-bridges use the active sites of the actin filaments as cogs of a *ratchet*.

Each one of the cross-bridges is believed to operate independently of all others, each attaching and pulling in a continuous, alternating ratchet cycle. Therefore, the greater the number of cross-bridges in contact with the actin filament at any given time, the greater, theoretically, is the force of contraction.

ATP as the Source of Energy for Contraction—Chemical Events in the Ratchet Cycle. When a muscle contracts against a load, work is performed, and energy is required. It is found that large amounts of ATP are cleaved to form ADP during the contraction process. Furthermore, the greater the amount of work performed by the muscle, the greater is the amount of ATP that is cleaved. However, unfortunately, it is still not known exactly how ATP is used to provide the energy for contraction. Yet, the following is a sequence of events that has been suggested as the means by which this occurs:

1. When the inhibitory effect of the troponin-tropomyosin complex has itself been inhibited by calcium ions, the heads of the cross-bridges that are in the nontilted position bind with uncovered sites on the actin filament, as illustrated in Figure 2–8.

2. It is assumed that the bond between the head of the cross-bridge and the active site of the actin filament causes a conformational change in the head, thus causing the head to tilt and to provide the power stroke for pulling the actin filament. This power stroke is believed to result from energy that has already been stored in the heavy meromyosin molecule and not from energy derived from ATP.

3. Once the head of the cross-bridge is tilted, the conformational change in the head exposes a reactive site in the head where ATP can bind. Therefore, one molecule of ATP binds with the head, and this binding in turn causes detachment of the head from the active site.

4. Once the head bound with ATP splits away from the active site, the ATP is itself cleaved by a very potent ATPase activity of the heavy meromyosin. The energy released supposedly tilts the head back to its normal perpendicular condition and theoretically "cocks" the head in this position.

5. Then, when the "cocked" head, with its stored energy derived from the cleaved ATP, binds with a new active site on the actin filament, it becomes uncocked and once again provides the power stroke.

6. Thus, the process proceeds again and again until the actin filament pulls the Z membrane up against the ends of the myosin filaments or until the load on the muscle becomes too great for further pulling to occur.

RELATIONSHIP BETWEEN ACTIN AND MYOSIN FILAMENT OVERLAP AND TENSION DEVELOPED BY THE CONTRACTING MUSCLE

Figure 2–9 illustrates the relationship between the length of sarcomere and the tension developed by the contracting muscle fiber. To the right are illustrated different degrees of overlap of the myosin and actin filaments at different sarcomere lengths. At point D on the diagram, the actin filament has pulled all the way out to the end of the myosin filament with no overlap at all. At this point, the tension developed by the activated muscle is zero. Then as the sarcomere shortens and the actin filament overlaps the myosin filament progressively more and more, the tension increases progressively until the sarcomere length decreases to

Figure 2–9. Length-tension diagram for a single sarcomere, illustrating maximum strength of contraction when the sarcomere is 2.0 to 2.2 microns in length. At the upper right are shown the relative positions of the actin and myosin filaments at different sarcomere lengths from point A to point D. (Modified from Gordon, Huxley, and Julian: *J. Physiol., 171:28P, 1964.*)

about 2.2 microns. At this point the actin filament has already overlapped all the cross-bridges of the myosin filament but has not yet reached the center of the myosin filament. Upon further shortening, the sarcomere maintains full tension until point B at a sarcomere length of approximately 2.0 microns. It is at this point that the ends of the two actin filaments begin to overlap. As the sarcomere length falls from 2 microns down to about 1.65 microns at point A, the strength of contraction decreases. It is at this point that the two Z membranes of the sarcomere abut the ends of the myosin filaments. Then, as contraction proceeds to still shorter sarcomere lengths, the ends of the myosin filaments are actually crumpled, but, as illustrated in Figure 2–9, the strength of contraction also decreases precipitously.

This diagram illustrates that maximum contraction occurs when there is maximum overlap between the actin filaments and the cross-bridges of the myosin filaments, and it supports the idea that the greater the number of cross-bridges pulling the actin filaments, the greater is the strength of contraction.

Relation of Force of Contraction of the Intact Muscle to Muscle Length. Figure 2–10 illustrates a diagram similar to that in Figure 2–9, but this time for the intact whole muscle rather than for the isolated muscle fiber. The whole muscle has a large amount of connective tissue in it; also the sarcomeres in different parts of the muscle do not necessarily contract exactly in unison. Therefore, the curve has

somewhat different dimensions from those illustrated for the individual muscle fiber, but it nevertheless exhibits the same form.

Note in Figure 2–10 that when the muscle is at its normal resting *stretched* length and is then activated, it contracts with maximum force of contraction. If the muscle is stretched to much greater than normal length prior to contraction, a large amount of *resting tension* develops in the muscle even before contraction takes place; that is, the two ends of the muscle are pulled toward each other by the elastic forces of the connective tissue, of the sarcolemma, the blood vessels, the nerves, and so forth. However, the *increase* in tension during contraction, called *active tension*, decreases as the muscle is stretched beyond its normal length.

Note also in Figure 2–10 that when the resting muscle is shortened to less than its normal fully stretched length, the maximum tension of contraction decreases progressively and reaches zero when the muscle has shortened to approximately 60 to 70 per cent of its maximum resting length.

RELATION OF VELOCITY OF CONTRACTION TO LOAD

A muscle contracts extremely rapidly when it contracts against no load—to a state of full contraction in approximately $1/20$ second for the average muscle. However, when loads are applied, the velocity of contraction becomes progressively less as the load increases, as illustrated in Figure 2–11. When the load increases

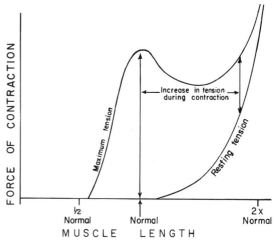

Figure 2–10. Relation of muscle length to force of contraction.

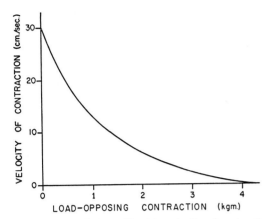

Figure 2–11. Relation of load to velocity of contraction in a skeletal muscle 8 cm. long.

to equal the maximum force that the muscle can exert, then the velocity of contraction becomes zero, and no contraction at all results, despite activation of the muscle fiber.

This decreasing velocity seems to be caused mainly by the fact that a load on a contracting muscle is a reverse force that opposes the contractile force caused by muscle contraction. Therefore, the net force that is available to cause velocity of shortening is correspondingly reduced.

INITIATION OF MUSCLE CONTRACTION: EXCITATION-CONTRACTION COUPLING

THE MUSCLE ACTION POTENTIAL

Initiation of contraction in skeletal muscle begins with action potentials in the muscle fibers. These elicit electrical currents that spread to the interior of the fiber where they cause release of calcium ions from the sarcoplasmic reticulum. It is the calcium ions that in turn initiate the chemical events of the contractile process.

Almost everything discussed in Chapter 1 regarding initiation and conduction of action potentials in nerve fibers applies equally well to skeletal muscle fibers, except for quantitative differences. Some of the quantitative aspects of muscle potentials are the following:

1. Resting membrane potential: Approximately −85 millivolts in skeletal muscle fibers—the same as in large myelinated nerve fibers of the type that excite skeletal muscle.

2. Duration of action potential: 1 to 5 milliseconds in skeletal muscle—about five times as long as in large myelinated nerves.

3. Velocity of conduction: 3 to 5 meters per second—about $1/18$ the velocity of conduction in the large myelinated nerve fibers that excite skeletal muscle.

Excitation of Skeletal Muscle Fibers by Nerves. In normal function of the body, skeletal muscle fibers are excited by large myelinated nerve fibers. These attach to the skeletal muscle fibers at the neuromuscular junction, which will be discussed in detail in the following chapter. Except for 2 per cent of the muscle fibers, there is only one neuromuscular junction to each muscle fiber; this junction is located near the middle of the fiber. Therefore, the action potential spreads from the middle of the fiber toward its two ends. This spreading is important because it allows nearly coincident contraction of all sarcomeres of the muscle so that they can all contract together rather than separately.

SPREAD OF THE ACTION POTENTIAL THROUGH THE T-TUBULE SYSTEM

Not only does the action potential spread along the muscle fiber membrane but it also spreads through the T tubule system of the muscle fiber. As discussed earlier, the T tubules are a system of *transverse* tubules that interconnect with each other and spread all the way through the muscle fiber. A whole plane of such tubules spreads crosswise through the skeletal muscle fiber at two points in each sarcomere: the two points where the actin and myosin filaments overlap. It is at these points where the excitation activates the contractile process, for reasons that have been discussed in the past few pages.

Figure 2–12 illustrates the spread of the action potential in the form of local circuits of current, as illustrated by the dashed arrows along the sarcolemma and also into the T tubule system. Note that a local circuit of current also flows around each one of the T tubules. Though the T tubules are only 300 Ångstroms in diameter, the extensiveness of the T tubule system in each half of the sarcomere allows tremendous flow of electrical current between each T tubule and the fluid in the substance of the muscle fiber. Remember that the fluid in the T tubule system is *extracellular fluid* that is continuous with the outside of the muscle fiber.

There is only one significant difference be-

Figure 2–12. Excitation-contraction coupling in the muscle, showing an action potential that causes release of calcium ions from the sarcoplasmic reticulum and then re-uptake of the calcium ions by a calcium pump.

tween the action potential that spreads through the T tubule system and that which spreads along the sarcolemma: the T tubule action potential spreads at a velocity of only 7 to 10 centimeters per second, which is about $\frac{1}{50}$ the velocity along the sarcolemma. Even so, the transverse distance across a muscle fiber is extremely slight, so that the action potential still reaches the deep recesses of the muscle fiber within less than 1 millisecond.

RELEASE OF CALCIUM IONS BY THE CISTERNAE OF THE SARCOPLASMIC RETICULUM

Figure 2–12 shows that the action potential of the T tubule causes current flow through the cisternae of the sarcoplasmic reticulum. In some way not yet known, this causes the cisternae to release calcium ions into the surrounding sarcoplasmic fluid. Where the cisternae abut the T tubule, they project *junctional feet* toward the tubule; these structures surround the tubule, presumably facilitating the passage of electrical current from the T tubule into the cisternae. The electrical circuit is then completed by passage of current outward through the lateral sides of the cisternae and thence back into the T tubule system, as illustrated by the dashed arrows in the figure. The current flow through the walls of the cisternae is postulated to be the stimulus that causes release of calcium ions from the cisternae.

The calcium ions that are thus released from the cisternae diffuse to the adjacent myofibrils where they bind strongly with troponin, as discussed in an earlier section, and this in turn supposedly elicits the muscle contraction, as has also been discussed. However, the calcium ions also bind less strongly with the myosin filaments, which could theoretically be another factor in initiating contraction.

The Calcium Pump for Removing Calcium Ions from the Sarcoplasmic Fluid. Once the calcium ions have been released from the cisternae and have diffused to the myofibrils, muscle contraction will then continue as long as the calcium ions are still present in high concentration in the sarcoplasmic fluid. However, a continually active calcium pump located in the walls of the longitudinal tubules of the sarcoplasmic reticulum pumps calcium ions out of the sarcoplasmic fluid back into the vesicular cavities of the longitudinal tubules. This pump can concentrate the calcium ions about 2000-fold inside the tubules, a condition which allows massive buildup of calcium in the sarcoplasmic reticulum and also causes almost total depletion of calcium ions in the fluid of the myofibrils. Therefore, except immediately after an action potential, the calcium ion concentration in the myofibrils is kept at an extremely low level.

The Excitatory "Pulse" of Calcium Ions. The normal concentration (less than 10^{-7} molar) of calcium ions in the sarcoplasm that bathes the myofibrils is too little to elicit contraction. Therefore, in the resting state, the troponin-tropomyosin complex keeps the actin filaments inhibited and maintains a relaxed state of the muscle.

On the other hand, full excitation of the T tubule–sarcoplasmic reticulum system causes enough release of calcium ions to increase the concentration in the myofibrillar fluid to as high as 2×10^{-4} molar concentration, which will cause maximum muscle contraction. Immediately thereafter, the calcium pump depletes the calcium ions again. The total duration of this calcium "pulse" in the usual skeletal muscle fiber lasts about $1/50$ of a second, though it may last several times as long as this in some skeletal muscle fibers and be several times shorter in others (in heart muscle the pulse lasts for as long as 0.3 second). It is during this calcium pulse that muscle contraction occurs. If the contraction is to continue without interruption for longer intervals, a series of such pulses must be initiated by a continuous series of repetitive action potentials, as will be discussed in more detail later in the chapter.

THE SOURCE OF ENERGY FOR MUSCLE CONTRACTION

We have already seen that muscle contraction is dependent upon energy supplied by ATP. Most of this energy is required to actuate the ratchet mechanism by which the cross-bridges pull the actin filaments, but small amounts are required for (1) pumping calcium from the sarcoplasm into the sarcoplasmic reticulum, and (2) pumping sodium and potassium ions through the muscle fiber membrane to maintain an appropriate ionic environment for the propagation of action potentials.

However, the amount of ATP that is present in the muscle fiber is sufficient to maintain full contraction for less than 1 second. Fortunately, after the ATP is broken into ADP, as was described in Chapter 2, the ATP is rephosphorylated to form new ATP within a fraction of a second. There are several sources of the energy required for this rephosphorylation:

The first source of energy that is used to reconstitute the ATP is the substance *creatine phosphate,* which carries a high energy phosphate bond similar to those of ATP. The high energy phosphate bond of the creatine phosphate is cleaved and the released energy causes bonding of a new phosphate ion to ADP to reconstitute the ATP. However, the total amount of creatine phosphate is also very little—only about five times as great as the ATP. Therefore, the combined energy of both the stored ATP and the creatine phosphate in the muscle is still capable of causing maximal muscle contraction for no longer than a few seconds.

The next source of energy used to reconstitute both the creatine phosphate and the ATP is energy released from the foodstuffs—from carbohydrates, fats, and proteins. Most of this energy is released in the course of oxidation of these foodstuffs. This oxidative release of energy takes place almost entirely in the mitochondria, which utilize the released energy to form new ATP. The ATP, in turn, provides the energy needed to re-form creatine phosphate. Thus, the ultimate source of energy for muscle contraction is the basic food substances and oxygen.

Relation of Muscle Energy Expenditure to Work Performed—the "Fenn" Effect. The shortening process of muscles can lift objects or move objects against force and thereby perform *work*. The amounts of oxygen and other nutrients consumed by the muscle increase greatly when the muscle performs work rather than simply contracting without causing work. This is called the "Fenn" effect. Though this seems to be an obvious effect that one would expect, nevertheless, the chemical basis for it has not been discovered. In some way the contraction of a muscle against a load causes the rate of breakdown of ATP to ADP to increase. This possibly results from the fact that increased numbers of reactive sites and cross-bridges must be activated to overcome the load.

Efficiency of Muscle Contraction. The "efficiency" of an engine or a motor is calculated as the percentage of energy input that is converted into work instead of heat. The percentage of the input energy to a muscle (the chemical energy in the nutrients) that can be converted into work is less than 20 to 25 per cent, the remainder becoming heat. Maximum efficiency can be realized only when the muscle contracts at a moderate velocity. If the muscle contracts very slowly, large amounts of *maintenance heat* are released during the process of contraction, thereby decreasing the efficiency. On the other hand, if contraction is too rapid, large proportions of the energy are used to overcome the viscous friction within the muscle itself, and this, too, reduces the efficiency of contraction. Ordinarily, maximum efficiency is developed when the velocity of contraction is about 30 per cent of maximum.

CHARACTERISTICS OF A SINGLE MUSCLE TWITCH

Many features of muscle contraction can be especially well demonstrated by eliciting single *muscle twitches.* This can be accomplished by instantaneously exciting the nerve to a muscle or by passing a short electrical stimulus through the muscle itself, giving rise to a single, sudden contraction lasting for a fraction of a second.

Isometric versus Isotonic Contraction. Muscle contraction is said to be *isometric* when the muscle does not shorten during contraction and *isotonic* when it shortens but the tension on the muscle remains constant. Systems for recording the two types of muscle contraction are illustrated in Figure 2–13.

To the right is the isometric system in which the muscle is suspended between a solid rod and a lever of an electronic force transducer. This transducer records force with almost zero movement of the lever; therefore, in effect, the muscle is bound between fixed points so that it cannot contract significantly. To the left is shown an isotonic recording system: the muscle simply lifts a pan of weights so that the force against which the muscle contracts remains constant, though the length of the muscle changes considerably.

There are several basic differences between isometric and isotonic contractions. First, isometric contraction does not require sliding of myofibrils among each other. Second, in isotonic contraction a load is moved, which involves the phenomenon of inertia. That is, the weight or other type of object being moved must first be accelerated, and once a velocity has been attained the load has momentum that causes it to continue moving even after the contraction is over. Therefore an isotonic contraction is likely to last considerably longer than an isometric contraction of the same muscle. Third, isotonic contraction entails the performance of external work. Therefore, in accordance with the Fenn effect discussed previously, a greater amount of energy is used by the muscle.

In comparing the rapidity of contraction of different types of muscle, isometric recordings such as those illustrated in Figure 2–14 are usually used instead of isotonic recordings because the duration of an isotonic recording is almost as dependent on the inertia of the recording system as upon the contraction itself, and this makes it difficult to compare time relationships of contractions from one muscle to another.

Muscles can contract both isometrically and iso-

tonically in the body, but most contractions are actually a mixture of the two. When a person stands, he tenses his quadriceps muscles to tighten the knee joints and to keep the legs stiff. This is isometric contraction. On the other hand, when a person lifts a weight using his biceps, this is mainly an isotonic contraction. Finally, contractions of leg muscles during running are a mixture of isometric and isotonic contractions—isometric mainly to keep the limbs stiff when the legs hit the ground and isotonic mainly to move the limbs.

The Series Elastic Component of Muscle Contraction. When muscle fibers contract against a load, those portions of the muscle that do not contract—the tendons, the sarcolemmal ends of the muscle fibers where they attach to the tendons, and perhaps even the hinged arms of the cross-bridges—will stretch slightly as the tension increases. Consequently, the muscle must shorten an extra 3 to 5 per cent to make up for the stretch of these elements. The elements of the muscle that stretch during contraction are called the *series elastic component* of the muscle.

Characteristics of Isometric Twitches Recorded from Different Muscles. The body has many different sizes of skeletal muscles—from the very small stapedius muscle of only a few millimeters length and a millimeter or so in diameter up to the very large quadriceps muscle. Furthermore, the fibers may be as small as 10 microns in diameter or as large as 80 microns. And, finally, the energetics of muscle contraction vary considerably from one muscle to another. These different physical and chemical characteristics often manifest themselves in the form of different characteristics of contraction, some muscles contracting rapidly while others contract slowly.

Fast versus Slow Muscle. Figure 2–14 illustrates isometric contractions of three different types of skeletal muscles: an ocular muscle, which has a duration of contraction of less than $1/100$ second; the gastrocnemius muscle, which has a duration of contraction of about $1/30$ second; and the soleus muscle, which has a duration of contraction of about $1/10$ second. It is interesting that these durations of contraction are adapted to the function of each of the respective muscles, for ocular movements must be extremely rapid to maintain fixation of the eyes upon specific objects, the gastrocnemius muscle must contract moderately rapidly to provide sufficient velocity of limb movement for running and jumping, while the soleus muscle is concerned principally with slow reactions for continual support of the body against gravity.

Thus, there is a wide range of gradations from *fast* to *slow* muscles. In general, the slow muscles are used more for prolonged performance of work. Their muscle fibers generally are smaller, are surrounded by more blood capillaries, and have far more mitochondria than the fast muscles. They also have a large amount of *myoglobin* in the sarcoplasm (myoglobin is a substance similar to the hemoglobin in red

Figure 2–13. Isotonic and isometric recording systems.

Figure 2–14. Duration of isometric contractions of different types of mammalian muscles, showing also a latent period between the action potential and muscle contraction.

blood cells and can combine with oxygen and store this oxygen inside the muscle cell until it is needed by the mitochondria). On the other hand, the fast muscles generally have a much more extensive sarcoplasmic reticulum, which allows very rapid release of calcium ions and then rapid re-uptake of the calcium ions so that the contraction can be rapid. The slow muscle is frequently called *red muscle* because of the reddish tint caused by the myoglobin as well as by the large amount of red blood cells in the capillaries; the fast muscle is called *white muscle* because of a whitish appearance caused by lack of these elements.

CONTRACTION OF SKELETAL MUSCLE IN THE BODY

THE MOTOR UNIT

Each motor neuron that leaves the spinal cord usually innervates many different muscle fibers, the number depending on the type of muscle. All the muscle fibers innervated by a single motor nerve fiber are called a *motor unit*. In general, small muscles that react rapidly and whose control is exact have few muscle fibers (as few as 2 to 3 in some of the laryngeal muscles) in each motor unit and have a large number of nerve fibers going to each muscle. On the other hand, the large muscles which do not require a very fine degree of control, such as the gastrocnemius muscle, may have as many as 1000 muscle fibers in each motor unit. An average figure for all the muscles of the body can be considered to be about 180 muscle fibers to the motor unit.

Usually muscle fibers of adjacent motor units

overlap, with small bundles of 10 to 15 fibers from one motor unit lying among similar bundles of the second motor unit. This interdigitation allows the separate motor units to contract in support of each other rather than entirely as individual segments.

Macromotor Units. Loss of some of the nerve fibers to a muscle belly causes the remaining nerve fibers to sprout forth and innervate many of the paralyzed muscle fibers. When this occurs, such as following poliomyelitis, one occasionally develops *macromotor units,* which can contain as many as 5 times the normal number of muscle fibers. This obviously decreases the degree of control that one has over his muscles, but, nevertheless, allows the muscle to regain function.

SUMMATION OF MUSCLE CONTRACTION

Summation means the adding together of individual muscle twitches to make strong and concerted muscle movements. In general, summation occurs in two different ways: (1) by increasing the number of motor units contracting simultaneously and (2) by increasing the rapidity of contraction of individual motor units. These are called, respectively, *multiple motor unit summation* and *wave summation* (or spatial summation and temporal summation).

Multiple Motor Unit Summation. Figure 2–15 illustrates multiple motor unit summation, showing that the force of contraction increases progressively as the number of contracting motor units increases from 1 to 8.

Even within a single muscle, the numbers of muscle fibers and their sizes in the different motor units vary tremendously, so that one motor unit may be as much as 50 times as strong as another. The smaller motor units are far more easily excited than are the larger ones be-

Figure 2–15. Multiple motor unit summation.

cause they are innervated by smaller nerve fibers whose cell bodies in the spinal cord have a naturally high level of excitability. This effect causes the gradations of muscle strength during weak muscle contraction to occur in very small steps, while the steps become progressively greater as the intensity of contraction increases.

Wave Summation. Figure 2–16 illustrates the principles of wave summation, showing in the lower left-hand corner a single muscle twitch followed by successive muscle twitches at various frequencies. When the frequency of twitches is 10 per second, the first muscle twitch is not completely over by the time the second one begins. Therefore, since the muscle is already in a partially contracted state when the second twitch begins, the degree of muscle shortening this time is slightly greater than that which occurs with the single muscle twitch. The third, fourth, and additional twitches add still more shortening.

At more rapid rates of contraction, the degree of summation of successive contractions becomes greater and greater, because the successive contractions appear at earlier times following the preceding contraction.

Tetanization. When a muscle is stimulated at progressively greater frequencies, a frequency is finally reached at which the successive contractions fuse together and cannot be distinguished one from the other. This state is called *tetanization,* and the lowest frequency at which it occurs is called the *critical frequency.*

Tetanization results partly from the viscous properties of the muscle and partly from the nature of the contractile process itself. The muscle fibers are filled with sarcoplasm, which is a viscous fluid, and the fibers are encased in fasciae and muscle sheaths that have a viscous resistance to change in length. Therefore, undoubtedly these viscous factors play a role in causing the successive contractions to fuse with each other.

But in addition to the viscous property of muscle, the activation process itself lasts for a definite period of time, and successive pulsatile states of activation of the muscle fiber can occur so rapidly that they fuse into a long continual state of activation; that is, free calcium ions persist continuously in the myofibrils and provide an uninterrupted stimulus for maintenance of contraction. Once the critical frequency for tetanization is reached, further increase in rate of stimulation increases the force of contraction only a few more per cent, as shown in Figure 2–16.

Asynchronous Summation of Motor Units. Actually it is rare for either multiple motor unit summation or wave summation to occur separately from each other in normal muscle function. Instead, special neurogenic mechanisms in the spinal cord normally increase both the impulse rate and the number of motor units firing at the same time. If a motor unit fires at all, it usually fires at least five times per second, but this can increase to as high as 50 per second for most muscles or much more than this for the very fast muscles—to frequencies sufficient to cause complete tetanization.

Yet, even when tetanization of individual motor units of a muscle is not occurring, the tension exerted by the whole muscle is still continuous and nonjerky because *the different motor units fire asynchronously;* that is, while one is contracting another is relaxing; then another fires, followed by still another, and so forth. Consequently, even when motor units fire as infrequently as five times per second, the muscle contraction, though weak, is nevertheless very smooth.

Maximum Strength of Contraction. The maximum strength of tetanic contraction of a muscle operating at a normal muscle length is about 3.5 kilograms per square centimeter of muscle, or 50 pounds per square inch. Since a quadriceps muscle can at times have as much as 16 square inches of muscle belly, as much as 800 pounds of tension may at times be applied to the patellar tendon. One can readily understand, therefore, how it is possible for muscles sometimes to pull their tendons out of the

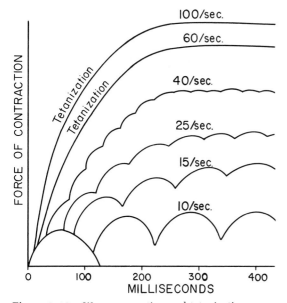

Figure 2–16. Wave summation and tetanization.

insertions in bones. This often occurs where the patellar tendon inserts in the tibia, and it occurs even more frequently where the Achilles tendon of the gastrocnemius muscle inserts at the heel.

Changes in Muscle Strength at the Onset of Contraction—The Staircase Effect (Treppe). When a muscle begins to contract after a long period of rest, its initial strength of contraction may be as little as one-half its strength 30 to 50 muscle twitches later. That is, the strength of contraction increases to a plateau, a phenomenon called the *staircase effect* or *treppe*. This phenomenon has interested physiologists greatly because it gives possible insights into the mechanism of muscle contraction.

Though all the possible causes of the staircase effect are not yet known, it is believed to be caused primarily by electrolyte changes that occur when a series of contractions begins. For instance, there is a net increase in calcium ions inside the muscle fiber because of movement of calcium ions inward through the membrane with each action potential. There is probably also further increase of calcium ions in the sarcoplasm because of release of these ions from the sarcoplasmic reticulum and failure to recapture the ions immediately. In addition, there is decreased potassium inside the cell as well as increased sodium; it has been suggested that the changes in these two ions increase the rate of liberation of calcium ions from the sarcoplasmic reticulum. Recalling the earlier discussion of the relationship of calcium ions to the contractile process, one can readily understand that progressive increase in calcium ion concentration in the sarcoplasm, caused either directly or as a consequence of sodium and potassium movement, could progressively increase the strength of muscle contraction, giving rise to the staircase effect.

SKELETAL MUSCLE TONE

Even when muscles are at rest, a certain amount of tautness usually remains. This residual degree of contraction in skeletal muscle is called *muscle tone*. Since skeletal muscle fibers do not contract without an actual action potential to stimulate the fibers except in certain pathological conditions, it is believed that skeletal muscle tone results entirely from nerve impulses coming from the spinal cord. These in turn are controlled partly by impulses transmitted from the brain to the appropriate anterior motor neurons and partly by impulses that originate in *muscle spindles* located in the muscle itself.

Muscle spindles are sensory receptors that exist throughout essentially all skeletal muscles to detect the degree of muscle contraction. These will be discussed in detail in Chapter 9, but, briefly, they transmit impulses almost continually through the posterior roots into the spinal cord, where they excite the anterior motor neurons, which in turn provide the necessary nerve stimuli for muscle tone. Simply cutting the posterior roots, thereby blocking the muscle spindle impulses, usually reduces muscle

tone to such a low level that the muscle becomes almost completely flaccid.

Many other neurogenic factors, originating especially in the brain, enter into the control of muscle tone. These will be discussed in detail in relation to muscle spindle and spinal cord function in Chapter 9.

MUSCLE FATIGUE

Prolonged and strong contraction of a muscle leads to the well-known state of muscle fatigue. This results simply from inability of the contractile and metabolic processes of the muscle fibers to continue supplying the same work output. The nerve continues to function properly, the nerve impulses pass normally through the neuromuscular junction into the muscle fiber, and even normal action potentials spread over the muscle fibers, but the contraction becomes weaker and weaker because of depletion of ATP in the muscle fibers themselves.

Interruption of blood flow through a contracting muscle leads to almost complete muscle fatigue in a minute or more because of the obvious loss of nutrient supply.

THE LEVER SYSTEMS OF THE BODY

Muscles obviously operate by applying tension to their points of insertion into bones, and the bones in turn form various types of lever systems. Figure 2–17 illustrates the lever system activated by the biceps muscle to lift the forearm. If we assume that a large biceps muscle has a cross-sectional area of 6 square inches, then the maximum force of contraction would be about 300 pounds. When the forearm is exactly at right angles with the upper arm, the tendon attachment of the biceps is about 2 inches anterior to the fulcrum at the elbow, and the total length of the forearm lever is about 14 inches. Therefore, the amount of lifting power that the biceps would have at the hand would be only one seventh of the 300 pounds force, or about 43 pounds. When the arm is in the fully extended position the attachment of the

Figure 2–17. The lever system activated by the biceps muscle.

biceps is much less than 2 inches anterior to the fulcrum, and the force with which the forearm can be brought forward is much less than 43 pounds.

In short, an analysis of the lever systems of the body depends on (a) a discrete knowledge of the point of muscle insertion and (b) its distance from the fulcrum of the lever, as well as (c) the length of the lever arm and (d) the position of the lever. Obviously, many different types of movement are required in the body, some of which need great strength and others large distances of movement. For this reason there are all varieties of muscles; some are long and contract a long distance and some are short but have large cross-sectional areas and therefore can provide extreme strengths of contraction over short distances. The study of different types of muscles, lever systems, and their movements is called *kinesiology* and is a very important phase of human physioanatomy.

Accommodation of Muscle Length to the Length of the Lever System. If a bone is broken and then heals in a shortened state, the force of contraction of the muscles lying along this broken bone would obviously become decreased because of the shortened lengths of muscles. However, muscles shortened in this manner undergo *physical shortening* during the next few weeks. That is, the muscle fibers actually shorten and re-establish new muscle lengths approximately equal to the maximum length of the lever system itself, thus re-establishing optimum force of contraction by the muscles.

The same shortening process also occurs in muscles of limbs immobilized for several weeks in casts if the muscles during this time are in a shortened position. When the cast is removed, the muscles must often be restretched over a period of weeks before full mobility is restored.

SPECIAL FEATURES AND ABNORMALITIES OF SKELETAL MUSCLE FUNCTION

MUSCULAR HYPERTROPHY

Forceful muscular activity causes the muscle size to increase, a phenomenon called hypertrophy. The diameters of the individual muscle fibers increase, and the fibers gain in total numbers of myofibrils as well as in various nutrient and intermediary metabolic substances, such as adenosine triphosphate, phosphocreatine, glycogen, and so forth. Briefly, muscular hypertrophy increases both the motive power of the muscle and the nutrient mechanisms for maintaining increased motive power.

Weak muscular activity, even when sustained over long periods of time, does not result in significant hypertrophy. Instead, hypertrophy results mainly from *very* forceful muscle activity, though the activity might occur for only a few minutes each day. For

this reason, strength can be developed in muscles much more rapidly when "resistive" or "isometric" exercise is used rather than simply prolonged mild exercise. Indeed, essentially no new myofibrils develop unless the muscle contracts to at least 75 per cent of its maximum tension.

MUSCULAR ATROPHY

Muscular atrophy is the reverse of muscular hypertrophy; it results any time a muscle is not used or even when a muscle is used only for very weak contractions. Atrophy is particularly likely to occur when limbs are placed in casts, thereby preventing muscular contraction. As little as one to two months of disuse can sometimes decrease the muscle size to one-half normal.

Atrophy Caused by Muscle Denervation. When a muscle is denervated it immediately begins to atrophy, and the muscle continues to decrease in size for several years. If the muscle becomes re-innervated during the first three to four months, full function of the muscle usually returns, but after four months of denervation some of the muscle fibers usually will have degenerated. Re-innervation after two years rarely results in return of any function at all. Pathological studies show that the muscle fibers have by that time been replaced by fat and fibrous tissue.

Prevention of Muscle Atrophy by Electrical Stimulation. Strong electrical stimulation of denervated muscles, particularly when the resulting contractions occur against loads, will delay and in some instances prevent muscle atrophy despite denervation. This procedure is used to keep muscles alive until re-innervation can take place.

Physical Contracture of Muscle Following Denervation. When a muscle is denervated, its fibers tend to shorten if the muscle is kept in a shortened position, and even the associated nerves and fasciae shorten. All this is a natural characteristic of protein fibers called "creep." That is, unless continual movement keeps stretching the muscle and other structures, they will creep toward a shortened length. This is one of the most difficult problems in the treatment of patients with denervated muscles, such as occur in poliomyelitis or nerve trauma. Unless passive stretching is applied daily to the muscles, they may become so shortened that even when re-innervated they will be of little value. But, more important, the shortening can often result in extremely contorted positions of different parts of the body.

RIGOR MORTIS

Several hours after death all the muscles of the body go into a state of *contracture* called rigor mortis; that is, the muscle contracts and becomes rigid even without action potentials. It is believed that this rigidity is caused by loss of all the ATP, which is required to cause separation of the cross-bridges from the actin filaments during the relaxation process. The muscles remain in rigor until the muscle proteins are destroyed, which usually results from autolysis caused by enzymes released from the lysosomes some 15 to 25 hours later.

FAMILIAL PERIODIC PARALYSIS

Occasionally, a hereditary disease called familial periodic paralysis occurs. In persons so afflicted, the extracellular fluid potassium concentration periodically falls to very low levels, causing various degrees of paralysis. The paralysis is caused in the following manner: A great decrease in extracellular fluid potassium increases the muscle fiber membrane potential to a very high value. This results in strong *hyperpolarization* of the membrane (a membrane potential more negative than the normal −85 millivolts) making the fiber almost totally inexcitable; that is, the membrane potential is so high that the normal stimulus at the neuromuscular junction is incapable of exciting the fiber.

THE ELECTROMYOGRAM

Each time an action potential passes along a muscle fiber a small portion of the electrical current spreads away from the muscle as far as the skin. If many muscle fibers contract simultaneously, the summated electrical potentials at the skin may be very great. By placing two electrodes on the skin or inserting needle electrodes into the muscle, an electrical recording called the electromyogram can be made when the muscle is stimulated. Figure 2–18 illustrates a typical electromyographic recording from the gastrocnemius muscle during a moderate contraction. Electromyograms are frequently used clinically to discern abnormalities of muscle excitation. Two such abnormalities are muscle *fasciculation* and *fibrillation*.

Muscle Fasciculation. When an abnormal impulse occurs in a motor nerve fiber its whole motor unit contracts. This often causes sufficient contraction in the muscle that one can see a slight ripple in the skin over the muscle. This process is called fasciculation.

Fasciculation occurs especially following destruction of anterior motor neurons in poliomyelitis or fol-

lowing traumatic interruption of a nerve. As the peripheral nerve fibers die, spontaneous impulses are generated during the first few days, and fasciculatory muscle movements result in the muscle. Typical electromyographic records of weak periodic potentials can be obtained from the skin overlying the muscle.

Muscle Fibrillation. After all nerves to a muscle have been destroyed and the nerve fibers themselves have become nonfunctional, which requires three to five days, spontaneous impulses begin to appear in the denervated muscle fibers. At first, these occur at a rate of once every few seconds, but, after a few more days or a few weeks, the impulses become as rapid as 3 to 10 times per second. Thus, skeletal muscle fibers, when released from innervation, develop an intrinsic rhythmicity. After several more weeks the muscle fibers atrophy to such an extent that the fibrillatory impulses finally cease. To record an electromyogram of fibrillation, minute bipolar needle electrodes must be inserted into the muscle belly itself because adjacent muscle fibers do not fire simultaneously and, therefore, do not summate. As a result, the potentials are not strong enough to record from the surface of the skin.

REFERENCES

Abbott, B. C., and Howarth, J. V.: Heat studies in excitable tissues. *Physiol. Rev.*, 53:120, 1973.

Astrand, P., and Rodahl, K.: Textbook of Work Physiology. New York, McGraw-Hill Book Company, 1968.

Basmajian, J. V.: Muscles Alive, 3rd Ed. Baltimore, The Williams & Wilkins Co., 1974.

Bourne, G. H. (ed.): The Structure and Function of Muscle, 2nd Ed. New York, Academic Press, Inc., 1973.

Buller, A. J.: The physiology of skeletal muscle. *In* Guyton, A. C. (ed.): MTP International Review of Science: Physiology. Baltimore, University Park Press, 1975, Vol. 3, p. 279.

Carlson, B. M.: The regeneration of skeletal muscle. A review. *Amer. J. Anat.*, 137:119, 1973.

Close, R. I.: Dynamic properties of mammalian skeletal muscles. *Physiol. Rev.*, 52:129, 1972.

Ebashi, S.: Calcium ions and muscle contraction. *Nature*, 240:217, 1972.

Ebashi, S.: Regulatory mechanism of muscle contraction with special reference to the Ca-troponin-tropomyosin system. *Essays Biochem.*, 10:1, 1974.

Falls, H. B.: Exercise Physiology. New York, Academic Press, Inc., 1968.

Fuchs, F.: Striated muscle. *Ann. Rev. Physiol.*, 36:461, 1974.

Grimby, G., and Saltin, B.: Physiological effects of physical training. *Scand. J. Rehabil. Med.*, 3:6, 1971.

Hess, A.: Vertebrate slow muscle fibers. *Physiol. Rev.*, 50:40, 1970.

Hill, A. L., et al.: Physiology of voluntary muscle. *Brit. Med. Bull.*, 12(Sept.): 1956.

Hoyle, G.: Comparative aspects of muscle. *Ann. Rev. Physiol.*, 31:43, 1969.

Hoyle, G.: How is muscle turned on and off? *Sci. Amer.*, 222:84, 1970.

Hughes, J. T.: Pathology of Muscle. Philadelphia, W. B. Saunders Company, 1975.

Huxley, H. E.: Muscular contraction and cell motility. *Nature*, 243:445, 1973.

Huxley, A. F., and Gordon, A. M.: Striation patterns in active and passive shortening of muscle. *Nature (Lond.)*, 193:280, 1962.

James, S. L., and Brubaker, C. E.: Biomechanics of running. *Orthop. Clin. North. Amer.*, 4:605, 1973.

50 mv.

Contraction

Figure 2–18. Electromyogram recorded during contraction of the gastrocnemius muscle.

Keul, J.: The relationship between circulation and metabolism during exercise. *Med. Sci. Sports, 5:*209, 1973.

Margaria, R.: The sources of muscular energy. *Sci. Amer., 226:*84, 1972.

Mommaerts, W. F. H. M.: Energetics of muscular contraction. *Physiol. Rev., 49:*427, 1969.

Murray, J. M., and Weber, A.: The cooperative action of muscle proteins. *Sci. Amer., 230:*58, 1974.

Nelson, P. G.: Nerve and muscle cells in culture. *Physiol. Rev., 55:*1, 1975.

Pearson, C. M. (ed.): The Striated Muscle. International Academy of Pathology, Monograph No. 2. Baltimore, The Williams & Wilkins Company, 1973.

Podolsky, R. J. (ed.): Mechanisms of Movement: A Symposium. Woods Hole, Mass., Sept. 1970. Englewood Cliffs, N.J., Prentice-Hall, Inc., 1972.

Sandow, A.: Skeletal muscle. *Ann. Rev. Physiol., 32:*87, 1970.

Spurway, N. C.: Mechanisms of anion permeation. A review of available data, principally on muscle cells, with the fixed charge concept in mind. *Biomembranes, 3:*363, 1972.

Taylor, E. W.: Chemistry of muscle contraction. *Ann. Rev. Biochem., 41:*577, 1972.

Tonomura, Y.: Muscle Proteins, Muscle Contraction, and Cation Transport. Baltimore, University Park Press, 1973.

Tonomura, Y., and Oosawa, F.: Molecular mechanism of contraction. *Ann. Rev. Biophys. Bioeng., 1:*159, 1972.

Walton, J. N. (ed.): Disorders of Voluntary Muscle. New York, Churchill Livingstone, Div. of Longman Inc., 1974.

Weber, A., and Murray, J. M.: Molecular control mechanisms in muscle contraction. *Physiol. Rev., 53:*612, 1973.

Zachar, J.: Electrogenesis and Contractility in Skeletal Muscle Cells. Baltimore, University Park Press, 1972.

3

Neuromuscular Transmission; Function of Smooth Muscle

TRANSMISSION OF IMPULSES FROM NERVES TO SKELETAL MUSCLE FIBERS: THE NEUROMUSCULAR JUNCTION

The skeletal muscles are innervated by large myelinated nerve fibers that originate in the large motoneurons of the anterior horns of the spinal cord. It was pointed out in the previous chapter that each nerve fiber normally branches many times and stimulates from 3 to 2000 skeletal muscle fibers. The nerve ending makes a junction, called the *neuromuscular junction* or the *myoneural junction,* with the muscle fiber approximately at the fiber's midpoint so that the action potential in the fiber travels in both directions. With the exception of about 2 per cent of the muscle fibers there is only one such junction per muscle fiber.

Physiologic Anatomy of the Neuromuscular Junction. Figure 3–1, Parts A and B, illustrates the neuromuscular junction between a large myelinated nerve fiber and a skeletal mus-

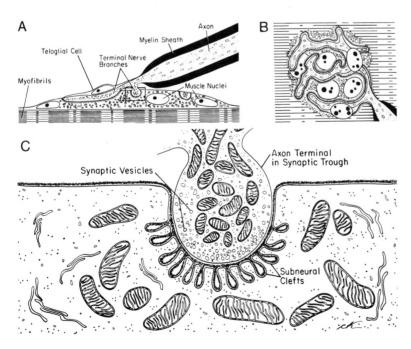

Figure 3–1. Different views of the motor end-plate. (A) Longitudinal section through the end-plate. (B) Surface view of the end-plate. (C) Electronmicrographic appearance of the contact point between one of the axon terminals and the muscle fiber membrane, representing the rectangular area shown in A. (From Bloom and Fawcett, as modified from R. Couteaux: A Textbook of Histology, 1975.)

cle fiber. The nerve fiber branches at its end to form a complex of branching nerve *terminals* called the *end-plate*, which invaginates into the muscle fiber but lies entirely outside the muscle fiber plasma membrane. The entire structure is covered by one or more Schwann cells that insulate the end-plate from the surrounding fluids.

Figure 3–1C shows an electronmicrographic sketch of the juncture between an axon terminal and the muscle fiber membrane. The invagination of the membrane is called the *synaptic gutter,* and the space between the terminal and the fiber membrane is called the *synaptic cleft.* The synaptic cleft is 200 to 300 Å wide and is filled with a gelatinous "ground" substance through which diffuses extracellular fluid. At the bottom of the gutter are numerous *folds* of the muscle membrane which form *secondary synaptic clefts* that greatly increase the surface area at which the synaptic transmitter can act. In the axon terminal are many mitochondria that supply energy mainly for synthesis of the excitatory transmitter *acetylcholine.* The acetylcholine is synthesized in the cytoplasm of the terminal, but is rapidly absorbed into many small synaptic vesicles, approximately 300,000 of which are normally in all the terminals of a single end-plate. On the surfaces of the folds in the synaptic gutter are aggregates of the enzyme *cholinesterase,* which is capable of destroying acetylcholine, as is explained in further detail below.

Secretion of Acetylcholine by the Axon Terminals.   When a nerve impulse reaches the neuromuscular junction, some 200 to 300 vesicles of acetylcholine are released by the terminals into the synaptic clefts between the terminals and the muscle fiber membrane. It has been postulated that the nerve action potential causes calcium ions to move from the extracellular fluid into the membranes of the terminal, and that it is these ions that in turn cause the vesicles of acetylcholine to rupture through the membrane. In the absence of calcium or in the presence of excess magnesium, the release of acetylcholine is greatly depressed.

Diffusion of the Released Acetylcholine Away from the Muscle Fiber Membrane, and Its Destruction by Cholinesterase.   Within approximately 2 to 3 milliseconds after acetylcholine is released by the axon terminal, some of it presumably diffuses out of the synaptic gutter and no longer acts on the muscle fiber membrane, and the remaining greater bulk of it is destroyed by the cholinesterase on the surfaces of the folds in the gutter. The very short period of time

that the acetylcholine remains in contact with the muscle fiber membrane—2 to 3 milliseconds—is almost always sufficient to excite the muscle fiber, and yet the rapid removal of the acetylcholine prevents re-excitation after the muscle fiber has recovered from the first action potential.

The "End-Plate Potential" and Excitation of the Skeletal Muscle Fiber.   Even though the acetylcholine released into the space between the end-plate and the muscle membrane lasts for only a minute fraction of a second, nevertheless, even during this period of time it can affect the muscle membrane sufficiently to make it very permeable to sodium ions, allowing rapid influx of sodium into the muscle fiber. As a result, the membrane potential rises *in the local area of the end-plate* as much as 50 to 75 millivolts, creating a *local potential* called the *end-plate potential.*

The mechanism by which acetylcholine increases the permeability of the muscle membrane is probably the following: It is believed that the muscle membrane contains a special protein molecule called an *acetylcholine receptor substance* to which the acetylcholine binds. Under the influence of the acetylcholine this receptor supposedly undergoes a conformational change that increases the permeability of the membrane to ions, most importantly to sodium ions. Rapid influx of sodium ions ensues, and this elicits the end-plate potential that is responsible for initiation of the action potential at the muscle fiber membrane.

A typical end-plate potential is illustrated at point A in Figure 3–2. This potential was recorded after the muscle had been poisoned with

Figure 3–2. End-plate potentials: *A,* normal end-plate potential recorded in a curarized muscle so that the muscle fiber itself could not generate an action potential; *B,* end-plate potential eliciting a muscle action potential; and *C,* end-plate potential too weak to elicit a muscle action potential.

curare, which made the end-plate potential too low to excite an action potential in the muscle fiber. However, in the normal muscle fiber, the effect shown at point B occurs: The end-plate potential begins, but before it can complete its course the intense local current flow created by this potential initiates an action potential; this in turn spreads in both directions along the muscle fiber. The threshold voltage at which the muscle fiber is stimulated is approximately −50 millivolts. Thus, if the resting membrane potential of the muscle is at the normal level of about −85 millivolts, then an end-plate potential of +35 millivolts is required to elicit an action potential in the muscle fiber.

At point C, another situation is illustrated in which only a small quantity of acetylcholine is released at the end-plate. This also causes an end-plate potential that is less than the threshold value required to cause an action potential. Note that the potential dies in a few milliseconds. Thus, failure to transmit a signal to the muscle fiber can result from either diminished receptivity of the muscle membrane or decreased release of acetylcholine.

"Safety Factor" for Transmission at the Neuromuscular Junction; Fatigue of the Junction. Ordinarily, each impulse that arrives at the neuromuscular junction creates an end-plate current flow about three to four times that required to stimulate the muscle fiber. Therefore, the normal neuromuscular junction is said to have a very high _safety factor_. However, artificial stimulation of the nerve fiber at rates greater than 150 times per second for many minutes often diminishes the number of vesicles of acetylcholine released with each impulse so that impulses then often fail to pass into the muscle fiber. This is called _fatigue_ of the neuromuscular junction, and it is analogous to fatigue of the synapse in the central nervous system. However, under normal functioning conditions, fatigue of the neuromuscular junction almost never occurs, because almost never do the spinal nerves stimulate even the most active neuromuscular junctions more than 150 times per second.

Drugs that Affect Transmission at the Neuromuscular Junction. _Drugs that Stimulate the Muscle Fiber by Acetylcholine-Like Action._ Many different compounds, including _methacholine, carbachol,_ and _nicotine,_ have the same effect on the muscle fiber as does acetylcholine. The difference between these drugs and acetylcholine is that they are not destroyed by cholinesterase or are destroyed very slowly, so that when once applied to the muscle fiber the action persists for many minutes to several hours. Moderate quantities of the above three drugs applied to a muscle fiber cause localized areas of depolarization, and every time the muscle fiber becomes repolarized elsewhere, these depolarized areas, by virtue of their leaking ions, cause new action potentials, thereby causing a state of spasm. On the other hand, when extreme dosages of these drugs are used, so much of the membranes becomes depolarized that the fibers can no longer pass impulses at all, and a state of flaccid paralysis exists instead of the spasm that occurs with moderate dosages.

Drugs that Block Transmission at the Neuromuscular Junction. One group of drugs, known as the _curariform drugs,_ can prevent passage of impulses from the end-plate into the muscle. Thus, D-tubocurarine affects the membrane, probably by competing with acetylcholine for the receptor sites of the membrane, so that the acetylcholine cannot increase the permeability of the membrane sufficiently to initiate a depolarization wave.

A second group of drugs prevents transmission of impulses into muscle fibers by a different mechanism. These, of which _decamethonium_ is a principal example, act in the same manner as _large doses_ of nicotine, methacholine, and carbachol to depolarize the muscle fibers completely. As a result, no impulses can be transmitted over the muscle fiber membranes even though the end-plate of the motor nerve fiber functions entirely normally.

Drugs that Stimulate the Neuromuscular Junction by Inactivating Cholinesterase. Three particularly well-known drugs, _neostigmine, physostigmine,_ and _diisopropyl fluorophosphate,_ inactivate cholinesterase so that the cholinesterase normally in the muscle fibers will not hydrolyze acetylcholine released at the end-plate. As a result, acetylcholine increases in quantity with successive nerve impulses so that extreme amounts of acetylcholine can accumulate and repetitively stimulate the muscle fiber. This causes _muscular spasm_ when even a few nerve impulses reach the muscle; this can cause death due to laryngeal spasm, which smothers the person.

Neostigmine and physostigmine combine with cholinesterase to inactivate it for several hours, after which they are displaced from the cholinesterase so that it once again becomes active. On the other hand, diisopropyl fluorophosphate, which has military potential as a very powerful "nerve" gas, actually inactivates cholinesterase for several weeks, which makes this a particularly lethal drug.

MYASTHENIA GRAVIS

The disease _myasthenia gravis,_ which occurs in rare instances in human beings, causes the person to become paralyzed because of inability of the neuromuscular junctions to transmit signals from the nerve fibers to the muscle fibers. Pathologically, the number of folds in the synaptic gutter is reduced and the synaptic cleft is widened. Also, antibodies that attack the muscle fibers have been demonstrated in the bloods of many of these patients. Therefore, it has been postulated that myasthenia gravis is an autoimmune disease in which the person has developed antibodies against his own muscles. And the antibodies in turn have damaged the muscle fibers—one of the effects being partial destruction of the receptor membrane of the neuromuscular junction.

Though it has not been possible to make precise neurophysiological measurements at the neuromuscular junctions in these patients, circumstantial evidence suggests that the end-plate potentials in these patients are greatly reduced, perhaps or probably because of the damaged receptor membrane of the junction. However, it is also possible that the axon terminals of the end-plate do not secrete adequate quantities of acetylcholine.

Regardless of the cause the end-plate potentials developed at the nerve endings are too weak to stimulate the muscle fibers adequately. If the disease is intense enough, the patient dies of paralysis—in particular, of paralysis of the respiratory muscles. However, the disease can usually be ameliorated with several different drugs, as follows:

Treatment with Drugs. When a patient with myasthenia gravis is treated with a drug, such as neostigmine, that is capable of inactivating or destroying cholinesterase, the acetylcholine secreted by the end-plate is not destroyed immediately. If a sequence of nerve impulses arrives at the end-plate, the quantity of acetylcholine present at the membrane increases progressively until finally the end-plate potential caused by the acetylcholine rises above threshold value for stimulating the muscle fiber. Thus, it is possible by diminishing the quantity of cholinesterase in the muscles of a patient with myasthenia gravis to allow even the inadequate quantities of acetylcholine secreted at the end-plates to effect almost normal muscular activity.

CONTRACTION OF SMOOTH MUSCLE

In the previous chapter and thus far in the present chapter, the discussion has been concerned with skeletal muscle. We now turn to smooth muscle that is composed of fibers far smaller than the skeletal muscle fibers—usually 2 to 5 microns in diameter and only 50 to 200 microns in length—in contrast to the skeletal muscle fibers that are as much as 20 times as large (in diameter) and thousands of times as long. Nevertheless, many of the same principles of contraction apply to both smooth muscle and skeletal muscle. Most important, the same chemical substances cause contraction in smooth muscle as in skeletal muscle, but the physical arrangement of smooth muscle fibers is entirely different, as we shall see.

TYPES OF SMOOTH MUSCLE

The smooth muscle of each organ is often distinctive from that of most other organs in several different ways: physical dimensions, organization into bundles or sheets, response to different types of stimuli, characteristics of its innervation, and function. Yet, for the sake of simplicity, smooth muscle can generally be divided into two major types, which are illustrated in Figure 3–3: *multiunit smooth muscle* and *visceral smooth muscle*.

Multiunit Smooth Muscle. This type of smooth muscle is composed of discrete smooth muscle fibers. Each fiber operates entirely independently of the others and is often innervated by a single nerve ending as occurs for skeletal muscle fibers. Furthermore, the outer surfaces of these fibers, like those of skeletal muscle fibers, are covered by a thin layer of "basement membrane–like" substance, a glycoprotein that helps to insulate the separate fibers from each other.

The most important characteristic of multiunit smooth muscle fibers is that their control is exerted almost entirely by nerve signals and very little by other stimuli such as local tissue factors. This is in contrast to a major share of the control of visceral smooth muscle. An additional characteristic is that they do not exhibit spontaneous contractions.

Some examples of multiunit smooth muscle found in the body are the smooth muscle fibers of the ciliary muscle of the eye, the iris of the eye, the nictitating membrane that covers the eyes in some lower animals, the piloerector muscles that cause erection of the hairs when stimulated by the sympathetic nervous system, and the smooth muscle of many of the larger blood vessels.

Visceral Smooth Muscle. Visceral smooth

VISCERAL   MULTIUNIT

Figure 3–3. Visceral and multiunit smooth muscle fibers.

muscle fibers are similar to multiunit fibers except that they are crowded together and lie in such close contact with each other that the cell membranes between adjacent cells either fuse or almost fuse. For this reason, this type of smooth muscle is also known as *unitary smooth muscle*. This type of muscle is found in most of the organs of the body, especially in the walls of the gut, the bile ducts, the ureters, the uterus, and so forth.

When one portion of a visceral muscle tissue is stimulated, the action potential ordinarily is conducted to the surrounding fibers by *ephaptic conduction*. This means that the action potential generated in one area of the muscle electrically excites the adjacent fibers without secretion of any excitatory substance. Visceral smooth muscle fibers can transmit action potentials one to another in this manner because the fiber membranes where the fibers contact each other form "tight junctions" with greatly enhanced permeability so that the electrical resistance between the inside of one fiber and the next is only a fraction of the normal membrane resistance. This obviously allows easy flow of current from the interior of one cell to the next and therefore allows ease of transmission of action potentials over the surface membranes of the muscle mass.

THE CONTRACTILE PROCESS IN SMOOTH MUSCLE

The Chemical Basis for Contraction. Smooth muscle contains exactly the same chemical substances as skeletal muscle, including both actin and myosin. However, the actin and myosin filaments do not have the same periodic spatial arrangement as that seen in the sarcomeres of skeletal muscle. Instead the filaments sometimes lie at odd angles to each other, though mostly oriented in the longitudinal direction of the muscle fibers. Typical actin filaments can be seen in electron micrographs; the tips of some of these are apparently attached to the cell membrane, thereby providing a method for mechanically coupling the contractile process inside the fiber with the tissues outside the fiber. On the other hand, typical myosin filaments as seen in striated muscle are rarely seen in smooth muscle, so that there is actually some doubt that myosin filaments of the type known to occur in skeletal muscle are necessary for smooth muscle contraction. Yet, chemically there is approximately the same ratio of myosin molecules to actin molecules in smooth muscle as in skeletal muscle. It is possible that some of the filaments that have tentatively been identified as actin filaments are instead myosin filaments, or it could be that unpolymerized myosin molecules too small to be seen with the electron microscope could provide binding forces between the actin filaments during contraction.

Nevertheless, the contractile process appears in many other ways to be the same as in skeletal muscle: that is, it is activated by calcium ions; ATP is converted to ADP, just as occurs in skeletal muscle; and contraction occurs after depolarization of the membrane and stops a fraction of a second to a few seconds following repolarization.

One significant difference between smooth muscle contraction and skeletal muscle contraction is the timing of the process; contraction develops only one-fourth to one-twentieth as rapidly in smooth muscle as in skeletal muscle. Also, relaxation at the end of the action potential is often very prolonged. This difference probably results from slowness of the activation and inactivation processes in smooth muscle, which will be discussed in subsequent sections.

It has also been suggested that the contractile filaments in smooth muscle tend to stick to each other so that they "drag" against each other during contraction and relaxation. This could explain a special ability of smooth muscle to maintain large amounts of tension over long periods of time without utilizing much ATP, an effect that is quite different from that in skeletal muscle.

MEMBRANE POTENTIALS AND ACTION POTENTIALS IN SMOOTH MUSCLE

Smooth muscle exhibits membrane potentials and action potentials similar to those that occur in skeletal muscle fibers. Furthermore, smooth muscle contraction is elicited by depolarization of the membrane in the same way that contraction is initiated by depolarization of skeletal muscle fibers. However, there are both quantitative and qualitative differences in the membrane potentials and action potentials of smooth muscle that require special attention.

Membrane Potentials in Smooth Muscle. The quantitative value of the membrane potential of smooth muscle is variable from one type of smooth muscle to another, and it also depends on the momentary condition of the muscle. However, in the normal resting state, the membrane potential is usually about −55 to

−60 millivolts, or about 25 millivolts less negative than in skeletal muscle.

Action Potentials in Visceral Smooth Muscle. Action potentials occur in visceral smooth muscle in the same way that they occur in skeletal muscle. However, action potentials probably do not normally occur in multiunit types of smooth muscle, as will be discussed in a subsequent section.

The action potentials of visceral smooth muscle occur in two different forms: (1) spike potentials and (2) action potentials with plateaus.

Spike potentials. Typical spike action potentials, such as those seen in skeletal muscle, occur in most types of visceral smooth muscle. The duration of this type of action potential is usually about 10 milliseconds, as illustrated in Figure 3–4A. Such action potentials can be elicited in many ways, such as by electrical stimulation, by the action of hormones on the smooth muscle, by the action of transmitter substances from nerve fibers, or as a result of spontaneous generation in the muscle fiber itself, as discussed below.

Slow Wave Potentials in Visceral Smooth Muscle and Spontaneous Generation of Spike Potentials. Some smooth muscle is self-excitatory. That is, action potentials arise within the smooth muscle itself without an extrinsic stimulus. This is usually associated with

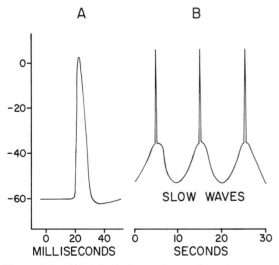

Figure 3–4. (A) A typical smooth muscle action potential (spike potential) elicited by an external stimulus. (B) A series of spike action potentials elicited by rhythmical slow electrical waves occurring spontaneously in the smooth muscle wall of the intestine.

a basic *slow wave rhythm* of the membrane potential. A typical slow wave of this type is illustrated in Figure 12–4B. The slow wave itself is not an action potential. It is not a self-regenerative process that spreads progressively over the membranes of the muscle fibers. Instead, it is a local property of the smooth muscle fibers that make up the muscle mass.

The cause of the slow wave rhythm is as yet unknown, though one suggestion for which there is considerable circumstantial evidence is that the slow waves are caused by waxing and waning of the pumping of sodium outward through the muscle fiber membrane; the membrane potential becomes more negative when sodium is pumped rapidly and less negative when the sodium pump becomes less active.

The importance of the slow waves lies in the fact that they can initiate action potentials. The slow waves themselves cannot cause muscle contraction, but when the potential of the slow wave rises above the level of approximately −35 millivolts (the approximate threshold for eliciting action potentials in visceral smooth muscle), an action potential develops and spreads over the visceral smooth muscle mass, and then contraction does occur. Figure 3–4B illustrates this effect, showing that at each peak of the slow wave, an action potential (a spike potential) occurs. Indeed, sometimes a series of action potentials occur on the peak while no action potentials at all occur during the trough. This effect can obviously promote a series of rhythmical contractions of the smooth muscle mass. Therefore, the slow waves are frequently called *pacemaker waves*. This type of activity is especially prominent in tubular types of smooth muscle masses, such as in the gut, the ureter, and so forth. Especially important, this type of activity controls the rhythmical contractions of the gut.

Action Potentials with Plateaus. Another type of action potential that occurs in some visceral smooth muscle is illustrated in Figure 3–5. The onset of this action potential is similar to that of the typical spike potential. However, instead of rapid repolarization of the muscle fiber membrane, the repolarization is delayed for several hundred milliseconds, mainly because of delay in the membrane inactivation process, as was explained in Chapter 1. This causes a plateau in the action potential before repolarization finally occurs and obviously provides a prolonged period of membrane depolarization that is also associated with prolonged contraction. This type of action potential

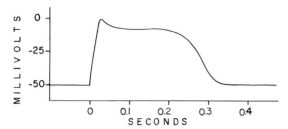

Figure 3–5. Monophasic action potential from a smooth muscle fiber of the rat uterus.

often occurs in the ureter and in the uterus under some conditions. It is also the type of action potential seen in cardiac muscle fibers, which also have a prolonged period of contraction.

Spread of Action Potentials Through Visceral Smooth Muscle. Because of the "tight junctions" that allow easy spread of electrical current between the smooth muscle fibers in visceral smooth muscle, once an action potential begins, it spreads slowly through the entire muscle mass. For instance, if it begins at the upper end of the gastrointestinal tract, it can spread downward along the intestinal wall, creating a constrictive ring that moves forward. The constrictive ring propels the intestinal contents forward. This process is called *peristalsis,* an important end result of smooth muscle function.

Excitation of Visceral Smooth Muscle by Stretch. When visceral smooth muscle is stretched sufficiently, spontaneous action potentials are usually generated. These result from a combination of the normal slow wave potentials plus a decrease in the membrane potential caused by the stretch itself. This response to stretch is an especially important function of visceral smooth muscle because it allows a hollow organ that is excessively stretched to contract automatically and therefore to resist the stretch. For instance, when the gut is overstretched by intestinal contents, a local automatic contraction sets up a peristaltic wave that moves the contents away from the super-stretched intestine.

Depolarization of Multiunit Smooth Muscle Without Action Potentials. The smooth muscle fibers of multiunit smooth muscle are normally contracted only in response to nerve stimuli. The nerve endings secrete acetylcholine in the case of some multiunit smooth muscles and norepinephrine in the case of others. In both instances, these transmitter

substances cause depolarization of the smooth muscle membrane, and this response in turn elicits the contraction. However, action potentials most often do not develop. The reason for this is presumably that the fibers are too small to generate an action potential. In fact, when action potentials are elicited in visceral smooth muscle, as many as 30 to 40 smooth muscle fibers must depolarize simultaneously before a self-propagating action potential ensues. Yet, even without an action potential in the multiunit smooth muscle fibers, the local depolarization caused by the nerve transmitter substance itself spreads "electrotonically" over the entire fiber and is all that is needed to cause the muscle contraction.

Role of Calcium Ions in Causing Smooth Muscle Action Potentials. It will be recalled from the discussion in Chapter 1 that the depolarization process during the action potential of nerve fibers (and also of skeletal muscle fibers) is caused almost entirely by rapid influx of sodium ions to the interior of the cell membrane. In the action potential of smooth muscle fibers, the rapid influx of ions includes not only sodium ions but also a large quantity of calcium ions. Indeed, it is believed that for many types of smooth muscle, the onset of depolarization is caused mainly by influx of calcium ions rather than of sodium ions. This is particularly important in view of the fact that influx of calcium ions seems also to be the major means by which muscle contraction itself is elicited, as will be discussed in the following section.

EXCITATION-CONTRACTION COUPLING—ROLE OF CALCIUM IONS

In the previous chapter it was pointed out that the actual contractile process in skeletal muscle is activated by calcium ions. This is also true in smooth muscle. However, the source of the calcium ions differs from smooth muscle to skeletal muscle because the sarcoplasmic reticulum of smooth muscle is poorly developed in contrast to the sarcoplasmic reticulum of skeletal muscle which is very extensive and is the source of the contraction-inducing calcium ions.

In smooth muscle, most of the calcium ions that cause contraction enter the muscle fiber from the extracellular fluid at the time of the action potential. There is a reasonably high concentration of calcium ions in the extracellular fluid, and as was pointed out in the previous section, the action potential is caused at least partly by influx of calcium ions into the muscle fiber. Because the smooth muscle fibers are extremely small (in contrast to the sizes of the skeletal muscle fibers), these calcium ions can diffuse to all parts of the smooth muscle and elicit the contractile process. The time required for this diffusion to occur is usually 200 to 300 milliseconds and is called the *latent period* before the contraction begins; this latent period is some 50 times as great as that for skeletal muscle contraction.

Yet, in some smooth muscle there are rudiments of a developing sarcoplasmic reticulum in which the cisternae of the reticulum abut the cell membrane. Therefore, it is believed that the membrane action potentials in these smooth muscle fibers cause additional release of calcium ions from these cisternae, thereby providing a greater degree of contraction than would occur on the basis of calcium ions entering through the cell membrane alone.

The Calcium Pump.   To cause relaxation of the smooth muscle contractile elements, it is necessary to remove the calcium ions. This removal is achieved by a calcium pump that pumps the calcium ions out of the smooth muscle fiber and back into the extracellular fluid, or perhaps also pumps calcium ions into the rudimentary sarcoplasmic reticulum when it is present. However, this pump is very slow-acting in comparison with the fast-acting sarcoplasmic reticulum pump in skeletal muscle. Therefore, the duration of smooth muscle contraction is often in the order of seconds rather than in tens of milliseconds as occurs for skeletal muscle.

GROSS CHARACTERISTICS OF SMOOTH MUSCLE CONTRACTION

From the foregoing discussion of the many different types of smooth muscle and the many different types of membrane depolarizations, one can readily understand why smooth muscle in different parts of the body has many different characteristics of contraction. For instance, the multiunit smooth muscle of the large blood vessels contracts mainly in response to nerve impulses, whereas, in many types of visceral smooth muscle—the smaller blood vessels, the ureter, the bile ducts, and other glandular ducts—a self-excitatory process causes continuous rhythmic contraction.

Tone of Smooth Muscle—Summation of Individual Contractions.   Smooth muscle can maintain a state of long-term, steady contrac-

tion that has been called either *tonus* contraction of smooth muscle or simply *smooth muscle tone*. This is an important feature of smooth muscle contraction because it allows prolonged or even indefinite continuance of the smooth muscle function. For instance, the arterioles are maintained in a state of tonic contraction almost throughout the entire life of the person. Likewise, tonic contraction in the gut wall maintains steady pressure on the contents of the gut, and tonic contraction of the urinary bladder wall maintains a moderate amount of pressure on the urine in the bladder.

The tonic contraction of smooth muscle is caused by summation of individual contractile pulses. That is, each time an action potential occurs, a small quantity of calcium ions enters the smooth muscle cell. If another action potential occurs before the first calcium ions have been pumped out, then the concentration of calcium ions will rise still further. In addition, since a pulse of calcium ions in smooth muscle usually lasts for a second or more, any time action potentials occur at frequencies greater than 1 per second, summation usually ensues and the strength of contraction increases. This effect is illustrated in Figure 3–6. Furthermore, rhythmic contractions can be superimposed on the tonic contraction, as also illustrated in the figure. The rhythmic contractions are caused by waxing and waning of the frequency of stimulation and, therefore, waxing and waning of the summation of the contractile process.

Degree of Shortening of Smooth Muscle During Contraction.   A special characteristic of smooth muscle—one that is also different from skeletal muscle—is its ability to shorten a far greater percentage of its length than can skeletal muscle. Skeletal muscle has a useful distance of contraction equal to only 25 to 35

Figure 3–6.   Record of rhythmic and tonic smooth muscle contraction.

per cent of its length, while smooth muscle can contract quite effectively from a length two times its normal length to as short as one-half its normal length, giving as much as a four-fold distance of contraction. This allows smooth muscle to perform important functions in the hollow viscera—for instance, allowing the gut, the bladder, blood vessels, and other internal structures of the body to change their lumen diameters from almost zero up to very large values.

Stress-Relaxation of Smooth Muscle. A very important characteristic of smooth muscle is its ability to change length greatly without marked changes in tension. This results from a phenomenon called stress-relaxation, which may be explained as follows:

If a segment of smooth muscle 1 inch long is suddenly stretched to 2 inches, the tension between the two ends increases tremendously at first, but the extra tension also begins to disappear immediately, and within a few minutes it has returned almost to its level prior to the stretch, even though the muscle is now twice as long. This probably results from the fact that the actin and myosin filaments are arranged randomly in smooth muscle. Over a period of time, the filaments of the stretched muscle presumably rearrange their bonds and gradually allow the sliding process to take place, thus allowing the tension to return almost to its original amount.

Exactly the converse effect occurs when smooth muscle is shortened. Thus, if the 2 inch segment of smooth muscle is shortened back to 1 inch, essentially all tension will be lost from the muscle immediately. Gradually, over a period of 1 minute or more, the tension returns, this again presumably resulting from slow sliding of the filaments. This is called *reverse stress-relaxation*.

NEUROMUSCULAR JUNCTIONS OF SMOOTH MUSCLE

Physiologic Anatomy of Smooth Muscle Neuromuscular Junctions. There are two major types of smooth muscle neuromuscular junctions: (1) the *contact* type, and (2) the *diffuse* type. The contact type of neuromuscular junctions is illustrated in Figure 3-7. This figure shows a nerve fiber arborizing into a reticulum of terminal fibrils that spread among smooth muscle fibers. These terminal fibrils are insulated by sheaths of Schwann cells, but

Figure 3-7. Junction of terminal nerve fibrils with smooth muscle fibers, showing a rare discrete terminal but many points where naked axons touch smooth muscle fibers, which points are also believed to act as transmission junctions.

where the fibers come in contact with muscle fibers the sheath is often interrupted, allowing the naked axons to touch the muscle fibers. Also, at these points the fibers form *varicosities* that contain acetylcholine or norepinephrine vesicles. In rare instances, a minute nerve terminal invaginates into the membrane of a smooth muscle fiber and is thus similar to the end-plate of the skeletal neuromuscular junction. However, it is believed that most transmission occurs at the points of contact between the varicosities and the smooth muscle fibers.

The diffuse type of smooth muscle neuromuscular junction is characterized by terminal nerve fibrils that never come into direct contact with the smooth muscle fibers. Instead, these terminal fibers either wend their way through the smooth muscle mass, partially protected by Schwann cells, or they even lie in the fibrous tissue adjacent to the smooth muscle mass, never penetrating at all. These fibers also have varicosities that release transmitter substances, and these substances then diffuse, often long distances, into the muscle mass. For instance, the innervation of portions of the gut and of some blood vessels is achieved in this way—simply secretion of the transmitter substances onto the surfaces of the smooth muscle masses or between layers of smooth muscle and the transmitter then diffusing to the other layers.

Excitatory and Inhibitory Transmitter Substances at the Smooth Muscle Neuromuscular Junction. Two different transmitter substances known to be secreted by the autonomic nerves innervating smooth muscle are *acetylcholine* and *norepinephrine*. Acetylcholine is an excitatory substance for smooth muscle fibers in some organs but an inhibitory substance for smooth muscle in other organs. And when acetylcholine excites a muscle fiber, norepinephrine ordinarily inhibits it, or when acetylcholine inhibits a fiber norepinephrine excites it.

It is believed that *receptor substances* in the membranes of the different smooth muscle fibers determine which will excite them, acetylcholine or norepinephrine. These receptor substances will be discussed in more detail in Chapter 15 in relation to function of the autonomic nervous system.

Excitation of Action Potentials in Smooth Muscle Fibers—The Junctional Potential. Transmission of impulses from terminal nerve fibers to smooth muscle fibers occurs in very much the same manner as transmission at the neuromuscular junction of skeletal muscle fibers except for temporal differences. When an action potential reaches the terminal of an excitatory nerve fibril, there is a latent period of about 50 milliseconds before any change in the membrane potential of the smooth muscle fiber can be detected. Then the potential rises to a maximal level in approximately 100 milliseconds. If an action potential does not occur, this potential gradually disappears at a rate of approximately one-half every 200 to 500 milliseconds. This complete sequence of potential changes is called the *junctional potential*; it is analogous to the end-plate potential of the skeletal muscle fibers except that its duration is 20 to 100 times as long.

If the junctional potential rises to the threshold level for discharge of the smooth muscle membrane, an action potential will occur in the smooth muscle fiber in exactly the same way that an action potential occurs in a skeletal muscle fiber. A typical smooth muscle fiber has a normal resting membrane potential of -55 to -60 millivolts, and the threshold potential at which the action potential occurs is about -30 to -40 millivolts.

Inhibition at the Smooth Muscle Neuromuscular Junction. When an inhibitory transmitter substance is released instead of an excitatory transmitter, the membrane potential of the muscle fiber becomes more negative than ever, for instance -70 millivolts; that is, it becomes *hyperpolarized* and therefore becomes much more difficult to excite than is usually the case.

Excitation of Smooth Muscle by Hormones. Many different hormones affect the degree of response of smooth muscle to nerve stimuli and other stimuli. Also, some hormones can cause direct stimulation of smooth muscle contrac-

tion. In addition to the usual transmitter substances acetylcholine and norepinephrine, the other hormonal factors that at times either excite or inhibit smooth muscle include epinephrine, serotonin, histamine, estrogens, progesterone, vasopressin, and oxytocin. The functions of these different substances will be discussed at different points in this text in relation to specific organs. To give an example, estrogens affect uterine muscle toward the end of pregnancy to decrease its membrane potential. This increases the excitability of the uterus, probably playing a role in the final onset of labor. On the other hand, progesterone has the opposite effect; it increases the membrane potential, causing a state of hyperpolarization and thus decreasing the excitability of the uterine musculature. Therefore, progesterone plays an important role in preventing expulsion of the fetus by the uterus during the early weeks and months of pregnancy.

REFERENCES

Barbeau, A.: Drugs affecting movement disorders. *Ann. Rev. Pharmacol.*, 14:91, 1974.

Barr, L.: Smooth muscle as an electrical syncytium. *In* Fishman, A. P., and Hecht, H. H. (eds.): The Pulmonary Circulation and Interstitial Space. Chicago, University of Chicago Press, 1969, p. 161.

Bennett, M. R., and Burnstock, G.: Electrophysiology of the innervation of intestinal smooth muscle. *In* Handbook of Physiology. Baltimore, The Williams & Wilkins Co., 1968, Vol. 4, Sec. 6, p. 1709.

Bohr, D. F., and Uchida, F.: Activation of vascular smooth muscle. *In* Fishman, A. P., and Hecht, H. H. (eds): The Pulmonary Circulation and Interstitial Space. Chicago, University of Chicago Press, 1969, p. 133.

Bozler, E.: Role of calcium in initiation of activity of smooth muscle. *Amer. J. Physiol.*, 216:671, 1969.

Bradley, P. B.: Pharmacology of the central nervous system. *Brit. Med. Bull.*, 21:1, 1965.

Bulbring, E.: Smooth Muscle. Baltimore, The Williams & Wilkins Co., 1970.

Bulbring, E., Kostyuk, P. G., and Shuba, M. F. (eds.): Physiology of Smooth Muscles; Twenty-sixth International Congress of Physiological Sciences. New York, Raven Press, 1975.

Cohen, L. B.: Changes in neuron structure during action potential propagation and synaptic transmission. *Physiol. Rev.*, 53:373, 1973.

De Robertis, E., and Schacht, J. (eds.): Neurochemistry of Cholinergic Receptors. New York, American Elsevier Publishing Co., Inc., 1974.

Gerschenfeld, H. M.: Chemical transmission in invertebrate central nervous systems and neuromuscular junctions. *Physiol. Rev.*, 53:1, 1973.

Ginsborg, B. L.: Electrical changes in the membrane in junctional transmission. *Biochim. Biophys. Acta*, 300:289, 1973.

Greengard, P., and Kebabian, J. W.: Role of cyclic AMP in synaptic transmission in the mammalian peripheral nervous system. *Fed. Proc.*, 33:1059, 1974.

Guyton, A. C., and MacDonald, M. A.: Physiology of botulinus toxin. *Arch. Neurol. Psychiat.*, 57:578, 1947.

Guyton, A. C., and Reeder, R. C.: The dynamics of curarization. *J. Pharmacol. Exp. Ther.*, 97:322, 1949.

Hall, Z. W., Hildebrand, J. G., and Kravitz, E. A.: Chemistry of synaptic transmission. Newton, Mass., Chiron Press, 1974.

Hebb, C.: CNS at the cellular level: identity of transmitter agents. *Ann. Rev. Physiol., 32*:165, 1970.

Hubbard, J. I.: Microphysiology of vertebrate neuromuscular transmission. *Physiol. Rev., 53*:674, 1973.

Hubbard, J. I., and Quastel, D. M.: Micropharmacology of vertebrate neuromuscular transmission. *Ann. Rev. Pharmacol., 13*:199, 1973.

Kandel, E. R., and Kupfermann, I.: The functional organization of invertebrate ganglia. *Ann. Rev. Physiol., 32*:193, 1970.

McGeachie, J. K.: Smooth Muscle Regeneration; a Review and Experimental Study. Basel, S. Karger, A. G., 1975.

Minton, S. A., Jr.: Venom Diseases. Springfield, Ill., Charles C Thomas, Publisher, 1974.

Nachmansohn, D.: Chemical events in conducting and synaptic membranes during electrical activity. *Proc. Natl. Acad. Sci. U.S.A., 68*:3170, 1971.

Prosser, C. L.: Smooth muscle. *Ann. Rev. Physiol., 36*:503, 1974.

Radouco-Thomas, S.: Cellular and molecular aspects of transmitter release: calcium monoamine dynamics. *Adv. Cytopharmacol., 1*:457, 1971.

Reuter, H.: Divalent cations as charge carriers in excitable membranes. *Prog. Biophys. Mol. Biol., 26*:1, 1973.

Ruegg, J. C.: Smooth muscle tone. *Physiol. Rev., 51*:201, 1971.

Simpson, L. L., and Curtis, D. R. (eds.): Neuropoisons. New York, Plenum Publishing Co., 1974.

Somlyo, A. P.: Excitation-contraction coupling in vertebrate smooth muscle: correlation of ultrastructure with function. *Physiologist, 15*:338, 1972.

Tauc, L: Transmission in invertebrate and vertebrate ganglia. *Physiol. Rev., 47*:521, 1967.

Yang, C. C.: Chemistry and evolution of toxins in snake venoms. *Toxicon, 12*:1, 1974.

PART II

THE CENTRAL
NERVOUS SYSTEM

4

Organization of the Central Nervous System; Basic Functions of Synapses

The nervous system, along with the endocrine system, provides most of the control functions for the body. In general, the nervous system controls the rapid activities of the body, such as muscular contractions, rapidly changing visceral events, and even the rate of secretion of some endocrine glands. The endocrine system, by contrast, regulates principally the metabolic functions of the body.

The nervous system is unique in the vast complexity of the control actions that it can perform. It receives literally thousands of bits of information from the different sensory organs and then integrates all these to determine the response to be made by the body. The purpose of this chapter is to present, first, a general outline of the overall mechanisms by which the nervous system performs such functions. Then we will discuss the function of central nervous system synapses, the basic structures that control the passage of signals into, through, and then out of the nervous system. In succeeding chapters we will analyze in detail the functions of the individual parts of the nervous system. Before beginning this discussion, however, the reader should refer to Chapters 1 and 3, which present, respectively, the principles of membrane potentials and transmission of impulses through neuromuscular junctions.

GENERAL DESIGN OF THE NERVOUS SYSTEM

THE SENSORY DIVISION— SENSORY RECEPTORS

Most activities of the nervous system are originated by sensory experience emanating from *sensory receptors,* whether these be visual receptors, auditory receptors, tactile receptors on the surface of the body, or other kinds of receptors. This sensory experience can cause an immediate reaction, or its memory can be stored in the brain for minutes, weeks, or years and then can help to determine the bodily reactions at some future date.

Figure 4–1 illustrates a portion of the sensory system, the *somatic* portion that transmits sensory information from the receptors of the entire surface of the body and deep structures. This information enters the nervous system through the spinal nerves and is conducted into (a) the spinal cord at all levels, (b) the reticular substance of the medulla, pons, and mesencephalon, (c) the cerebellum, (d) the thalamus, and (e) the somesthetic areas of the cerebral cortex. But in addition to these "primary sensory" areas, signals are then relayed to essentially all other segments of the nervous system.

THE MOTOR DIVISION— THE EFFECTORS

The most important ultimate role of the nervous system is control of bodily activities. This is achieved by controlling (a) contraction of skeletal muscles throughout the body, (b) contraction of smooth muscle in the internal organs, and (c) secretion of both exocrine and endocrine glands in many parts of the body. These activities are collectively called *motor functions* of the nervous system, and the muscles and glands are called *effectors* because they perform the functions dictated by the nerve signals. That portion of the nervous system directly

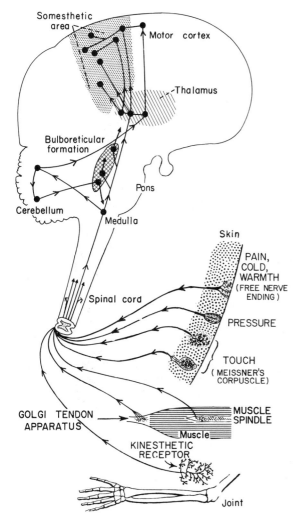

Figure 4–1. The somatic sensory axis of the nervous system.

plays its own specific role in the control of body movements, the lower regions being concerned primarily with automatic, instantaneous responses of the body to sensory stimuli and the higher regions with deliberate movements controlled by the thought processes of the cerebrum.

PROCESSING OF INFORMATION

The nervous system would not be at all effective in controlling bodily functions if each bit of sensory information caused some motor reaction. Therefore, one of the major functions of the nervous system is to process incoming information in such a way that *appropriate* motor responses occur. Indeed, more than 99 per cent of all sensory information is continually discarded by the brain as unimportant. For instance, one is ordinarily totally unaware of the parts of his body that are in contact with his clothes and is also unaware of the pressure on his seat when he is sitting. Likewise, his attention is drawn only to an occasional object in his field of vision, and even the perpetual noise of

concerned with transmitting signals to the muscles and glands is called the motor division of the nervous system.

Figure 4–2 illustrates the *motor axis* of the nervous system for controlling skeletal muscle contraction. Operating parallel with this axis is another similar system for control of the smooth muscles and glands; it is the *autonomic nervous system,* which will be presented in detail in Chapter 15. Note in Figure 4–2 that the skeletal muscles can be controlled from many different levels of the central nervous system, including (a) the spinal cord, (b) the reticular substance of the medulla, pons, and mesencephalon, (c) the basal ganglia, (d) the cerebellum, and (e) the motor cortex. Each of these different areas

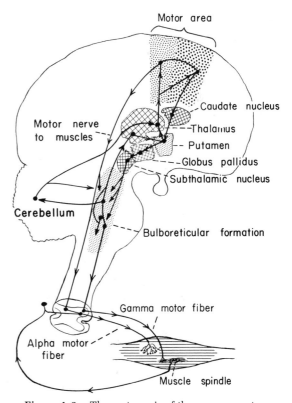

Figure 4–2. The motor axis of the nervous system.

his surroundings is usually relegated to the background.

After the important sensory information has been selected, it must be channeled into proper motor regions of the brain to cause the desired responses. Thus, if a person places his hand on a hot stove, the desired response is to lift the hand, plus other associated responses, such as moving the entire body away from the stove and perhaps even shouting with pain. Yet even these responses represent activity by only a small fraction of the total motor system of the body.

Role of Synapses in Processing Information. The synapse is the junction point from one neuron to the next and, therefore, is an advantageous site for control of signal transmission. Later in this chapter we will discuss the details of synaptic function. However, it is important to point out here that the synapses determine the directions that the nervous signals spread in the nervous system. Some synapses transmit signals from one neuron to the next with ease, whereas others transmit signals only with difficulty. Also, facilitatory and inhibitory signals from other areas in the nervous system can control synaptic activity, sometimes opening the synapses for transmission and other times closing them. In addition, some postsynaptic neurons respond with large numbers of impulses, whereas others respond with only a few. Thus, the synapses perform a selective action, often blocking the weak signals while allowing the strong signals to pass, often selecting and amplifying certain weak signals, and often channeling the signal in many different directions rather than simply in one direction. The basic principles of this processing of information by the synapses are so important that they are discussed in detail in the latter part of this chapter and in the entire following chapter.

STORAGE OF INFORMATION—MEMORY

Only a small fraction of the important sensory information causes an immediate motor response. Much of the remainder is stored for future control of motor activities and for use in the thinking processes. Most of this storage occurs in the *cerebral cortex*, but not all, for even the basal regions of the brain and perhaps even the spinal cord can store small amounts of information.

The storage of information is the process we call *memory,* and this too is a function of the synapses. That is, each time a particular sensory signal passes through a sequence of synapses, the respective synapses become more capable of transmitting the same signal the next time, which process is called *facilitation.* After the sensory signal has passed through the synapses a large number of times, the synapses become so facilitated that signals from the "control center" of the brain can also cause transmission of impulses through the same sequence of synapses even though the sensory input has not been excited. This gives the person a perception of experiencing the original sensation, though in effect it is only a memory of the sensation.

Unfortunately, we do not know the precise mechanism by which facilitation of synapses occurs in the memory process, but what is known about this and other details of the memory process will be discussed in Chapter 13.

Once memories have been stored in the nervous system, they become part of the processing mechanism. The thought processes of the brain compare new sensory experiences with the stored memories; the memories help to select the important new sensory information and to channel this into appropriate storage areas for future use or into motor areas to cause bodily responses.

THE THREE MAJOR LEVELS OF NERVOUS SYSTEM FUNCTION

The human nervous system has inherited specific characteristics from each stage of evolutionary development. From this heritage, there remain three major levels of the nervous system that have special functional significance: (1) the spinal cord level, (2) the lower brain level, and (3) the higher brain or cortical level.

THE SPINAL CORD LEVEL

The spinal cord of the human being still retains many functions of the multisegmental animal. Sensory signals are transmitted through the spinal nerves into each *segment* of the spinal cord, and these signals can cause localized motor responses either in the segment of the body from which the sensory information is received or in adjacent segments. Essentially all the spinal cord motor responses are automatic and occur almost instantaneously in response to

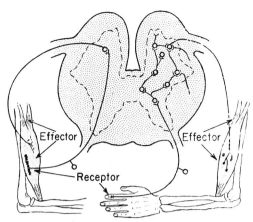

Figure 4–3. *Left:* The simple stretch reflex. *Right:* A withdrawal reflex.

the sensory signal. In addition, they occur in specific patterns of response called *reflexes*.

Figure 4–3 illustrates two of the simpler cord reflexes. To the left is the neural control of the *muscle stretch reflex*. If a muscle suddenly becomes stretched, a sensory nerve receptor in the muscle called the *muscle spindle* becomes stimulated and transmits nerve impulses through a sensory nerve fiber into the spinal cord. This fiber synapses directly with a motoneuron in the anterior horn of the cord gray matter, and the motoneuron in turn transmits impulses back to the muscle to cause the muscle, the effector, to contract. The muscle contraction opposes the original muscle stretch. Thus, this reflex acts as a *feedback* mechanism, operating from a receptor to an effector, to prevent sudden changes in length of the muscle. This allows a person to maintain his limbs and other parts of his body in desired positions despite sudden outside forces that tend to move the parts out of position.

To the right in Figure 4–3 is illustrated the neural control of another reflex called the *withdrawal reflex*. This is a protective reflex that causes withdrawal of any part of the body from an object that is causing pain. For instance, let us assume that the hand is placed on a sharp object. Pain signals are transmitted into the gray matter of the spinal cord, and, after appropriate selection of information by the synapses, signals are channeled to the appropriate motoneurons to cause flexion of the biceps muscle. This obviously lifts the hand away from the sharp object.

We see, then, that the withdrawal reflex is much more complex than the stretch reflex, for it involves many neurons in the gray matter of the cord, and signals are transmitted to many adjacent segments of the cord to cause contraction of the appropriate muscles.

Cord Functions After the Brain Is Removed. The many reflexes of the spinal cord will be discussed in Chapter 9; however, the following list of important cord reflex functions that occur even after the brain is removed illustrates the many capabilities of the spinal cord:

1. The animal can under certain conditions be made to stand up. This is caused primarily by reflexes initiated from the pads of the feet. Sensory signals from the pads cause the extensor muscles of the limbs to tighten, which in turn allows the limbs to support the animal's body.

2. A spinal animal held in a sling so that its feet hang downward often begins walking or galloping movements involving one, two, or all its legs. This illustrates that the basic patterns for causing the limb movements of locomotion are present in the spinal cord.

3. A flea crawling on the skin of a spinal animal causes reflex to-and-fro scratching by the paw, and the paw can actually localize the flea on the surface of the body.

4. Cord reflexes exist to cause emptying of the urinary bladder and of the rectum.

5. Segmental temperature reflexes are present throughout the body. Local cooling of the skin causes vasoconstriction, which helps to conserve heat in the body. Conversely, local heating in the skin causes vasodilatation, resulting in loss of heat from the body.

This list of some of the segmental and multisegmental reflexes of the spinal cord demonstrates that many of our day-by-day and moment-by-moment activities are controlled locally by the respective segmental levels of the spinal cord, and the brain plays only a modifying role in these local controls.

THE LOWER BRAIN LEVEL

Many if not most of what we call subconscious activities of the body are controlled in the lower areas of the brain—in the medulla, pons, mesencephalon, hypothalamus, thalamus, cerebellum, and basal ganglia. Subconscious control of arterial blood pressure and respiration is achieved primarily in the reticular substance of the medulla and pons. Control of equilibrium is a combined function of the older portions of the cerebellum and the reticular substance of the medulla, pons, and mesencephalon. The coordinated turning movements of the head, of the entire body, and of the eyes are controlled by specific centers located in the mesencephalon, paleocerebellum, and lower basal ganglia. Feeding reflexes, such as salivation in response to taste of food and licking of the lips, are controlled by areas in the medulla, pons, mesencephalon, amygdala, and hypothalamus. And many emotional patterns, such as anger, excitement, sexual activities, reactions to pain, or reactions of pleasure, can occur in animals without a cerebral cortex.

In short, the subconscious but coordinate functions of the body, as well as many of the life processes themselves—arterial pressure and respiration, for instance—are controlled by the lower regions of the brain, regions that usually, but not always, operate below the conscious level.

THE HIGHER BRAIN OR CORTICAL LEVEL

We have seen from the above discussion that many of the intrinsic life processes of the body are controlled by subcortical regions of the brain or by the spinal cord. What then is the function of the cerebral cortex? The cerebral cortex is primarily a vast information storage area. Approximately three quarters of all the neuronal cell bodies of the entire nervous system are located in the cerebral cortex. It is here that most of the memories of past experiences are stored, and it is here that many of the patterns of motor responses are stored, which information can be called forth at will to control motor functions of the body.

Relation of the Cortex to the Thalamus and Other Lower Centers. The cerebral cortex is actually an outgrowth of the lower regions of the brain, particularly of the thalamus. For each area of the cerebral cortex there is a corresponding and connecting area of the thalamus, and activation of a minute portion of the thalamus activates the corresponding and much larger portion of the cerebral cortex. It is presumed that in this way the thalamus can call forth cortical activities at will. Also, activation of regions in the mesencephalon transmits diffuse signals to the cerebral cortex, partially through the thalamus and partially directly, to activate the entire cortex. This is the process that we call *wakefulness*. On the other hand, when these areas of the mesencephalon become inactive, the thalamic and cortical regions also become inactive, which is the process we call *sleep*.

Function of the Cerebral Cortex in Thought Processes. Some areas of the cerebral cortex are not directly concerned with either sensory or motor functions of the nervous system—for example, the prefrontal lobe and large portions of the temporal and parietal lobes. These areas are set aside for the more abstract processes of thought, but even they also have direct nerve connections with the lower regions of the brain.

Large areas of the cerebral cortex can be destroyed without blocking the subconscious, and even some of the involuntary conscious, activities of the body. For instance, destruction of the somesthetic cortex does not destroy one's ability to feel objects touching his skin, but it does destroy his ability to distinguish the shapes of objects, their character, and the precise points on the skin where the objects are touching. Thus, the cortex is not required for perception of sensation, but it does add immeasurably to its depth of meaning. Likewise, destruction of the prefrontal lobe does not destroy one's ability to think, but it does destroy his ability to think in abstract terms. In other words, each time a portion of the cerebral cortex is destroyed, a vast amount of information is lost to the thinking process and some of the mechanisms for processing this information are also lost. Therefore, total loss of the cerebral cortex causes a vegetative type of existence rather than a "living" existence.

Telencephalization. In the process of evolution, the higher regions of the human nervous system have taken over many sensory and motor functions performed by lower regions of the brain in lower animals. For instance, if the spinal cord of an opossum is cut in the midthoracic region, the opossum can still walk perfectly well on both his forelimbs and hindlimbs, except that the hindlimbs are then unsynchronized with the forelimbs. A similar transection of the spinal cord in the human being causes complete loss of ability to use the legs for locomotion.

This process by which the progressively higher centers of the brain have taken over more and more of the function of the lower centers is called *telencephalization*. Yet, despite telencephalization, some of the very basic functions of the lower centers still remain active or at least partially active in the human being, such as many of the cord reflexes and the stereotyped control systems of the basal regions of the brain that were just discussed.

COMPARISON OF THE NERVOUS SYSTEM WITH AN ELECTRONIC COMPUTER

When electronic computers were first developed in many different laboratories of the world by as many different engineers, it soon became apparent that all these machines have many features in common with the nervous system. First, they all have input circuits which are comparable to the sensory portion of the nervous system and output circuits which are comparable to the motor portion of the nervous system. In the conducting pathway between the inputs and the outputs are the mechanisms for performing the different types of computations.

In simple computers, the output signals are controlled directly by the input signals, operating in a manner similar to that of the simple reflexes of the spinal cord. But, in the more complex computers, the output is determined both by the input signals and by information that has already been stored in the computer, which is analogous to the more complex reflex and processing mechanisms of our nervous system. Furthermore, as the computers become even more complex it is necessary to add still another unit, called the *programming unit,* which determines the sequence of computational operations. This unit is analogous to the mechanism in our brain that allows us to direct our attention first to one thought, then to another, and so forth, until complex sequences of thought take place.

Figure 4–4 illustrates a simple block diagram of a modern computer. Even a rapid study of this diagram will demonstrate its similarity to the nervous system. Furthermore, general purpose computers designed and built by many different scientific groups have ended up with almost identically the same basic components. The fact that these components are analogous to those of the human nervous system demonstrates that the brain is basically a computer that continuously collects sensory information and uses this along with stored information to compute the daily course of bodily activity.

FUNCTION OF NEURONAL SYNAPSES

Every medical student is aware that information is transmitted in the central nervous system through a succession of neurons, one after another. However, it is not immediately apparent that the impulse may be (a) blocked in its transmission from one neuron to the next, (b) changed from a single impulse into repetitive impulses, or (c) integrated with impulses from other neurons to cause highly intricate patterns of impulses in successive neurons. All these

Figure 4–4. Block diagram of a general-purpose electronic computer, showing the basic components and their interrelationships.

functions can be classified as *synaptic functions of neurons.*

PHYSIOLOGIC ANATOMY OF THE SYNAPSE

The juncture between one neuron and the next is called a *synapse.* Figure 4–5 illustrates a typical *motoneuron* in the anterior horn of the spinal cord. It is comprised of three major parts, the *soma,* which is the main body of the neuron; a single *axon,* which extends from the soma into the peripheral nerve; and the *dendrites,* which

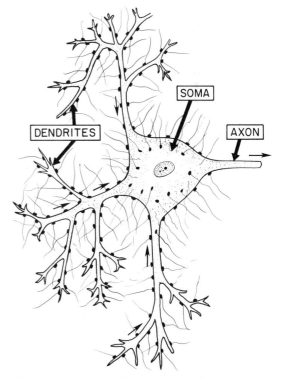

Figure 4–5. A typical motoneuron, showing synaptic knobs on the neuronal soma and dendrites. Note also the single axon.

are thin projections of the soma that extend up to 1 mm. into the surrounding areas of the cord.

It should be noted, also, that literally hundreds to many thousands of small knobs called *synaptic knobs* lie on the surfaces of the dendrites and soma, approximately 80 to 90 per cent of them on the dendrites. These knobs are the terminal ends of nerve fibrils that originate in many other neurons, and usually not more than a few of the knobs are derived from any single previous neuron. Later it will become evident that many of these synaptic knobs are *excitatory* and secrete a substance that excites the neuron, whereas still others are *inhibitory* and secrete a substance that inhibits the neuron.

Neurons in other parts of the cord and brain differ markedly from the motoneuron in (1) the size of the cell body, (2) the length, size, and number of dendrites, ranging in length from almost none at all up to as long as one meter (the peripheral sensory nerve fiber), (3) the length and size of the axon, and (4) the number of synaptic knobs, which may range from only a few up to many thousand. It is these differences that make neurons in different parts of the nervous system react differently to incoming signals and therefore to perform different functions, as will be explained in subsequent chapters.

The Synaptic Knobs. Electron microscope studies of the synaptic knobs show that they have varied anatomical forms, but most resemble small round or oval knobs and therefore are frequently called *terminal knobs, boutons, end-feet,* or simply *presynaptic terminals.*

Figure 4–6 illustrates the basic structure of the synaptic knob (presynaptic terminal). It is separated from the neuronal soma by a *synaptic cleft* having a width usually of 200 to 300 Ångstroms. The knob has two internal struc-

tures important to the excitatory or inhibitory functions of the synapse: the *synaptic vesicles* and the *mitochondria*. The synaptic vesicles of the excitatory knobs contain an *excitatory transmitter,* which, when released into the synaptic cleft, excites the neuron; the vesicles of the inhibitory knobs contain an *inhibitory transmitter* that inhibits the neuron. The mitochondria provide ATP, which is required to synthesize new transmitter substance. This transmitter must be synthesized extremely rapidly because the amount stored in the vesicles is sufficient to last for only a few seconds to a few minutes of maximum activity.

When an action potential spreads over a presynaptic terminal, the membrane depolarization causes emptying of a small number of vesicles into the cleft; and the released transmitter in turn causes an immediate change in the permeability characteristics of the subsynaptic neuronal membrane, which leads to excitation or inhibition of the neuron, depending on the type of transmitter substance.

Mechanism by Which the Synaptic Knob Action Potential Causes Release of Transmitter Vesicles. Unfortunately, we can only guess at the mechanism by which an action potential on reaching the synaptic knob causes the vesicles to release transmitter substance into the synaptic cleft. However, the number of vesicles released with each action potential is greatly reduced (a) when the quantity of calcium ions in the extracellular fluid is diminished, (b) when the quantity of sodium ions in the extracellular fluid is diminished, (c) when the quantity of magnesium ions in the extracellular fluids is increased, or (d) when the membrane of the synaptic knob has already been partially depolarized prior to transmission of the action potential so that the action potential is weaker than usual. On the basis of these characteristics, it has been suggested that the spread of the action potential over the membrane of the knob causes small amounts of calcium ions to leak into the knob. The calcium ions then supposedly attract the transmitter vesicles to the membrane and simultaneously cause one or more of them to rupture, thus allowing spillage of their contents into the synaptic cleft.

At any rate, it is known that each time an action potential travels over the surface of the synaptic knob, one or more vesicles of transmitter substance are emptied into the synaptic cleft. It may be only one vesicle, which is the average, or several vesicles, depending upon the factors mentioned above.

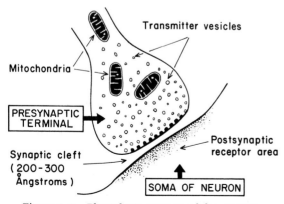

Figure 4–6. Physiologic anatomy of the synapse.

One transmitter substance that occurs in certain parts of the nervous system is acetylcholine, as is discussed later. It has been calculated that about 3000 molecules of acetylcholine are present in each vesicle, and enough vesicles are present in the synaptic knob on a neuron to transmit about 10,000 impulses.

Synthesis of New Transmitter Substance. Fortunately, the synaptic knobs have the capability of continually synthesizing new transmitter substance. Were it not for this ability, synaptic transmission would become completely ineffective within a few minutes. The synthesis is believed to occur mainly in the cytoplasm of the synaptic knobs, and then the newly synthesized transmitter is immediately absorbed into the vesicles and stored until needed. Thus, each time a vesicle empties its contents into the synaptic cleft, soon thereafter it becomes filled again with new transmitter. It is also possible that the vesicle wall itself plays a role in the synthesis of some of the transmitters.

In the case of the synthesis of acetylcholine, this substance is synthesized from acetyl-CoA and choline in the presence of the enzyme *choline acetyltransferase,* an enzyme that is present in abundance in the cytoplasm of the cholinergic type of synaptic knob. When acetylcholine is released from the knob into the synaptic cleft, it is rapidly split again to acetate and choline by the enzyme cholinesterase that is adherent to the outer surface of the knob. Then the choline is actively transported back into the knob to be used once more for synthesis of new acetylcholine. Thus, the vesicles are used again and again. But even so, both the vesicles and the mitochondria that supply the energy for transmitter synthesis eventually disintegrate. Fortunately, new vesicles and mitochondria are continually transported from the cell soma down the axon to the synaptic knob, moving along the axon at a velocity of about 10 cm. per day, and replenishing the supply in the knobs.

The formation, release, and re-uptake of norepinephrine by the presynaptic terminals of the sympathetic nervous system will be discussed in detail in Chapter 15 in relation to function of the autonomic nervous system.

Action of the Transmitter Substance on the Postsynaptic Neuron. The membrane of the postsynaptic neuron where a synaptic knob abuts it is believed to contain specific receptor molecules that bind the transmitter substance. These receptors are probably proteins that respond to the transmitter by changing their shapes or activities in such a way that they increase the membrane permeability especially to sodium ions when the transmitter is excitatory and increase the permeability to potassium and chloride ions when the transmitter is inhibitory.

The ribosomes and the endoplasmic reticulum are both increased in the area immediately beneath the synapse, as illustrated by the density of the postsynaptic area in Figure 4–6. It is possible that the degree of development of this postsynaptic receptor area increases with the intensity of activity of the synapse; therefore, this is possibly a means by which the synapse can subserve the memory function, as will be discussed in detail in Chapter 13.

CHEMICAL NATURES OF THE TRANSMITTER SUBSTANCES

The Excitatory Transmitters. From the discussion in Chapter 3 on the neuromuscular junction, a peripheral type of synapse, it will be recalled that the excitatory transmitter at that synapse is acetylcholine. It is also almost certain that the excitatory transmitter at the synapses in the autonomic ganglia is *acetylcholine.* The major reasons for believing this are: (a) acetylcholine-like substances will stimulate the postganglionic neurons in the autonomic ganglia, (b) substances that prevent the destruction of acetylcholine by cholinesterase at the synapses will potentiate the transmission through the autonomic ganglia, and (c) measurable quantities of acetylcholine can be recovered from fluids perfusing the autonomic ganglia after strong stimulation of the preganglionic neurons.

In the case of the central nervous system, at least several, and perhaps many, different excitatory transmitter substances are secreted by different types of excitatory synaptic knobs. At least one of these excitatory transmitters is acetylcholine, but how extensively this transmitter is used throughout the nervous system is not certain. It is known that synaptic knobs in widespread areas of the nervous system do contain vesicles of acetylcholine as well as choline acetyltransferase, which is required for synthesis of acetylcholine. They also contain cholinesterase for splitting the acetylcholine after it is secreted into the synaptic clefts.

Other excitatory substances for which specific synthesizing enzymes have been proved in different central nervous system neurons include:

1. Norepinephrine
2. Dopamine
3. Serotonin

The Inhibitory Transmitters. At least two substances appear to be important inhibitory transmitters:

1. Gamma aminobutyric acid (GABA), which is present especially in many brain nerve terminals but to less extent also in the spinal cord. This substance has been proved to be an inhibitory transmitter in some lower animals, thereby making it almost certain that it also acts as an inhibitory transmitter in mammals.

2. Glycine, one of the simple amino acids. This is highly concentrated in some synaptic knobs in the spinal cord and probably functions as an inhibitory transmitter at many synapses in that area.

Other Possible Transmitter Substances. To find an explanation for the many varied functions of synapses in different parts of the central nervous system, a vast search is under way for still other transmitter substances. Many substances that will excite or inhibit neurons have been found, but none of these has been proved with real certainty to be a functional transmitter. Indeed, the exact function of even several of the substances already mentioned is in doubt with the probable exception of acetylcholine, norepinephrine, and dopamine. Among the still newer substances that have been suggested as possible transmitters are:

1. Excitatory transmitters: L-*glutamate* and L-*aspartate*

2. Inhibitory transmitters: *taurine* and *alanine*

3. Possible excitatory or inhibitory transmitters under different circumstances: *histamine, prostaglandins,* and *P-substances,* which are a series of polypeptides that are found in the nervous system and that may have long-term excitatory or inhibitory effects on neurons.

It is especially to be noted that some of the transmitter substances might have prolonged effects of neuronal excitation or inhibition, perhaps lasting for minutes or hours. The presence of these effects gives an entirely new dimension to synaptic control over postsynaptic neuronal function. For instance, some of the small polypeptides when injected into the brain can at times cause prolonged sleep.

Excitatory versus Inhibitory Neurons. A single neuron can secrete only one type of transmitter substance at its nerve terminals. Therefore, even though the axon from a neuron divides a thousand times it will still secrete only the one type of transmitter substance. For this reason a neuron that secretes an excitatory transmitter substance will cause excitation wherever the terminal fibrils synapse with the next neuron. These neurons are therefore called *excitatory neurons.* Likewise, the terminals of neurons that secrete inhibitory substance can cause only inhibition, and these neurons are called *inhibitory neurons.*

ELECTRICAL EVENTS DURING NEURONAL EXCITATION

The electrical events in neuronal excitation have been studied mainly in the large motoneuron of the anterior horn of the spinal cord. Therefore, the events to be described in the following few sections pertain essentially to these neurons. However, except for some quantitative differences, they also apply to most other neurons of the nervous system as well.

Resting Membrane Potential of the Neuronal Soma. Figure 4–7 illustrates the soma of a motoneuron, showing the resting membrane potential to be about −70 millivolts. This is somewhat less than the −85 millivolts found in large peripheral nerve fibers and in skeletal muscle fibers; the lower voltage is important, however, because it allows both positive and negative control of the degree of excitability of the neuron. That is, decreasing the voltage to a less negative value makes the membrane of the neuron more excitable, whereas increasing this voltage to a more negative value makes the neuron less excitable. This is the basis of the two modes of function of the neuron—either excitation or inhibition—as we will explain in detail in the following sections.

Concentration Differences of Ions Across the Neuronal Somal Membrane. Figure 4–7 also illustrates the concentration differences across the neuronal somal membrane of the three ions that are most important for neuronal function: sodium ions, potassium ions, and chloride ions.

At the top, the sodium ion concentration is shown to be very great in the extracellular fluid but very low inside the neuron. This sodium concentration gradient is caused by a very strong sodium pump that continually pumps sodium out of the neuron. The capability of the pump to move sodium ions through the membrane is so great that it is the dominant factor in determining the distribution of sodium ions across the membrane; that is, the sodium pump maintains a very low sodium concentration inside the neuron despite slight back leakage of sodium through the pores, as illustrated in the figure.

The figure also shows that the potassium ion concentration is very great inside the neuronal soma but very low in the extracellular fluid. It illustrates that there is a weak potassium pump that tends to pump potassium to the interior while there is a very high degree of permeability to potassium. The pump is relatively unimportant because potassium ions leak through the neuronal somal pores so readily that this nullifies most of the effectiveness of the pump. Therefore, for most purposes one can consider the membrane to be relatively highly permeable to potassium and the potassium pump to be of only slight importance.

Figure 4–7 shows the chloride ion to be of high concentration in the extracellular fluid but of low concentration inside the neuron. It also shows that the membrane is highly permeable to chloride ions and that there is no chloride pump. Therefore, the chloride ions become distributed across the membrane passively. The reason for the low concentration of chloride ions inside the neuron is the −70 millivolts in the neuron. That is, this negative voltage repels the negatively charged chloride ions, forcing them outward through the pores until the concentration difference is so great that its tendency to move chloride ions inward exactly balances the tendency of the electrical difference to move them outward. That is, the chloride ions become distributed across the membrane in accordance with the Nernst equation for equilibrium conditions. This equation was discussed in detail in Chapter 1.

Origin of the Resting Membrane Potential of the Neuronal Soma.   The basic cause of the −70

millivolt resting membrane potential of the neuronal soma is the sodium pump. This pump causes the extrusion of positively charged sodium ions to the exterior. Since there are large numbers of negatively charged ions inside the soma that cannot diffuse through the membrane—protein ions, phosphate ions, and many others—extrusion of the positively charged sodium ions to the exterior leaves all these nondiffusible negative ions unbalanced by positive ions on the inside. Therefore, the interior of the neuron becomes negatively charged as the result of the sodium pump. This principle was discussed in more detail in Chapter 1 in relation to the resting membrane potential of nerves.

Uniform Distribution of the Potential Inside the Soma.   The interior of the neuronal soma contains a very highly conductive electrolytic solution, the intracellular fluid of the neuron. Furthermore, the diameter of the neuronal soma is very large (from 10 to 80 microns in diameter) causing there to be almost no resistance to conduction of electrical current from one part of the somal interior to another part. Therefore, any change in potential in any part of the soma causes an almost exactly equal change in potential at all other points in the soma. This is an important principle because it plays a major role in the summation of signals entering the neuron from multiple sources, as we shall see in subsequent sections of this chapter.

Effect of Excitatory Transmitter on the Postsynaptic Membrane—the Excitatory Postsynaptic Potential.   Figure 4–8A illustrates the resting neuron with an unexcited synaptic knob resting upon its surface. The resting membrane potential everywhere in the soma is −70 millivolts.

Figure 4–8B illustrates an excitatory knob

Figure 4–7. Distribution of sodium, potassium, and chloride ions across the neuronal somal membrane; origin of the intrasomal membrane potential.

Figure 4–8. Three states of a neuron: (A) a resting neuron, (B) a neuron in an excited state, with increased intraneuronal potential caused by sodium influx, and (C) a neuron in an inhibited state, with decreased intraneuronal membrane potential caused by potassium ion efflux.

that has secreted an excitatory transmitter into the cleft between the knob and the neuronal somal membrane. This excitatory transmitter acts on the membrane receptor to increase the membrane's permeability to all ions. This causes sodium ions in particular to flow to the interior of the neuron because of the large electrochemical gradient that tends to move sodium inward.

The rapid influx of the positively charged sodium ions to the interior of the neuron neutralizes part of the negativity of the resting membrane potential. Thus, in Figure 4–8B the resting membrane potential has been increased from −70 millivolts to −59 millivolts. This increase in voltage above the normal resting neuronal potential—that is, to a less negative value—is called the *excitatory postsynaptic potential* because when this potential rises high enough it will elicit an action potential in the neuron, thus exciting it.

However, we need to issue a word of warning at this point. Discharge of a single excitatory synaptic knob can never increase the neuronal potential from −70 millivolts up to −59 millivolts. Instead, an increase of this magnitude requires the simultaneous discharge of many excitatory knobs—tens to hundreds, usually—

at the same time. This occurs by a process called *summation,* which will be discussed in detail in the following sections.

Excitation at the Initial Segment of the Axon—Threshold for Excitation. When the membrane potential inside the neuron rises high enough, there comes a point that this increase initiates an action potential in the neuron. However, the action potential does not begin on the somal membrane adjacent to the excitatory knobs. Instead, it begins in the initial segment of the axon. This may be explained as follows: Any factor that increases the potential inside the soma at any single point also increases this potential everywhere in the soma at the same time. Yet, because of physical differences in the membrane and differences in geometrical arrangement of the membrane in different parts of the neuron, the intrasomal voltage that will elicit an action potential is also different at different points on the neuronal membrane. The most excitable part of the neuron by far is the initial segment of the axon—that, is the first 50 to 100 microns of the axon beyond the point where it leaves the neuronal soma. The excitatory postsynaptic potential that will elicit an action potential at this point on the neuron is approximately 11 millivolts. This is in contrast to approximately 30 millivolts required to elicit an action potential on the soma itself. Therefore, the new action potential originates in the initial segment of the axon and not on the soma. Once the action potential begins, it travels peripherally along the axon and also travels backwards over the soma of the neuron (it usually does not travel backwards very far into the dendrites, however).

Thus, in Figure 4–8B, it is shown that under normal conditions the *threshold* for excitation of the neuron is −59 millivolts, which represents an excitatory postsynaptic potential of +11 millivolts—that is, 11 millivolts more positive than the normal resting neuronal potential of −70 millivolts.

ELECTRICAL EVENTS IN NEURONAL INHIBITION

Effect of Inhibitory Transmitter on the Postsynaptic Membrane—the Inhibitory Postsynaptic Potential. It was pointed out above that the excitatory transmitter increases the permeability of the somal membrane to all ions—including sodium, potassium, and chloride. The inhibitory transmitter, in contrast, increases the permeability of the postsynaptic membrane only to potassium and chloride ions. Therefore, influx of sodium ions does not occur. However, potassium efflux does occur, as illustrated in Figure 4–8C. The reason potassium flows outward through the membrane is the following: In the resting state, a weak potassium pump has been pumping a slight excess of potassium ions to the interior of the neuron. Therefore, there are a few too many potassium ions on the inside to be in an exact equilibrium state as described by the Nernst equation for equilibrium conditions. Consequently, opening of the pores causes outward diffusion of some of the excess potassium ions, thereby decreasing the positive ions inside the neuron and leaving still more of the nondiffusible negative ions of the neuron (protein ions, phosphate ions, and others). This concentration of negative ions makes the internal potential of the neuron more negative than ever, as illustrated by the −75 millivolt potential inside the neuron in Figure 4–8C. This is called a *hyperpolarized state.* And the 5 millivolt decrease in intraneuronal voltage below the normal resting potential of −70 millivolts caused by the inhibitory transmitter is called the *inhibitory postsynaptic potential.*

Obviously, the increased negativity of the membrane potential (−75 millivolts) makes the neuron less excitable than it is normally. Since the potential must rise to −59 millivolts to excite the neuron, an excitatory postsynaptic potential must now be 16 millivolts instead of the normal 11 millivolts to cause excitation. Thus, in this way the inhibitory transmitter inhibits the neuron.

"Clamping" of the Resting Membrane Potential as a Means to Inhibit Neurons. Sometimes, excitation of the inhibitory synaptic knobs does not cause an inhibitory postsynaptic potential, but it still inhibits the neuron. The reason that the potential does not change is that in some neurons the concentration differences across the membrane for both the potassium and the chloride ions are already exactly in equilibrium states in accord with the Nernst equation. That is, the normal resting potential is exactly the voltage that each of these concentration differences will create when the membrane becomes permeable to the ions. Therefore, when the inhibitory pores open, there is no net outward flow of potassium ions to cause an inhibitory postsynaptic potential. Yet, both the potassium and the chloride ions do diffuse bidirectionally through the wide open pores many times as rapidly as normally, and this high

flux of these two ions inhibits the neuron in the following way: When excitatory knobs fire and sodium ions flow into the neuron, this raises the intraneuronal voltage far less than usual because any tendency for the membrane potential to change to a value that is not equal to the Nernst potential for the potassium and chloride ions is immediately opposed by rapid flux of these ions in the appropriate directions through the inhibitory pores to bring the potential back to the Nernst value. Therefore, the amount of influx of sodium ions required to cause excitation may be increased to as much as 5 to 20 times normal.

This tendency for the potassium and chloride ions to maintain a membrane potential near the resting value when the inhibitory pores are wide open is called "clamping" of the potential.

To express the phenomenon for clamping more mathematically, one needs to recall the Goldman equation from Chapter 1. This equation indicates that the membrane potential is determined by summation of the tendencies for the different ions to carry electrical charges through the membrane in the two directions. The membrane potential will approach the Nernst equilibrium potential for those ions that permeate the membrane to the greatest extent. When the inhibitory pores are wide open, the chloride and potassium ions permeate the membrane very greatly. Therefore, when the excitatory knobs fire, it is difficult to raise the neuronal potential up to the threshold value for excitation.

Presynaptic Inhibition

In addition to the inhibition caused by inhibitory knobs operating at the synapses, called *postsynaptic inhibition,* another type of inhibition often occurs before the signal reaches the synapse. This type of inhibition, called *presynaptic inhibition,* is believed to occur in the following way:

In presynaptic inhibition, instead of the postsynaptic neuron being inhibited, the presynaptic terminal fibrils and synaptic knobs are inhibited. This inhibition is caused by the presence of inhibitory knobs lying directly on the terminal fibrils and excitatory knobs themselves. These presynaptic inhibitory knobs are believed to come from interneurons that are excited by the incoming afferent signals; they secrete a transmitter substance that partially depolarizes the terminal fibrils and excitatory synaptic knobs. Consequently, the voltage of the action potential that occurs at the membrane of the excitatory knob is depressed, and, as has already been pointed out, this greatly decreases the amount of excitatory transmitter released by the knob. Therefore, the degree of excitation of the neuron is greatly suppressed.

The nature of the transmitter substance released by the interneurons to cause presynaptic inhibition is not known. However, presynaptic inhibition is blocked by *picrotoxin* and also by *bicuculline*. Since these two substances also block the action of the inhibitory transmitter substance, GABA, it has been suggested that the transmitter substance of the knobs that cause the presynaptic inhibition is GABA. On the other hand, since GABA normally causes hyperpolarization rather than depolarization, some neurophysiologists believe that the transmitter substance from these interneurons is one of the excitatory transmitters.

Presynaptic inhibition occurs especially at the more peripheral synapses of the sensory pathways. For instance, when an incoming sensory fiber to the spinal cord excites the second neuron in the sensory pathway, it simultaneously causes presynaptic inhibition of the surrounding neurons. This "sharpens" the spatial boundaries of the signal transmitted to the brain; that is, it decreases or eliminates other signals on each side of the major signal so that the major signal stands out more clearly at its terminus in the brain. We shall see the importance of this sharpening process, also called "contrast enhancement," in discussions of subsequent chapters.

SUMMATION OF POSTSYNAPTIC POTENTIALS

Time Course of Postsynaptic Potentials. When the excitatory transmitter is released from an excitatory synaptic knob, the neuronal membrane becomes highly permeable for only about 1 millisecond. During this time sodium ions diffuse rapidly to the interior of the cell to increase the intraneuronal potential, thus creating the *excitatory postsynaptic potential*. This potential then persists for about 15 milliseconds because this is the time required for the sodium ions to be pumped out or for potassium ions to leak out to reestablish the normal resting membrane potential. In the large anterior motoneuron, the potential disappears with a half-time of approximately 4 milliseconds. That is, each 4 milliseconds it decreases by one-half.

Precisely the same effect occurs for the inhibitory postsynaptic potential. That is, the inhibitory transmitter increases the permeability of the membrane to potassium and chloride ions

for approximately one millisecond, and this effect usually decreases the intraneuronal potential to a more negative value than normal, thereby creating the *inhibitory postsynaptic potential*. This potential also persists for about 15 milliseconds, disappearing with a half-time of approximately 4 milliseconds.

Spatial Summation of the Postsynaptic Potentials. It has already been pointed out that excitation of a single synaptic knob on the surface of a neuron will almost never excite the neuron. The reason for this is that sufficient excitatory transmitter substance is released by a single knob to cause an excitatory postsynaptic potential usually no more than a fraction of a millivolt instead of the required 10 millivolts or more that is the usual threshold for excitation. However, during an excitatory state in a neuronal pool of the nervous system, many excitatory knobs are usually stimulated at the same time, and even though these knobs are spread over wide areas of the neuron, their effects can still summate. The reason for this summation is the following: It has already been pointed out that a change in the potential at any single point within the soma will cause the potential to change everywhere in the soma almost exactly equally. Therefore, for each excitatory knob that discharges simultaneously, the intrasomal potential rises another fraction of a millivolt. When the excitatory postsynaptic potential becomes great enough, the threshold for firing will be reached, and an action potential will generate at the axon hillock. This effect is illustrated in Figure 4–9, which shows several excitatory postsynaptic potentials. The bottom postsynaptic potential in the figure was *theoretically* caused by stimulation of only four ex-

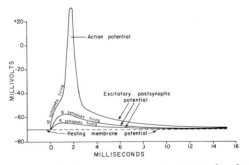

Figure 4–9. Excitatory postsynaptic potentials, showing that simultaneous firing of only a few synapses will not cause sufficient summated potential to elicit an action potential, but that simultaneous firing of many synapses will raise the summated potential to the threshold for excitation and cause a superimposed action potential. (The exact number of synapses firing is hypothetical.)

citatory knobs; then the next higher potential was caused by stimulation of two times as many knobs; finally, a still higher excitatory postsynaptic potential was caused by stimulation of four times as many knobs. This time an action potential was generated at the axon hillock.

This effect of summing simultaneous postsynaptic potentials created by excitation of multiple knobs on widely spaced areas of the membrane is called *spatial summation.*

Temporal Summation. Most synaptic knobs can fire in rapid succession only a few milliseconds apart. Each time a knob fires, the released transmitter substance opens the membrane pores for a millisecond or so. Since the postsynaptic potential lasts for up to 15 milliseconds, a second opening of the same pore can increase the postsynaptic potential to a still greater level so that the more rapid the rate of knob stimulation, the greater the effective postsynaptic potential. Thus, successive postsynaptic potentials of individual synaptic knobs, if they occur rapidly enough, can summate in the same way that postsynaptic potentials can summate from widely distributed knobs over the surface of the neuron. This summation of rapidly repetitive postsynaptic potentials is called *temporal summation.*

Simultaneous Summation of Inhibitory and Excitatory Postsynaptic Potentials. Obviously, if an inhibitory postsynaptic potential is tending to decrease the membrane potential to a more negative value while an excitatory postsynaptic potential is tending to increase the potential to a more positive value at the same time, these two effects can either completely nullify each other or partially nullify each other. Also, inhibitory "clamping" of the membrane potential can nullify much of an excitatory potential. Thus, if a neuron is currently being excited by an excitatory postsynaptic potential, then an inhibitory signal from another source can easily reduce the postsynaptic potential below the threshold value for excitation, thus turning off the activity of the neuron.

Facilitation of Neurons. Often the summated postsynaptic potential is excitatory in nature but has not risen high enough to reach the threshold for excitation. When this happens the neuron is said to be *facilitated.* That is, its membrane potential is nearer the threshold for firing than normally, but it is not yet to the level of firing. Nevertheless, a signal entering the neuron from some other source can then excite the neuron very easily. Diffuse signals in the nervous system often facilitate large groups of neurons so that they can respond quickly and easily to signals arriving from secondary sources.

SPECIAL FUNCTIONS OF DENDRITES IN EXCITING NEURONS

The Large Spatial Field of Excitation of the Dendrites. The dendrites of the anterior motoneurons extend for one-half to one millimeter in all directions from the neuronal soma. Therefore, these dendrites can receive signals from a fairly large spatial area around the motoneuron. This provides vast opportunity for summation of signals from many separate presynaptic neurons.

It is also important to note that between 80 and 90 per cent of all the synaptic knobs terminate on the dendrites of the anterior motoneuron in contrast to only 10 to 20 per cent terminating on the neuronal soma. Therefore, the preponderant share of the excitation of the neuron is provided by signals transmitted over the dendrites.

Failure of Many Dendrites to Transmit Action Potentials. Many dendrites fail to transmit action potentials because their thresholds for excitation are very high. Yet they do transmit *electrotonic current* down the dendrites to the soma. (Transmission of electrotonic current means the direct spread of current by electrical conduction in the fluids of the dendrites with no generation of new current by action potentials.) Stimulation of the neuron by this current has special characteristics, as follows:

Decrement of Electrotonic Conduction in the Dendrites—Greater Excitation Near the Soma. In Figure 4–10 a number of excitatory and inhibitory knobs are shown stimulating the dendrites of a neuron. On the two dendrites to the left in the figure are shown excitatory effects near the ends of the dendrites; note the high levels of the excitatory postsynaptic potentials at these ends. However, a large share of the excitatory postsynaptic potential is lost before it reaches the soma. The reason for this is that the dendrites are long and thin, and their membranes are also very leaky to electrical current. Therefore, before the excitatory potentials can reach the soma, a large share of the potential is lost by leakage through the membrane. This decrease in membrane potential as it spreads along dendrites toward the soma is called *decremental conduction* in the dendrites.

It is also obvious that the nearer the excitatory knob is to the soma of the neuron, the less will be the decrement of conduction from that point to the soma. Therefore, those knobs that lie near the soma have far more excitatory effect than those that lie far away from the soma. This is a very important principle necessary to an understanding of the function of neurons in neuronal pools, because knobs from presynaptic fibrils that terminate near the soma of the postsynaptic neuron always have a much higher chance of causing the postsynaptic neuron to fire than do knobs that terminate on the dendrites at a distance from the soma.

Rapid Re-excitation of the Neuron by the Dendrites After the Neuron Fires. When an action potential is generated in a neuron, this action potential spreads back over the soma but not always over the dendrites. Furthermore, the postsynaptic potentials in the dendrites often remain relatively undisturbed by the action potential. Therefore, just as soon as the action potential is over, the electrical charges still existing in the dendrites are ready and waiting to flow into the soma of the neuron and, therefore, ready to re-excite the neuron. Thus, the dendrites have a "holding capacity" for the excitatory signal from presynaptic sources.

Summation of Excitation and Inhibition in Dendrites. The uppermost dendrite of Figure 4–10 is shown to be stimulated by both excitatory and inhibitory knobs. At the tip end of the dendrite there is a strong excitatory postsynaptic potential, but much of this is lost by decremental conduction along the dendrite. Then near the soma two inhibitory knobs are stimulating the same dendrite. These inhibitory

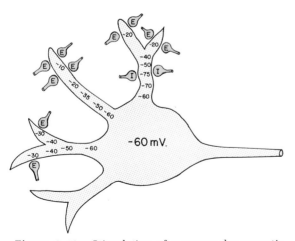

Figure 4–10. Stimulation of a neuron by synaptic knobs located on dendrites, showing, especially, decremental conduction of electrotonic potentials in the two dendrites to the left and inhibition of dendritic excitation in the dendrite that is uppermost.

knobs provide a hyperpolarizing voltage in the dendrite that completely nullifies the excitatory effect and indeed transmits a small amount of inhibition, by decremental conduction, toward the soma. Thus, dendrites can summate excitatory and inhibitory postsynaptic potentials in the same way that the soma can. In those instances when action potentials do develop in dendrites, inhibitory knobs located near the soma can completely block the action potentials and can prevent their ever entering the soma of the neuron. It is especially interesting that the inhibitory knobs tend to terminate on or near the soma.

RELATION OF STATE OF EXCITATION OF THE NEURON TO THE RATE OF FIRING

The "Central Excitatory State." The "central excitatory state" of a neuron is defined as the degree of excitatory drive to the neuron. If there is a higher degree of excitation than inhibition of the neuron at any given instant, then it is said that there is a *central excitatory state*. On the other hand, if there is more inhibition than excitation, then it is said that there is a *central inhibitory state*.

A quantitative definition of the central excitatory state is the increase in postsynaptic potential above the resting membrane potential of the soma that *would* develop in the neuron if action potentials did not occur to interfere with this postsynaptic potential. Thus, a postsynaptic potential of 5 millivolts above the resting membrane potential would be a central excitatory state of 5 millivolts. A postsynaptic potential of 50 millivolts above the resting membrane potential would be a central excitatory state of 50 millivolts. Unfortunately, however, when a postsynaptic potential this high occurs, an action potential supervenes immediately so that the central excitatory state is then in reality a theoretical potential rather than an actual potential.

When the central excitatory state of a neuron rises above the threshold for excitation, then the neuron will fire repetitively as long as the excitatory state remains at this level. However, the rate at which it will fire is determined by how much above threshold value the central excitatory state is. To explain this, we must first consider what happens to the neuronal somal potential during and following the action potential.

Changes in Neuronal Somal Potential During and Following the Action Potential.

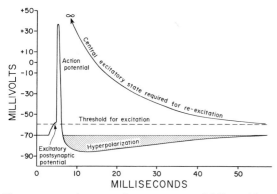

Figure 4–11. A neuronal action potential followed by a prolonged period of neuronal hyperpolarization. Also shown is the central excitatory state required for re-excitation of the neuron at given intervals after the action potential is over.

Figure 4–11 illustrates an action potential which is initiated by an excitatory postsynaptic potential that rises above the threshold level of −59 millivolts. Following the action potential there is a very long *positive after-potential* lasting for many milliseconds. This is a state of hyperpolarization during which the somal membrane potential falls below the normal resting membrane potential of −70 millivolts. It is caused by a very high degree of permeability of the neuronal membrane to potassium ions that persists for many milliseconds after the action potential is over. Potassium ions from inside the neuron diffuse to the exterior carrying positive charges out of the neuron and, therefore, creating an excessively high degree of negativity inside the neuron.

The importance of this state of hyperpolarization after the action potential is that the neuron remains in an *inhibited state* during this period of time. Therefore, a far greater central excitatory state is required during this period of time than normally to cause re-excitation of the neuron.

Relationship of Central Excitatory State to Rate of Firing. The curve shown at the top of Figure 4–11, labeled "central excitatory state required for re-excitation," depicts the level of the central excitatory state required at each instant after an action potential is over to re-excite the neuron. Note that very soon after an action potential is over a very high central excitatory state is required to cause re-excitation. That is, a very large number of excitatory synaptic knobs must be firing simultaneously. Then, after many milliseconds have passed and the state of hyperpolarization of the neuron has begun to disappear, the central excitatory state

required for re-excitation becomes greatly reduced.

Therefore, it is immediately evident that when the central excitatory state is high a second action potential will appear very soon after a previous one. Still a third action potential will appear soon after the second, and this process will continue indefinitely. Thus, at a very high central excitatory state the rate of firing of the neuron is great.

On the other hand, when the central excitatory state is only barely above threshold, the neuron must recover for many milliseconds before it can fire again. Therefore, the rate of neuronal firing is very slow.

(Note that the increase in the central excitatory state that is required for re-excitation is far greater than the decrease in the neuronal potential during the state of hyperpolarization. The reason for this is that at the same time that the neuron is hyperpolarized its voltage is also "clamped" to a great extent by the high permeability of the membrane to potassium and chloride ions. This clamping mechanism of neuronal inhibition was discussed earlier in the chapter.)

Response Characteristics of Different Neurons to Increasing Levels of Central Excitatory State. Histological study of the nervous system immediately convinces one of the widely varying types of neurons in different parts of the nervous system. And, physiologically, the different types of neurons perform different functions. Therefore, as would be expected, the ability to respond to stimulation by the presynaptic knobs varies from one type of neuron to another.

Figure 4–12 illustrates theoretical responses

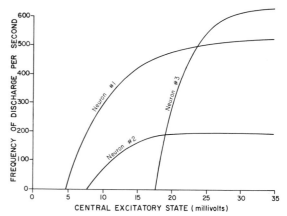

Figure 4–12. Response characteristics of different types of neurons to progressively increasing central excitatory states.

of three different types of neurons to varying levels of central excitatory state. Note that neuron number 1 will not discharge at all until the excitatory state rises to 5 millivolts. Then, as the excitatory state rises progressively to 35 millivolts the frequency of discharge rises to slightly over 500 per second.

Neuron number 2 is quite a different type, having a threshold for excitation of 8 millivolts and a maximum rate of discharge of only 190 per second. Finally, neuron number 3 has a high threshold for excitation, about 18 millivolts, but its discharge rate rises rapidly to over 600 per second as the central excitatory state rises only slightly above threshold.

Thus, different neurons respond differently, have different thresholds for excitation, and have widely differing maximal frequencies of discharge. With a little imagination one can readily understand the importance of having neurons with many different types of response characteristics to perform the widely varying functions of the nervous system.

SOME SPECIAL CHARACTERISTICS OF SYNAPTIC TRANSMISSION

Forward Conduction through Synapses. From the above discussion, it should be evident by now that impulses are conducted through synapses only from the synaptic knobs to the successive neurons and never in the reverse direction. This is called the *principle of forward conduction*.

Synaptic Delay. In transmission of an impulse from a synaptic knob to a postsynaptic neuron, a certain amount of time is consumed in the process of (a) discharge of the transmitter substance by the knob, (b) diffusion of the transmitter to the subsynaptic neuronal membrane, (c) action of the transmitter on the membrane, and (d) inward diffusion of sodium to raise the excitatory postsynaptic potential to a high enough value to elicit an action potential. The *minimal* period of time required for all these events to take place, even when large numbers of presynaptic terminals are stimulated simultaneously, is approximately 0.5 millisecond. This is called the *synaptic delay*. It is important for the following reason: Neurophysiologists can measure the *minimal* delay time between an input volley of impulses and an output volley and from this can estimate the number of series neurons in the circuit.

Fatigue of Synaptic Transmission. When the presynaptic knobs are repetitively stimu-

lated at a rapid rate, the number of discharges by the postsynaptic neuron is at first very great but becomes progressively less in succeeding milliseconds or seconds. This is called *fatigue* of synaptic transmission. Fatigue is an exceedingly important characteristic of synaptic function, for when areas of the nervous system become overexcited, fatigue causes them to lose this excess excitability after a while. For example, fatigue is probably the most important means by which the excess excitability of the brain during an epileptic fit is finally subdued so that the fit ceases. Thus, the development of fatigue is a protective mechanism against excess neuronal activity. This will be discussed further in the description of reverberating neuronal circuits in the following chapter.

The mechanism of fatigue is mainly exhaustion of the stores of transmitter substance in the synaptic knobs, particularly since it has been calculated that the excitatory knobs can store enough excitatory transmitter for only 10,000 normal synaptic transmissions, an amount that can be exhausted in only a few seconds to a few minutes.

Post-Tetanic Facilitation. When a rapidly repetitive (tetanizing) stimulus is applied to the synaptic knobs for a period of time and then a rest period is allowed, the neuron will usually be even more responsive to subsequent stimulation than normally. This is called *post-tetanic facilitation*.

One of the most likely explanations of post-tetanic facilitation is that the repetitive stimulation alters the membranes of the knobs to cause more rapid emptying of transmitter vesicles.

The physiological significance of post-tetanic facilitation is still very doubtful, and it may have no real significance at all. However, since post-tetanic facilitation can last from a few seconds in some neurons to many hours in others, it is immediately apparent that neurons could possibly store information by this mechanism. Therefore post-tetanic facilitation might well be a mechanism of "short-term" memory in the central nervous system. This possibility will be discussed at further length in Chapter 13 in relation to the memory function of the cerebral cortex.

Effect of Acidosis and Alkalosis on Synaptic Transmission. The neurons are highly responsive to changes in pH of the surrounding interstitial fluids. *Alkalosis greatly increases neuronal excitability.* For instance, a rise in arterial pH from the normal of 7.4 to about 7.8 often causes cerebral convulsions because of increased excitability of the neurons. This can be demonstrated especially well by having a person who is normally predisposed to epileptic fits overbreathe. The overbreathing elevates the pH of the blood only momentarily, but even this short interval can often precipitate an epileptic convulsive attack.

On the other hand, *acidosis greatly depresses neuronal activity;* a fall in pH from 7.4 to below 7.0 usually causes a comatose state. For instance, in very severe diabetic or uremic acidosis, coma always develops.

Effect of Hypoxia on Synaptic Transmission. Neuronal excitability is also highly dependent on an adequate supply of oxygen. Cessation of oxygen supply for only a few seconds can cause complete inexcitability of the neurons. This is often seen when the cerebral circulation is temporarily interrupted, for within 3 to 5 seconds the person becomes unconscious.

Effect of Drugs on Synaptic Transmission. Many different drugs are known to increase the excitability of neurons, and others are known to decrease the excitability. For instance, caffeine, theophylline, and theobromine, which are found in coffee, tea, and cocoa, respectively, all increase neuronal excitability, presumably by reducing the threshold for excitation of the neurons. However, strychnine, which is one of the best known of all the agents that increase the excitability of neurons, does not reduce the threshold for excitation of the neurons at all but, instead, *inhibits the action of at least some of the inhibitory transmitters* on the neurons, probably especially the inhibitory effect of glycine in the spinal cord. In consequence, the effects of the excitatory transmitter from the excitatory knobs become overwhelming, and the neurons become so excited that they go into rapidly repetitive discharge, resulting in severe convulsions.

The hypnotics and anesthetics have long been believed to increase the threshold for excitation of the neurons and thereby to decrease neuronal activity throughout the body. This is based principally on the fact that most of the volatile anesthetics are chemically inert compounds but are lipid soluble. Therefore, it has been reasoned that these substances might change the physical characteristics of the neuronal membranes, making them less excitable to excitatory agents. It still remains a possibility, however, that at least some hypnotics and anesthetics cause their anesthetic actions by (a) reducing the quantity of excitatory transmitter released or (b) enhancing the inhibitory effects of the inhibitory transmitter.

REFERENCES

Baldessarini, R. J., and Karobath, M.: Biochemical physiology of central synapses. *Ann. Rev. Physiol.,* 35:273, 1973.

Barondes, S. H.: Synaptic macromolecules: identification and metabolism. *Ann. Rev. Biochem.,* 43:147, 1974.

Bennett, M. V. L. (ed.): Synaptic Transmission and Neuronal Interaction (Society of General Physiologists Series, Vol. 28). New York, Raven Press, 1974.

Calvin, W. H.: Generation of spike trains in CNS neurons. *Brain Res.,* 84:1, 1975.

Costa, E., Gessa, G. L., and Sandler, M. (eds.): Serotonin, New Vistas: Biochemistry and Behavioral and Clinical Studies. New York, Raven Press, 1974.

Costa, E., Iversen, L. L., and Paoletti, R. (eds.): Studies of Neurotransmitters at the Synaptic Level. (Advances in Biochemical Psychopharmacology Series, Vol. 6.) New York, Raven Press, 1972.

Costa, E., and Meek, J. L.: Regulation of biosynthesis of catecholamines and serotonin in the CNS. *Ann. Rev. Pharmacol.,* 14:491, 1974.

Curtis, D. R.: Bicuculline, GABA, and central inhibition. *Proc. Aust. Assoc. Neurol.,* 9:145, 1973.

De Robertis, E., and Schacht, J. (eds.): Neurochemistry of Cholinergic Receptors. New York, Raven Press, 1974.

Fink, B. R. (ed.): Molecular Mechanisms of Anesthesia. Vol. 1: Progress in Anesthesiology. New York, Raven Press, 1975.

Fonnum, F.: Recent developments in biochemical investigations of cholinergic transmission. *Brain Res.,* 62:497, 1973.

Gerschenfeld, H. M.: Chemical transmissions in invertebrate central nervous systems and neuromuscular junctions. *Physiol. Rev.,* 53:1, 1973.

Hebb, C.: Biosynthesis of acetylcholine in nervous tissue. *Physiol. Rev.,* 52:918, 1972.

Hubbard, J. I., Linas, R., and Quastel, D. M.: Electrophysiological Analysis of Synaptic Transmission. Baltimore, The Williams & Wilkins Company, 1969.

Johnson, J. L.: Glutamic acid as a synaptic transmitter in the nervous system. A review. *Brain Res.,* 37:1, 1972.

Kandel, E. R.: Nerve cells and behavior. *Sci. Amer.,* 223:57, 1970.

Karlin, A.: The acetylcholine receptor: progress report. *Life Sci.,* 14:1385, 1974.

Kuno, M.: Quantum aspects of central and ganglionic transmission in vertebrates. *Physiol. Rev.,* 51:647, 1971.

Leibovic, K. N.: Nervous System Theory: An Introductory Study. New York, Academic Press, Inc., 1973.

Noback, C. R.: The Human Nervous System; Basic Principles of Neurobiology, 2nd Ed. New York, McGraw-Hill Book Company, 1975.

Obata, K.: The inhibitory action of –aminobutyric acid, a probable synaptic transmitter. *Inter. Rev. Neurobiol.,* 15:167, 1972.

Pappas, G. D., and Purpura, D. P. (eds.): Structure and Function of Synapses. New York, Raven Press, 1972.

Roberts, E., Chase, T., and Tower, D. B. (eds.): GABA in Nervous System Function. New York, Raven Press, 1975.

Sidman, R. L., and Rakic, P.: Neuronal migration, with special reference to developing human brain: a review. *Brain Res.,* 62:1, 1973.

Somjen, G. G.: Electrophysiology of neuroglia. *Ann. Rev. Physiol.,* 37:163, 1975.

Storm-Mathisen, J.: Proceedings: GABA as a transmitter in the central nervous system of vertebrates. *J. Neural Transm.,* 11:227, 1974.

Torda, C.: Model of molecular mechanism able to generate a depolarization-hyperpolarization cycle. *Inter. Rev. Neurobiol.,* 16:1, 1974.

Werman, R.: CNS cellular level. *Ann. Rev. Physiol.,* 34:337, 1972.

Willows, A. O. D.: Giant brain cells in mollusks. *Sci. Amer.,* 224:68, 1971.

5

Transmission and Processing of Information in the Nervous System

INFORMATION, SIGNALS, AND IMPULSES

The term *information,* as it applies to the nervous system, means a variety of different things, such as knowledge, facts, quantitative values, intensity of pain, intensity of light, temperature, and any other aspect of the body or its immediate surroundings that has meaning. Thus, pain from a pin prick is information, pressure on the bottom of the feet is information, degree of angulation of the joints is information, and a stored memory in the brain is information.

The primary function of the nervous system is (a) to transmit information from one point to another and (b) to process this information so that it can be used advantageously or so that its meaning can become clear to the mind. However, information cannot be transmitted in its original form but only in the form of nerve impulses. Thus, a part of the body that is subjected to pain must first convert this information into *nerve impulses;* and specific areas of the brain convert abstract thoughts also into nerve impulses that are then transmitted either elsewhere in the brain or into peripheral nerves to motor effectors throughout the body. The retina of the eye converts vision into nerve impulses, the nerve endings of the joints convert degree of angulation of the joints into nerve impulses, and so forth. The nerve impulses in turn are transmitted to the opposite ends of the neurons where they cause subsequent effects either at the synapses of other neurons or at the ends of motor nerves. This is what is meant by the transmission of information.

Signals. In the transmission of information, it is frequently not desirable to speak in terms of the individual impulses but instead in terms of the overall pattern of impulses; this pattern is called a *signal.* As an example, when pressure is applied to a large area of skin, impulses are transmitted by large numbers of parallel nerve fibers, and the total pattern of impulses transmitted by all these fibers is called a signal. Thus, we can speak of visual signals, auditory signals, somesthetic sensory signals, motor signals, and so forth.

TRANSMISSION OF SIGNALS IN NERVE TRACTS

A signal is almost never transmitted only in a single nerve fiber but instead it is transmitted in a group of parallel fibers bound together in peripheral nerves or in *nerve tracts* in the central nervous system.

SIGNAL STRENGTH

Spatial Summation (Multiple Fiber Summation). Figure 5–1 illustrates a sensory nerve leading from a segment of skin, showing extensive arborization of pain nerve fibers in the skin. A pin or other object stimulates nerve

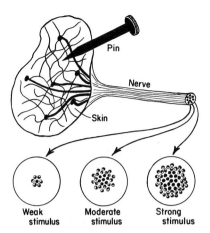

Figure 5–1. Pattern of stimulation of pain fibers in a nerve trunk leading from an area of skin pricked by a pin.

endings from a large number of different fibers, because each separate fiber divides and spreads over an area of skin sometimes as large as 5 cm. in diameter called the *receptive field*. The number of nerve endings from each fiber is large in the very center of its "field" but becomes less and less toward the periphery. Therefore, in Figure 5–1, a pin pricking the skin stimulates the nerve fiber strongly if the point of stimulation is in the center of its field of reception, but it stimulates the fiber only weakly if the point of stimulus is in the periphery of the field.

In the lower part of Figure 5–1 is shown a cross-section of the nerve leading from the skin, showing also the fibers stimulated by the pin-prick. Note in the left-hand circle that if the pinprick is slight, only a single fiber is stimulated strongly (the black fiber in the center), and several immediately adjacent fibers are stimulated moderately (half-black fibers), while all other fibers are not stimulated at all. When the stimulus becomes more intense, the number of fibers strongly stimulated becomes progressively greater. Thus, the signal spreads to more and more fibers. This phenomenon is called *spatial summation*, which means simply that one of the means by which signals of increasing strength are transmitted in the nervous system is by utilization of progressively greater numbers of fibers. The increase in number of fibers as the strength of signal increases is called *recruitment* of the additional fibers.

Temporal Summation (Frequency Modulation). A second means by which signals of increasing strength are transmitted through nerve tracts is by increasing the *frequency* of nerve impulses in each fiber. This occurs in ad-

dition to the increase in number of excited fibers. This process is called *temporal summation,* which means simply that during any given interval of time, the number of impulses transmitted is directly related to the strength of the signal.

Figure 5–2 illustrates temporal summation, showing in the upper part a changing strength of signal and in the lower part the actual impulses transmitted by the nerve fiber. This figure demonstrates that the frequency increases and decreases with the strength of the signal. Thus, this is actually a process of frequency modulation, the frequency of impulses being "modulated" in proportion to the strength of the signal.

DETECTION OF A SIGNAL AT THE TERMINUS OF THE NERVE PATHWAY

The nerve signals obviously are nothing more than a series of pulses rather than a smooth signal. However, all terminal points in the nervous system have means for averaging impulses and thereby smoothing out the signal. Let us consider as an example skeletal muscles. Impulses controlling a skeletal muscle are transmitted through large numbers of parallel nerve fibers. If 50 nerve fibers innervate a muscle and one impulse is transmitted per second, but nonsynchronously, the 50 separate impulses cause a weak but smooth contraction because the pulses in the different nerve fibers are spread out over a period of time. If each nerve fiber transmits 200 impulses per second, making a total of 10,000 pulses per second, the 10,000 pulses give a strong and still smooth contraction.

Similar averaging processes occur in the

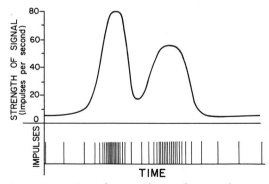

Figure 5–2. Translation of signal strength into a frequency-modulated series of nerve impulses, showing *above* the strength of signal and *below* the separate nerve impulses.

central nervous system; most postsynaptic neurons in the nervous system receive literally hundreds to thousands of impulses each second from the presynaptic terminals, and the synaptic membrane is capable of summating and averaging these impulses to give smooth changes in the excitatory state of the neuron, as was explained in the previous chapter.

"Granularity" of the Detected Signal. Despite the ability of the muscles and synapses in the central nervous system to average impulse rates, under some conditions the detected signal has unwanted ripples, which is called *granularity* of the signal. Two causes of this are, first, slow impulse rates and, second, synchrony of impulses in the parallel fibers through which the signal is transmitted.

A slow impulse rate causes granularity of the signal because of the nature of the averaging system itself. The synapses in the nervous system, the skeletal muscle, and the other signal detectors react to an impulse for a given period of time. Thus, the contractile twitch of a typical muscle lasts about one-twentieth second. If a second impulse comes along before this twitch is over, it causes the process of contraction to continue. Therefore, rapidly successive impulses cause smooth contraction of the muscle called *tetanization*. On the other hand, if the impulse rate is less than 30 per second, the muscle contracts in a series of twitches, and the signal is said to be granular. The same principles apply to the averaging mechanism of the central nervous system synapses.

The second cause of granularity is *synchrony* of impulses in the parallel fibers transmitting the signal. For instance, if 100 fibers are transmitting one impulse per second and the impulses are spread out in time in the different fibers, the signal will be smooth despite the low impulse frequency. But if all these impulses are transmitted in synchrony, a very granular signal will reach the detector at a frequency of one per second.

Fidelity of the Temporal Pattern of a Signal. The "temporal pattern" of a signal means the changes in signal strength with time. Unfortunately, extremely rapid changes in signal strengths cannot be transmitted through nerve pathways. The reason for this is that the averaging mechanisms of the detectors require a considerable number of impulses before the average can be determined. Therefore, the change in signal strength in the detector always *lags* a few milliseconds behind the change in signal strength in the nerve tract itself.

The fidelity of the temporal pattern is different for different types of nerve fibers. The large type A myelinated nerve fibers that can transmit as many as 2000 impulses per second are usually associated with rapidly responding sensory receptors and rapidly responding detectors. Therefore, they can transmit changes in signal strengths that occur as rapidly as 700 cycles per second (particularly those nerve fibers associated with the pacinian corpuscles). On the other hand, the minute unmyelinated type C fibers that transmit only a few impulses per second are usually associated with slowly responding receptors and detectors. The frequency of varying signals transmitted through these pathways is often limited to as little as one or less than one cycle per second (as is the case for autonomic signals controlling the internal organs).

SPATIAL ORIENTATION OF SIGNALS IN FIBER TRACTS

How does the brain detect the precise position on the body that is receiving a sensory stimulus, and how does the brain transmit impulses precisely to individual skeletal muscle bundles? The answer to this is by transmitting their signals in a precise spatial pattern through the nerve tracts. All the different nerve tracts, both in the peripheral nerves and in the fiber tracts of the central nervous system, are spatially organized. For instance, in the dorsal columns of the spinal cord the sensory fibers from the feet lie toward the midline, while those fibers entering the dorsal columns at higher levels of the body lie progressively more toward the lateral sides of the dorsal columns. This spatial organization is maintained with precision throughout the sensory pathway all the way to the somesthetic cortex. Likewise, the fiber tracts within the brain and those extending into motor nerves are spatially oriented in the same way.

As an example, Figure 5–3 illustrates to the left three separate pins stimulating the skin; to the right the spatial orientation of the stimulated fibers in the nerve are shown. Each pin in this example stimulates a single fiber strongly and adjacent fibers less strongly. This spatial orientation of the three separate bundles of fibers is maintained all the way to the cerebral cortex and obviously allows the brain to localize the three different pinpricks to their points of stimulation.

TRANSMISSION AND PROCESSING OF SIGNALS IN NEURONAL POOLS

The central nervous system is made up of literally hundreds of separate neuronal pools, some of which are extremely small and some very large. For instance, the entire cerebral cortex could be considered to be a single large neuronal pool. If all the surface area of the cerebral cortex were flattened out, including the

Figure 5–3. Spatial pattern of nerve fiber stimulation in a nerve trunk following stimulation of the skin by three separate but simultaneous pinpricks.

surfaces of the penetrating folds, the total area of this large flat pool would be several square feet. It has many separate fiber tracts coming to it (afferent fibers) and others leaving it (efferent fibers). Furthermore it maintains the same quality of spatial orientation as that found in the nerve bundles, individual points of the cortex connecting with specific points elsewhere in the nervous system or connecting through the peripheral nerves with specific points in the body. However, within this pool of neurons are large numbers of short nerve fibers whereby signals spread horizontally from neuron to neuron within the pool itself.

Other neuronal pools include the different basal ganglia and the specific nuclei in the thalamus, cerebellum, mesencephalon, pons, and medulla. Also, the entire dorsal gray matter of the spinal cord could be considered to be one long pool of neurons, and the entire anterior gray matter another long neuronal pool. Each pool has its own special characteristics of organization which cause it to process signals in its own special way. It is these special characteristics of the different pools that allow the multitude of functions of the nervous system. Yet, despite their differences in function, the pools also have many similarities of function which are described in the following pages.

Organization of Neurons in the Neuronal Pools. Figure 5–4 is a schematic diagram of the organization of neurons in a neuronal pool, showing "input" fibers to the left and "output" fibers to the right. Each input fiber divides hundreds to thousands of times and provides an average of a thousand or more terminal fibrils that spread over a large area in the pool to synapse with the dendrites or cell bodies of the neurons in the pool. The area into which the endings of each incoming nerve fiber spread is called its *stimulatory field*. Note that each input fiber arborizes so that large numbers of its

synaptic knobs lie on the centermost neurons in its "field," but progressively fewer knobs lie on the neurons farther from the center of the field.

Threshold and Subthreshold Stimuli— Facilitation. Going back to the discussion of synaptic function in the previous chapter, it will be recalled that stimulation of a single excitatory synaptic knob almost never stimulates the postsynaptic neuron. Instead, large numbers of knobs must discharge on the same neuron either simultaneously or in rapid succession to cause excitation. For instance, let us assume that 6 separate knobs must discharge simultaneously or in rapid succession to excite any one of the neurons in Figure 5–4. Note that input fiber 1 contributes a total of 10 synaptic knobs to neuron *a*. Therefore, an incoming impulse in fiber 1 will cause neuron *a* to discharge. This same incoming fiber has two knobs on neuron *b* and three on neuron *c*. Neither of these two neurons will fire.

Incoming nerve fiber 2 has 12 synaptic knobs on neuron *d*, three on neuron *c*, and two on neuron *b*. In this case, an impulse in fiber 2 excites only neuron *d*.

Though fiber 1 fails to stimulate neurons *b* and *c*, discharge of the synaptic knobs changes the membrane potentials of these neurons so that they can be more easily excited by other incoming signals. Thus, there are two types of stimuli that enter a neuronal pool, *excitatory stimuli* and *subthreshold stimuli*. A sub-

Figure 5–4. Basic organization of a neuronal pool.

threshold stimulus fails to excite the neuron but does make the neuron more excitable to impulses from other sources. The neuron that is made more excitable but does not discharge is said to be *facilitated*.

"Convergence" of Subthreshold Stimuli to Cause Excitation. Let us now assume that both fibers 1 and 2 in Figure 5–4 transmit concurrent impulses into the neuronal pool. In this case, neuron *c* is stimulated by six synaptic knobs simultaneously, which is the required number to cause excitation. Thus, subthreshold stimuli can *converge* from several sources and *summate* at a neuron to cause an excitatory stimulus.

Summation of Facilitation. Now, let us consider neuron *b* of Figure 5–4 when both input nerve fibers are stimulated. In this case each fiber excites two synaptic knobs on neuron *b*, but the total of four excited knobs still is not up to the threshold value required to excite the neuron. However, the degree of facilitation does become greatly increased so that now only two additional knobs excited from another source need fire to cause discharge.

The "Field" of Terminals. It must be recognized that Figure 5–4 represents a highly condensed version of the neuronal pool, for each input nerve fiber gives off terminals that spread to perhaps 100 or more separate neurons, and the surface of each neuron is covered by many hundred or many thousand synapses. In the centralmost portion of this *field* of terminals, almost all the neurons are stimulated by the incoming fiber; whereas farther toward the periphery of the field, the neurons are facilitated but do not discharge. Figure 5–5 illustrates this effect, showing the field of a single input nerve fiber. The area in the neuronal pool in which all the neurons discharge is called the *discharge* or *excited* or *liminal zone,* and the area to either side in which the neurons are facilitated but do not discharge is called the *facilitated* or *subthreshold* or *subliminal* zone.

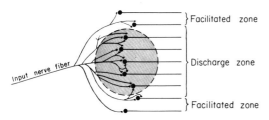

Figure 5–5. "Discharge" and "facilitated" zones of a neuronal pool.

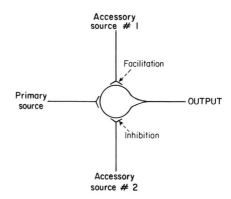

Figure 5–6. Basic neuronal circuit for facilitation or inhibition.

Facilitation of the Neuronal Pool by Signals from Accessory Sources. A neuronal pool frequently receives input nerve fibers from many different sources. Thus, in Figure 5–6 a neuron in a given pool receives impulses from a *primary source* and from two *accessory sources.* The nerve fiber from accessory source #1 is an excitatory fiber which secretes excitatory transmitter at its synaptic knobs. If enough knobs from this source are stimulated, the postsynaptic neuron discharges. However, in many parts of the nervous system the accessory sources supply only a few nerve fibers to the pool, not enough usually to cause excitation but yet enough to *facilitate* the neurons. Thus, in Figure 5–6, if a facilitatory signal is entering the pool from accessory source #1, a much weaker than usual signal from the primary source is able to excite the postsynaptic neuron. In this way the signal from accessory source #1 controls the ease with which signals pass from the primary source to the output, which explains one of the means by which different parts of the nervous system control the degree of activity of other parts.

Inhibition of a Neuronal Pool by Signals from an Accessory Source. It will be recalled from the previous chapter that some neurons of the central nervous system secrete an inhibitory transmitter substance instead of an excitatory transmitter substance. Thus, in Figure 5–6, stimulation of the inhibitory fibers from accessory source #2 strongly inhibits the neuronal pool so that a strong signal from the primary source is required to cause normal output.

Mechanism By Which a Single Input Signal Can Cause both Excitation and Inhibition— The Inhibitory Circuit. Figure 5–7 illustrates the so-called inhibitory circuit which can

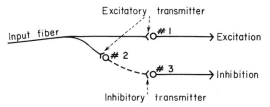

Figure 5–7. Inhibitory circuit. Neuron #2 is an inhibitory neuron.

change an excitatory signal into an inhibitory signal. In this figure the input fiber divides and secretes excitatory transmitter at both its endings. This causes excitation of both neurons 1 and 2. However, neuron 2 is an inhibitory neuron that secretes inhibitory transmitter at its terminal nerve endings. Excitation of this neuron therefore inhibits neuron 3.

In short, the usual means, if not the only means, to cause inhibition is for a signal *to be transmitted through an inhibitory neuron,* which then secretes the inhibitory transmitter substance.

Convergence. The term "convergence" means control of a single neuron by the converging signals from two or more separate input nerve fibers. One type of convergence was illustrated in Figure 5–4 in which two excitatory input nerve fibers from the same source converged upon several separate neurons to stimulate them. This type of convergence from a single source is illustrated again in Figure 5–8A.

However, convergence can also result from input signals (excitatory or inhibitory) from several different sources, which is illustrated in Figure 5–8B. For instance, the interneurons of the spinal cord receive converging signals from

(a) peripheral nerve fibers entering the cord, (b) propriospinal fibers passing from one segment of the cord to another, (c) corticospinal fibers from the cerebral cortex, and (d) probably several other long pathways descending from the brain into the spinal cord. Then the signals from the interneurons converge on the motoneurons to control muscle function.

Such convergence allows summation of information from different sources, and the resulting response is a summated effect of all these different types of information. Obviously, therefore, convergence is one of the important means by which the central nervous system correlates, summates, and sorts different types of information.

Divergence. Divergence means that excitation of a single input nerve fiber stimulates multiple output fibers from the neuronal pool. The two major types of divergence are illustrated in Figure 5–9 and may be described as follows:

An *amplifying* type of divergence often occurs, illustrated in Figure 5–9A. This means simply that an input signal spreads to an increasing number of neurons as it passes through successive pools of a nervous pathway. This type of divergence is characteristic of the corticospinal pathway in its control of skeletal muscles as follows: Stimulation of a single large pyramidal cell in the motor cortex transmits a single impulse into the spinal cord. Yet, under appropriate conditions, this impulse can stimulate perhaps several hundred interneurons, and these in turn stimulate perhaps an equal number of anterior motoneurons. Each of these then stimulates as many as 100 to 300 muscle fibers. Thus, there is a total divergence, or amplification, of as much as 10,000-fold.

Figure 5–8. "Convergence" of multiple input fibers on a single neuron: (A) Input fibers from a single source. (B) Input fibers from multiple sources.

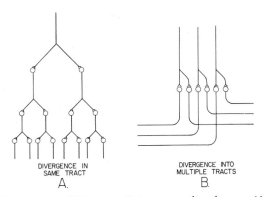

Figure 5–9. "Divergence" in neuronal pathways: (A) Divergence within a pathway to cause "amplification" of the signal. (B) Divergence into multiple tracts to transmit the signal to separate areas.

The second type of divergence, illustrated in Figure 5–9B, is *divergence into multiple tracts*. In this case, the signal is transmitted in two separate directions from the pool. This allows the same information to be transmitted to several different parts of the nervous system where it is needed. For instance, information transmitted in the dorsal columns of the spinal cord takes two courses in the lower part of the brain, (1) into the cerebellum and (2) on through the lower regions of the brain to the thalamus and cerebral cortex. Likewise, in the thalamus almost all sensory information is relayed both into deep structures of the thalamus and to discrete regions of the cerebral cortex.

TRANSMISSION OF SPATIAL PATTERNS THROUGH SUCCESSIVE NEURONAL POOLS

Most information is transmitted from one part of the nervous system to another through several successive neuronal pools. For instance, sensory information from the skin passes first through the peripheral nerve fibers, then through second order neurons that originate either in the spinal cord or in the cuneate and gracile nuclei of the medulla, and finally through third order neurons originating in the thalamus to the cerebral cortex. Such a pathway is illustrated at the top of Figure 5–10. Note that the sensory nerve endings in the skin overlap each other tremendously; and the terminal fibrils of each nerve fiber, on entering each neuronal pool, spread to many adjacent neurons, innervating perhaps 100 or more separate neurons. On first thought, one would expect signals from the skin to become completely mixed up by this haphazard arrangement of terminal fibrils in each neuronal pool. For statistical reasons, however, this does not occur, which can be explained as follows:

First, if a single point is stimulated in the skin, the nerve fiber with the most nerve endings in that particular spot becomes stimulated to the strongest extent, while the immediately adjacent nerve fibers become stimulated less strongly, and the nerve fibers still farther away become stimulated only weakly. When this signal arrives at the first neuronal pool, the stimulus spreads in many directions in the terminal fibrils of the neuronal pool. Yet the *greatest number* of *excited presynaptic terminals* lies very near the point of entry of the most excited input nerve fiber. Therefore, the neuron closest to this central point is the one that be-

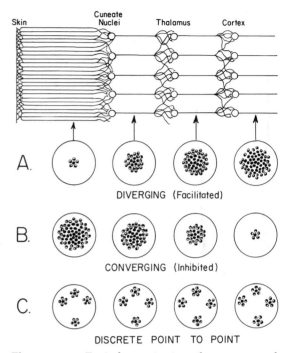

Figure 5–10. Typical organization of a sensory pathway from the skin to the cerebral cortex. *Below:* The patterns of fiber stimulation at different points in the pathway following stimulation by a pinprick when the pathway is (A) facilitated, (B) inhibited, and (C) normally excitable.

comes stimulated to the greatest extent. Exactly the same effect occurs in the second neuronal pool in the thalamus and again when the signal reaches the cerebral cortex.

Yet, it is true that a signal passing through *highly facilitated neuronal pools* could diverge so much that the spatial pattern at the terminus of the pathway would be completely obscured. This effect is illustrated in Figure 5–10A, which shows successively expanding spatial patterns of neuron stimulation in such a facilitated, diverging pathway.

However, the degree of facilitation of the different neuronal pools varies from time to time. Under some conditions the degree of facilitation is so low that the pathway becomes converging, as illustrated in Figure 5–10B. In this case, a broad area of the skin is stimulated, but the signal loses part of its fringe stimuli as it passes through each successive pool until the breadth of the stimulus becomes contracted at the opposite end. One can achieve this type of stimulation by pressing ever so lightly with a flat object on the skin. The signal converges to give the person a sensation of almost a point contact.

In Figure 5–10C, four separate points are simultaneously stimulated on the skin, and the degree of excitability in each neuronal pool is exactly that amount required to prevent either divergence or convergence. Therefore, a reasonably true spatial pattern of each of the four points of stimulation is transmitted through the entire pathway.

Centrifugal Control of Neuronal Facilitation in the Sensory Pathways. It is obvious from the above discussion that the degree of facilitation of each neuronal pool must be maintained at exactly the proper level if faithful transmission of the spatial pattern is to occur. Recent discoveries have demonstrated that the degrees of facilitation of most—indeed, probably all—neuronal pools in the different pathways are controlled by *centrifugal nerve fibers* that pass from the respective sensory areas of the cortex downward to the separate neuronal pools. Thus, these nerve fibers undoubtedly help to control the faithfulness of signal transmission.

Inhibitory Circuits to Provide Contrast in the Spatial Pattern. When a single point of the skin or other sensory area is stimulated, not only is a single fiber excited but a number of "fringe" fibers are excited less strongly at the same time, as already explained above. Therefore, the spatial pattern is blurred even before the signal begins to be transmitted through the pathway. However, in many pathways—if not all—such as in the visual pathway and in the somesthetic pathway, lateral *inhibitory circuits* inhibit the fringe neurons and re-establish a truer spatial pattern.

Figure 5–11A illustrates this circuit, showing that the nerve fibers of a pathway give off collateral fibers that excite inhibitory neurons. These inhibitory neurons in turn inhibit the less

excited fringe neurons in the signal pathway. The effect of this on transmission of the spatial pattern is illustrated in Figure 5–11B, which shows the same point-to-point transmission pattern that was illustrated in Figure 5–10C. The left-hand pattern illustrates four strongly excited fibers; penumbras of fringe excitation surround each of these. To the right is illustrated removal of the penumbras by the lateral inhibitory circuits; and obviously, this increases the contrast in the signal and helps the faithfulness of transmission of the spatial pattern. Unfortunately, we still know too little about this lateral inhibitory mechanism to be sure how effective it actually is. Furthermore, much of the lateral inhibition results from presynaptic inhibition; this was discussed in the previous chapter. The presynaptic type of lateral inhibition is probably the more prevalent mechanism in more peripheral areas of the nervous system, whereas postsynaptic inhibition is the mechanism in the cortical area.

Relationship of Numbers of Fibers in a Pathway to the Total Amount of Spatial Information that Can Be Transmitted. The upper part of Figure 5–10 illustrates that far more sensory nerve receptors transmit information into the spinal cord than there are nerve fibers to transmit the same information upward from the spinal cord to the cortex. Furthermore, the total number of points that can be recognized as individual and separate areas on the surface of the body is probably many times the number of nerve fibers in the sensory pathways ascending the spinal cord. The question must be asked, can a transmission system carry more discrete bits of spatial information than there are nerve fibers themselves?

In considering once again the organization of the transmission pathway shown in the top of Figure 5–10, we see that each sensory nerve fiber leads to a particular *place* in the first neuronal pool. Some fibers end almost directly on a second order neuron while others end *between* second order neurons. If a fiber lies directly on the neuron, that neuron is stimulated far more than the adjacent one. If the fiber lies between two neurons, both neurons are stimulated approximately equally. If the fiber lies three-quarters the way toward one neuron but one-quarter toward the second, the first neuron is stimulated perhaps three times as much as the second neuron. Thus, the spatial position of the incoming neuron can be transmitted by the second order neurons by the *ratios* of signal strengths in the output fibers. One ratio means one position, another ratio another position, and so forth. In this way, a large amount of information from many different sensory receptors probably can be condensed into much fewer nerve fibers. Here again, we do not know how highly this principle of transmission is developed in the nervous system. But, to give an example, each eye has about 125,000,000 re-

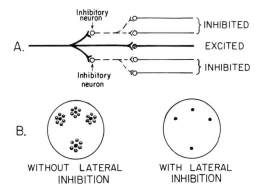

Figure 5–11. (A) Lateral inhibitory circuit by which an excited fiber of a neuronal pool can cause inhibition of adjacent fibers. (B) Increase in contrast of the stimulus pattern caused by the inhibitory circuit.

ceptors, and it can detect about 5,000,000 individual point areas in the visual field. Yet the total number of nerve fibers transmitting information in the optic nerve is believed to be only one million, many of which are probably concerned with other functions besides transmission of the spatial pattern. Therefore, we can guess that the fibers in this tract can carry 10 or more times as many bits of spatial information as there are fibers.

PROLONGATION OF A SIGNAL BY A NEURONAL POOL— "AFTER-DISCHARGE"

Thus far, we have considered signals that are transmitted instantaneously through a neuronal pool. However, in many instances, a signal entering a pool causes a prolonged output discharge, called *after-discharge*, even after the incoming signal is over. The three basic mechanisms by which after-discharge occurs are as follows:

Synaptic After-Discharge. When presynaptic terminals discharge on the surfaces of dendrites or the soma of a neuron, a postsynaptic potential develops in the neuron and lasts for many milliseconds—in the anterior motoneuron for about 15 milliseconds, though perhaps much longer in other neurons. As long as this potential lasts it can excite the neuron, causing it to transmit output impulses as was explained in the previous chapter. Thus, as a result of this synaptic after-discharge mechanism alone, it is possible for a single instantaneous input to cause a sustained signal output (a series of repetitive discharges) lasting as long as 15 milliseconds.

The Parallel Circuit Type of After-Discharge. Figure 5–12 illustrates a second type of neuronal circuit that can cause short periods of after-discharge. In this case, the input signal spreads through a series of neurons in the neuronal pool, and from many of these neurons impulses keep converging on an output

neuron. It will be recalled that a signal is delayed at each synapse for at least 0.5 millisecond, which is called the *synaptic delay*. Therefore, signals that pass through a succession of intermediate neurons reach the output neuron one by one after varying periods of delay. Therefore, the output neuron continues to be stimulated for many milliseconds.

It is doubtful that more than a few dozen successive neurons ordinarily enter into a parallel after-discharge circuit. Therefore, one would suspect that this type of after-discharge circuit could cause after-discharges that last for no more than perhaps 25 to 50 milliseconds. Yet, this circuit does represent a means by which a single input signal, lasting less than 1 millisecond, can be converted into a sustained output signal lasting many milliseconds.

The Reverberating (Oscillatory) Circuit as a Cause of After-Discharge. Probably one of the most important of all circuits in the entire nervous system is the reverberating, or oscillatory, circuit, several different varieties of which are illustrated in Figure 5–13. The simplest

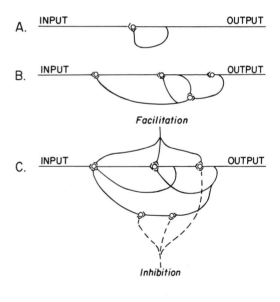

Figure 5–13. Reverberatory circuits of increasing complexity.

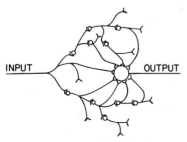

Figure 5–12. The parallel after-discharge circuit.

theoretical reverberating circuit, even though such may not actually exist in the nervous system, is that illustrated in Figure 5–13A, which involves a single neuron. In this case, the output neuron simply sends a collateral nerve fiber back to its own dendrites or soma to restimulate itself; therefore, once the neuron should discharge, the feedback stimuli could theoretically keep the neuron discharging for a long time thereafter.

Figure 5–13B illustrates a few additional neurons in the feedback circuit, which would give a longer period of time between the initial discharge and the feedback signal. Figure 5–13C illustrates a still more complex system in which both facilitatory and inhibitory fibers impinge on the reverberating pool. A facilitatory signal increases the ease with which reverberation takes place, while an inhibitory signal decreases the ease with which reverberation takes place.

Figure 5–13D illustrates that most reverberating pathways are constituted of many parallel fibers, and at each cell station the terminal fibrils diffuse widely. In such a system the total reverberating signal can be either weak or strong, depending on how many parallel nerve fibers are momentarily involved in the reverberation.

Finally, reverberation need not occur only in a single neuronal pool, for it can occur through a circuit of successive pools.

Characteristics of After-Discharge from a Reverberating Circuit. Figure 5–14 illustrates postulated output signals from a reverberating after-discharge circuit. The input stimulus need last only 1 millisecond or so, and yet the output can last for many milliseconds or even minutes. The figure demonstrates that the intensity of the output signal increases to a reasonably high value early in the reverberation, then decreases to a critical point, and suddenly ceases entirely. Furthermore, the duration of the after-discharge is determined by the degree of inhibition or facilitation of the neuronal pool. In this way, signals from other parts of the brain can control the reaction of the pool to the input stimulus.

Almost these exact patterns of output signals can be recorded from the motor nerves exciting a muscle involved in the flexor reflex (discussed in Chap. 9), which is believed to be caused by a reverberating type of after-discharge following stimulation of a pain fiber.

Importance of Synaptic Fatigue in Determining the Duration of Reverberation. It was pointed

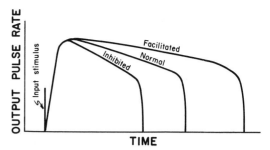

Figure 5–14. Typical pattern of the output signal from a reverberatory circuit following a single input stimulus, showing the effects of facilitation and inhibition.

out in the previous chapter that synapses fatigue if stimulated for prolonged periods of time. Therefore, one of the most important factors that determines the duration of the reverberatory type of after-discharge is probably the rapidity with which the involved synapses fatigue. Rapid fatigue would obviously tend to shorten the period of after-discharge and slow fatigue to lengthen it.

Furthermore, the greater the number of neurons in the reverberatory pathway and the greater the number of collateral feedback fibrils, the easier it would be to keep the reverberation going. Therefore, it is to be expected that longer reverberating pathways would in general sustain after-discharges for longer periods of time.

Duration of Reverberation. Typical after-discharge patterns of different reverberatory circuits have durations from as short as 10 milliseconds to as long as several minutes, or perhaps even hours. Indeed, as will be explained in Chapter 12, wakefulness may be an example of reverberation of neuronal circuits in the basal region of the brain. In this theory of wakefulness, ''arousal impulses'' are postulated to set off the wakefulness reverberation at the beginning of each day and thereby to cause sustained excitability of the brain, this excitability lasting 14 or more hours.

CONTINUOUS SIGNAL OUTPUT FROM NEURONAL POOLS

Some neuronal pools emit output signals continuously even without excitatory input signals. At least two different mechanisms can cause this effect, (1) intrinsic neuronal discharge and (2) reverberatory signals.

Continuous Discharge Caused by Intrinsic Neuronal Excitability. Neurons, like other excitable tissues, discharge repetitively if their membrane potentials rise above certain threshold levels. The membrane potentials of some neurons are even normally high enough to cause these neurons to emit impulses continually. This occurs especially in some of the cells of the cerebellum and in some of the interneurons of the spinal cord. The rates at which these cells emit impulses can be increased by facilitatory signals or decreased by inhibitory signals; the latter can sometimes decrease the rate to extinction.

Continuous Signals Emitted from Reverberation Circuits. Obviously, a reverberating circuit that never fatigues to extinction could also be a source of continual impulses. Facilitatory impulses entering the reverberating pool, as illustrated in Figure 5–13C, could increase the output signal, and inhibition could decrease or even extinguish the output signal.

Figure 5–15 illustrates a continual output signal from a pool of neurons, whether it be a pool emitting impulses because of intrinsic neuronal excitability or as a result of reverberation. Note that an excitatory (or facilitatory) input signal greatly increases the output signal, whereas an inhibitory input signal greatly decreases the output. Those students who are familiar with radio transmitters will recognize this to be a *carrier wave* type of information transmission. That is, the excitatory and inhibitory control signals are not the *cause* of the output signal, but they do *control* it. Note that this carrier wave system allows decrease in signal intensity as well as increase, whereas, up to this point, the types of information transmission that we have discussed have been only positive information rather than negative information. This type of information transmission is used by the autonomic nervous system to control such

functions as vascular tone, gut tone, degree of constriction of the iris, heart rate, and others.

RHYTHMIC SIGNAL OUTPUT

Many neuronal circuits emit rhythmic output signals—for instance, the rhythmic respiratory signal originating in the reticular substance of the medulla and pons. This repetitive rhythmic signal continues throughout life, while other rhythmic signals, such as those that cause scratching movements by the hind leg of a dog or the walking movements in an animal, require input stimuli into the respective circuits to initiate the signals.

Rhythmic signals probably result from reverberating pathways. One can readily understand that each time a signal passes around a reverberatory loop, collateral impulses could be transmitted into the output pathway. Thus, the rhythmic respiratory signals could result from such a reverberatory mechanism. Indeed, a reverberating circuit in the medulla probably does provide the control signals for respiration.

Obviously, facilitatory or inhibitory signals can affect rhythmic signal output in the same way that they can affect continual signal outputs. Figure 5–16, for instance, illustrates the rhythmic respiratory signal in the phrenic nerve. However, when the carotid body is stimulated by arterial oxygen deficiency, the frequency and amplitude of the rhythmic signal pattern increase progressively.

INSTABILITY AND STABILITY OF NEURONAL CIRCUITS

Almost every part of the brain connects either directly or indirectly with every other part, and this creates a serious problem. If the first part excites the second, the second the third, the third the fourth, and so on until finally the signal re-excites the first part, it is clear that an excitatory signal entering any part of the brain would set off a continuous cycle of re-excitation of all parts. If this should occur, the brain would be inundated by a mass of uncontrolled reverberating signals—signals that would be transmitting no information but, nevertheless, would be consuming the circuits of the brain so that none of the informational signals could be transmitted. Such an effect actually occurs in widespread areas of the brain during *epileptic fits.*

How does the central nervous system prevent this from happening all the time? The answer

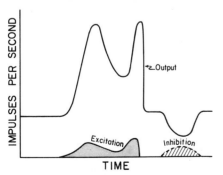

Figure 5–15. Continuous output from either a reverberating circuit or from a pool of intrinsically discharging neurons. This figure also shows the effect of excitatory or inhibitory input signals.

Figure 5–16. The oscillatory output from the respiratory center, showing that progressively increasing stimulation of the carotid body increases both the intensity and frequency of oscillation.

seems to lie in two basic mechanisms that function throughout the central nervous system: (1) inhibitory circuits, and (2) decremental transmission through synapses.

INHIBITORY CIRCUITS AS A MECHANISM FOR STABILIZING NERVOUS SYSTEM FUNCTION

The phenomenon of lateral inhibition that was discussed earlier in the chapter prevents signals in an informational pathway from spreading diffusely everywhere. In addition, two other types of inhibitory circuits in widespread areas of the brain help to prevent excessive spread of unwanted signals: (a) inhibitory feedback circuits that return from the termini of pathways back to the initial excitatory neurons of the same pathways—these inhibit the input neurons when the termini become overly excited, and (b) some neuronal pools that exert gross inhibitory control over widespread areas of the brain—for instance, many of the basal ganglia exert inhibitory influences throughout the motor control system.

It is easy to understand how the inhibitory feedbacks can provide negative feedback signals for limiting the degree of excitability when an area of the brain tends to become too excited. Unfortunately, the inhibitory circuits do not seem to be widespread enough to stabilize nervous system function by themselves. Instead, the equally as important (if not even much more important) phenomenon of decremental conduction through synapses stabilizes nervous system function.

DECREMENTAL CONDUCTION THROUGH SYNAPSES AS A MEANS FOR STABILIZING THE NERVOUS SYSTEM (HABITUATION, FATIGUE)

Decremental conduction through synapses means simply that the signal becomes progressively weaker the more prolonged the period of excitation. This phenomenon has often been called *fatigue,* which is similar to the fatigue of synapses that was discussed in the previous chapter, and it has also been called *habituation.* Figure 5–17 illustrates typical decremental conduction, showing a muscle response during the so-called flexor reflex. That is, stimulation of the pain sensory endings in a limb causes reflex contraction of the flexor muscles of the limb, leading to withdrawal of the limb from the painful stimulus. However, if this stimulus is repeated at close intervals, as was done in Figure 5–17, the response progressively decreases. But how does this decremental conduction, as illustrated by the decreasing response of the flexor reflex, play a role in stabilizing nervous system function? The answer to this is the following: When any given synapse is excited too much, the phenomenon of decremental conduction progressively depresses the signal pathway. Therefore, any tendency for reverberatory feedbacks to occur becomes automatically blocked before reverberation can become widespread.

Synaptic Pathways That Exhibit Decremental Conduction; Those That Do Not. Fortunately, some synaptic pathways exhibit very little decremental conduction, whereas others exhibit extreme degrees. One type of pathway that exhibits almost no decremental conduction

Figure 5–17. Successive flexor reflexes illustrating decrement in conduction of the signals through the reflex pathway.

is the fast-conducting sensory pathways from the peripheral parts of the body to the brain, such as the pathways through the dorsal columns to the thalamus and thence to the somesthetic cortex. This seems to be of purposeful benefit to nervous function because it allows faithful transmission of sensory information into the brain.

On the other hand, the interconnecting links through the short interneurons between the sensory system and the motor system frequently exhibit extreme degrees of decremental conduction. This was illustrated in Figure 5–17 for the flexor reflex pathway, because it is the interneurons between the sensory input and the motor output of the spinal cord that fatigue. At least in certain parts of the nervous system, this decremental conduction has been shown to result from exhaustion of transmitter substance in the synaptic knobs.

Obviously, if the connecting links between major portions of the nervous system exhibit decremental conduction, reverberatory instability in the nervous system is generally prevented.

Recovery From Decremental Conduction. After a major degree of decrement has occurred in the conductive properties of a synapse, the conduction recovers if an adequate period of rest between stimuli is allowed. Thus, when a pathway is not used often, it becomes progressively more excitable until full conduction returns.

Automatic Adjustment of Sensitivity of Pathways by the Decremental Conduction Mechanism. It is clear by now that if the excitability of a pathway in the nervous system is too great, then too many impulses will be transmitted and the mechanism of decremental conduction will automatically adjust the sensitivity of the pathway to a lower level. Conversely, if the sensitivity is too low, then too few impulses will be transmitted, and the sensitivity of the system will automatically adjust to a higher level. Therefore, this decremental conduction mechanism, and its recovery during rest, is probably an extremely important mechanism for maintaining a proper balance among the sensitivities of the respective pathways throughout the brain.

ALERTING SIGNALS ("DIFFERENTIAL" SIGNALS)

A special type of output signal that occurs commonly in neuronal pools of the nervous system is the *alerting signal*. The alerting signal is a very strong output signal from a neuronal pool that occurs immediately after the input signal enters the pool; the alerting signal then dies away, however, even though the input signal continues indefinitely. When the input signal is suddenly removed, a second alerting response is likely to occur.

Figure 5–18 illustrates typical alerting signals that occur in the output from a retinal ganglion cell in response to changes in degree of retinal receptor stimulation. Thus, when light first impinges on the eye and the rods and cones become excited, the ganglion cells, which fire normally at a slow rate of about 5 per second, suddenly begin to fire at a much higher rate. However, once the signal from the rods and cones reaches a steady state level, the output signal from the ganglion cell falls back essentially to its original level. Nevertheless, the brain has been "alerted" to the onset of the light stimulus. Then, when the light is turned off, the signal from the ganglion cell falls below normal (actually all the way to zero, at times), but this too lasts for only a short time. Therefore, once again the brain is alerted to the change in the light stimulus.

Similar alerting responses occur in response to changes in pressure on the surface of the body: to noise, to movement of images across the retinal field, to changes in pitch in the auditory signal, to onset of a new taste sensation, to onset of smell stimuli, and so forth.

Decremental Conduction as the Cause of the Alerting Response. The alerting response almost certainly occurs from *very fast* decremental conduction through synapses. That is, at the

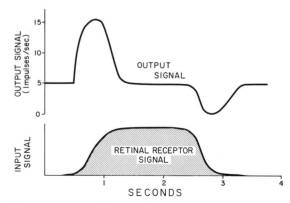

Figure 5–18. "Differentiation" of the signal from the retinal receptors (rods and cones) as it passes through the retinal neuronal circuit.

onset of the input signal conduction is very great, but then it fades very quickly.

Differentiation of Signals

The two curves in Figure 5–18 illustrate that the output curve is very nearly the *differential* of the input curve that depicts the retinal receptor signal, though there is always a very slight lag in the differential signal. Nevertheless, it is clear that the nervous system does have the capability of "differentiating" input signals, which is a simple mathematical way of depicting *changes* in signals without being bothered by the continuous signal that lasts thereafter. In this way the brain can become alerted, but still, it can discard a tremendous amount of chaff or noise in the incoming signals to the nervous system after extracting most of their meaningful information.

The nervous system can also differentiate spatial signal patterns as well as time signal patterns. For instance, everywhere that a sharp boundary in light intensity occurs on the retina of the eye, the retinal neuronal circuit transmits a very powerful signal to the brain, whereas it transmits only weak signals from areas of the retina that are illuminated with noncontrasting borders. Here again, this alerts the person to the important features of the signal. Indeed, it explains how it is possible for one to recognize a person's image simply from a line drawing even though the line drawing is certainly not a true picture of the person. It just so happens that the "mind's eye" actually sees images almost as if they were line drawings even when the object is not a series of lines.

REFERENCES

Bennett, M. V. L. (ed.): Synaptic Transmission and Neuronal Interaction. New York, Raven Press, 1975.

Blumenthal, R., Homsy, Y. M., Katchalsky, A. K., and Rowland, V. (eds.): Dynamic Patterns of Brain Cell Assemblies. Neurosciences Research Program Bulletin. Vol. 12, No. 1. Cambridge, Mass., Massachusetts Institute of Technology, 1974.

Chung, S. H.: In search of the rules for nerve connections. *Cell,* 3:201, 1974.

Freides, D.: Human information processing and sensory modality: cross-modal functions, information complexity, memory, and deficit. *Psychol. Bull.,* 81:284, 1974.

Heimer, L.: Pathways in the brain. *Sci. Amer.,* 225:48, 1971.

Kater, S. B., Heyer, C. B., and Kaneko, C. R. S.: Identifiable neurons and invertebrate behavior. *In* Guyton, A. C. (ed.): MTP International Review of Science: Physiology. Vol. 3. Baltimore, University Park Press, 1974, p. 1.

Kennedy, D.: Crayfish interneurons. *Physiologist,* 14:5, 1971.

Kreutzberg, G. W. (ed.): Physiology and Pathology of Dendrites. (Advances in Neurology, Vol. 12.) New York, Raven Press, 1975.

Martin, A. R.: Synaptic transmissions. *In* Guyton, A. C. (ed.): MTP International Review of Science: Physiology. Vol. 3. Baltimore, University Park Press, 1974, p. 53.

Nicholls, J. C., and Van Essen, D.: The nervous system of the leech. *Sci. Amer.,* 230:38, 1974.

Shepherd, G. M.: The Synaptic Organization of the Brain: an Introduction. New York, Oxford University Press, 1974.

Simpson, L. L.: The use of neuropoisons in the study of cholinergic transmission. *Ann. Rev. Pharmacol.,* 14:305, 1974.

Stenevi, U., Björklund, A., and Moore, R. Y.: Morphological plasticity of central adrenergic neurons. *Brain Behav. Evol.,* 8:110, 1973.

Szentagothai, J., Arbib, M. A., and Homsy, Y. M. (eds.): Conceptual Models of Neural Organization. Neurosciences Research Program. Cambridge, Mass., Massachusetts Institute of Technology, 1974.

Ungar, G., and Irwin, L. N.: Chemical correlates of neural function. *Neurosci. Res.,* 1:73, 1968.

Zippel, H. P. (ed.): Symposium on Memory and Transfer of Information, Göttingen, Mercksche Gesellschaft für Kunst und Wissenschaft, 1972.

Zippel, H. P. (ed.): Memory and Transfer of Information. New York, Plenum Publishing Corporation, 1973.

See also bibliographies at the ends of Chapters 4 and 9.

6

Sensory Receptors and Their Basic Mechanisms of Action

Input to the nervous system is provided by the sensory receptors that detect such sensory stimuli as touch, sound, light, cold, warmth, and so forth. The purpose of the present chapter is to discuss the basic mechanisms by which these receptors change sensory stimuli into nerve signals and, also, how both the type of sensory stimulus and its strength are detected by the brain.

TYPES OF SENSORY RECEPTORS AND THE SENSORY STIMULI THEY DETECT

The student of medical physiology will have already studied many different anatomical types of nerve endings, and Table 6–1 gives a list and classification of most of the body's sensory receptors. This table shows that there are basically five different types of sensory receptors: (1) *mechanoreceptors*, which detect mechanical deformation of the receptor or of cells adjacent to the receptors; (2) *thermoreceptors*, which detect changes in temperature, some receptors detecting cold and others warmth; (3) *nociceptors*, which detect damage in the tissues, whether it be physical damage or chemical damage; (4) *electromagnetic receptors*, which detect light on the retina of the eye; and (5) *chemoreceptors*, which detect taste in the mouth, smell in the nose, oxygen level in the arterial blood, osmolality of the body fluids, carbon dioxide concentration, and perhaps other factors that make up the chemistry of the body.

This chapter will discuss especially the function of specific types of receptors, primarily the peripheral mechanoreceptors, to illustrate some of the basic principles by which receptors in general operate. Other receptors will be discussed in relation to the sensory systems that they subserve, which will be presented mainly in the next few chapters. Figure 6–1 illustrates some of the different types of mechanoreceptors found in the skin or in the deep structures of the body, and Table 6–1 gives their respective sensory functions. All of these receptors will be discussed in the following chapters in relation to the respective sensory systems. However, the functions of some of these are described briefly, as follows:

Free nerve endings are found in all parts of the body. A very large proportion of these detect pain. However, other free nerve endings detect warmth, cold, and crude touch sensations.

Several of the more complex receptors listed in Figure 6–1 detect tissue deformation. These include the *Merkel's discs*, the *tactile hairs, pacinian corpuscles, Meissner's corpuscles, Krause's corpuscles,* and *Ruffini's end-organs*. In the skin, it is these receptors that detect the tactile sensations of touch and pressure. In the deep tissues, they detect stretch, deep pressure, or any other type of tissue deformation—even the stretch of joint capsules and ligaments to determine the angulation of a joint.

The *Golgi tendon apparatus* detects degree of tension in tendons, and the *muscle spindle* detects the length of muscle. These receptors will be discussed in Chapter 9 in relation to the muscle and tendon reflexes.

TABLE 6–1. Classification of Sensory Receptors

Mechanoreceptors

Skin tactile sensibilities (epidermis and dermis)
  Free nerve endings
  Expanded tip endings
    Ruffini's endings
    Merkel's discs
    Plus several other variants
  Encapsulated endings
    Meissner's corpuscles
    Krause's corpuscles
    Pacinian corpuscles
  Hair end-organs
Deep tissue sensibilities
  Free nerve endings
  Expanded tip endings
    Ruffini's endings
    Plus a few other variants
  Encapsulated endings
    Pacinian corpuscles
    Plus a few other variants
  Specialized endings
    Muscle spindles
    Golgi tendon receptors
Hearing
  Sound receptors of cochlea
Equilibrium
  Vestibular receptors
Arterial pressure
  Baroreceptors of carotid sinuses and aorta

Thermoreceptors

Cold
  Probably free nerve endings
Warmth
  Probably free nerve endings

Nociceptors

Pain
  Free nerve endings

Electromagnetic Receptors

Vision
  Rods
  Cones

Chemoreceptors

Taste
  Receptors of taste buds
Smell
  Receptors of olfactory epithelium
Arterial oxygen
  Receptors of aortic and carotid bodies
Osmolality
  Probably neurons of supraoptic nuclei
Blood CO_2
  Receptors in or on surface of medulla and in aortic and
    carotid bodies
Blood glucose, amino acids, fatty acids
  Receptors in hypothalamus

DIFFERENTIAL SENSITIVITY OF RECEPTORS

The first question that must be answered is how do two types of sensory receptors detect different types of sensory stimuli? The answer to this: By virtue of differential sensitivities. That is, each type of receptor is very highly sensitive to one type of stimulus for which it is designed and yet is almost nonresponsive to normal intensities of the other types of sensory stimuli. Thus, the rods and cones are highly responsive to light but are almost completely nonresponsive to heat, cold, pressure on the eyeballs, or chemical changes in the blood. The osmoreceptors of the supraoptic nuclei in the hypothalamus detect minute changes in the osmolality of the body fluids but yet have never been known to respond to sound. Finally, pain receptors in the skin are almost never stimulated by usual touch or pressure stimuli but do become highly active the moment tactile stimuli become severe enough to damage the tissues.

Modality of Sensation—Law of Specific Nerve Energies. Each of the principal types of sensation that we can experience—pain, touch, sight, sound, and so forth—is called a *modality* of sensation. Yet, despite the fact that we experience these different modalities of sensation, nerve fibers transmit only impulses. Therefore, how is it that different nerve fibers transmit different modalities of sensation?

The answer to this is that each nerve tract terminates at a specific point in the central nervous system, and the type of sensation felt when a nerve fiber is stimulated is determined by this specific area in the nervous system to which the fiber leads. For instance, if a pain fiber is stimulated, the person perceives pain regardless of what type of stimulus excites the fiber. This stimulus can be electricity, heat, crushing, or stimulation of the pain nerve ending by damage to the tissue cells. Yet, whatever the means of stimulation, the person still perceives pain. Likewise, if a touch fiber is stimulated by exciting a touch receptor electrically or in any other way, the person perceives touch because touch fibers lead to specific touch areas in the brain. Similarly, fibers from the retina of the eye terminate in the vision areas of the brain, fibers from the ear terminate in the auditory areas of the brain, and temperature fibers terminate in the temperature areas.

This specificity of nerve fibers for transmitting only one modality of sensation is called the *law of specific nerve energies*.

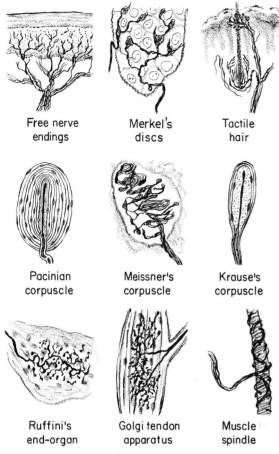

Free nerve
endings

Merkel's
discs

Tactile
hair

Pacinian
corpuscle

Meissner's
corpuscle

Krause's
corpuscle

Ruffini's
end-organ

Golgi tendon
apparatus

Muscle
spindle

Figure 6–1. Several types of somatic sensory nerve endings. (Modified from Ramon y Cajal: Histology. William Wood and Co.)

TRANSDUCTION OF SENSORY STIMULI INTO NERVE IMPULSES

LOCAL CURRENTS AT NERVE ENDINGS—RECEPTOR POTENTIALS

All sensory receptors studied thus far have one feature in common. Whatever the type of stimulus that excites the ending, it first causes a local potential called a *receptor potential* in the neighborhood of the nerve endings, and it is *local flow of current* caused by the receptor potential that in turn excites action potentials in the nerve fiber.

There are two different ways in which receptor potentials can be elicited. One of these is to deform or chemically alter the terminal nerve ending itself. This causes ions to diffuse through the nerve membrane, thereby setting up the receptor potential.

The second method for causing receptor potentials involves specialized receptor cells that lie adjacent to the nerve endings. For instance, when sound enters the cochlea of the ear, specialized *receptor cells* called *hair cells* that lie on the basilar membrane develop local potentials which are receptor potentials that stimulate the terminal nerve fibrils entwining the hair cells.

(Some physiologists prefer to use the term *generator potentials* to designate the receptor potentials elicited in terminal nerve endings because the nerve fibers themselves actually "generate" the potentials, and they reserve the term "receptor potentials" only for those potentials that arise in specialized receptor cells of non-nervous tissue origin such as taste cells, hair cells of the ear, and so forth. However, because both of these potentials subserve the same function and because of the confusion that has developed by use of two separate terms, it is probably best to use the single term "receptor potentials" as we shall do here.)

The Receptor Potential of the Pacinian Corpuscle. The pacinian corpuscle is a very large and easily dissected sensory receptor. For this reason, one can study in detail the mechanism by which tactile stimuli excite it and by which it causes action potentials in the sensory fiber leading from it. Note in Figure 6–1 that the pacinian corpuscle has a central non-myelinated tip of a nerve fiber extending through its core. Surrounding this fiber are many concentric capsule layers so that compression on the outside of the corpuscle tends to elongate, shorten, indent, or otherwise deform the central core of the fiber, depending on how the compression is applied. The deformation causes a sudden change in membrane potential, as illustrated in Figure 6–2. This perhaps results from stretching the nerve fiber membrane, thus increasing its permeability and allowing

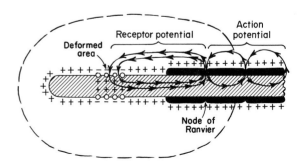

Figure 6–2. Excitation of a sensory nerve fiber by a generator potential produced in a pacinian corpuscle. (Modified from Loewenstein: *Ann. N.Y. Acad. Sci.,* 94:510, 1961.)

positively charged sodium ions to leak to the interior of the fiber. This change in local potential causes a local circuit of current flow that spreads along the nerve fiber to its myelinated portion. At the first node of Ranvier, which itself lies inside the capsule of the pacinian corpuscle, the local current flow initiates action potentials in the nerve fiber. That is, the current flow through the node depolarizes it, and this then sets off a typical saltatory transmission of an action potential along the nerve fiber toward the central nervous system, as was explained in Chapter 1.

Electrotonic Nature of the Receptor Potential. Note especially that the receptor potential has a different electrical character from the action potential. It will be recalled from Chapter 1 and also from Chapter 4 that the action potential is a self-regenerative cyclic event that begins with a resting negative potential, then changes to a positive potential and finally returns back to a negative potential. On the other hand, the receptor potential is an "electrotonic" potential that causes "tonic" flow of current without proceeding through the regenerative events of an action potential. It is a local potential just as are the end-plate potential of muscle fibers and the postsynaptic potential of neurons. If the receptor potential is great enough, it will elicit one or more action potentials at the first node of Ranvier. On the other hand, if the potential does not reach *threshold* level for excitation of an action potential, it will simply exist locally and will spread only a short distance along the fiber; the spreading will be by the process of electrotonic conduction, not by means of a self-regenerative action potential.

Relationship Between Receptor Potential and Stimulus Strength. Figure 6–3 illustrates the effect on the amplitude of the receptor potential caused by progressively stronger stimuli applied to the central core of the pacinian corpuscle. Note that the amplitude increases rapidly at first but then progressively less rapidly at high stimulus strengths. The maximum amplitude that can be achieved by receptor potentials is around 100 millivolts. That is, a receptor potential can have almost as high a voltage as an action potential.

Receptor Potentials Recorded from Other Sensory Receptors. Receptor potentials have been recorded from many other sensory receptors, including most notably the muscle spindles, the hair cells of the ear, and the rods and cones of the eyes and many others. In all of these, the amplitude of the potential increases as the strength of stimulus increases, but the additional response usually becomes progressively less as the strength of stimulus becomes great.

Figure 6–3. Relationship of amplitude of receptor (generator) potential to strength of a stimulus applied to a pacinian corpuscle. (From Loewenstein: *Ann. N.Y. Acad. Sci.*, 94:510, 1961.)

Yet, the mechanism for causing the receptor potential is not the same in different receptors. For instance, in the rods and cones of the eye changes in certain intracellular chemicals caused by exposure to light alter the membrane potential, resulting in the receptor potential. In this case, the basic mechanism eliciting the receptor potential is a chemical one in contrast to mechanical deformation that causes the receptor potential in the pacinian corpuscle. In the case of thermal receptors, it is believed that changes in rates of chemical reaction at or near the membrane alter the membrane potential and thereby create a receptor potential. In the case of the hair cells of the ear, bending of cilia protruding from the hairs probably causes the receptor potentials. Thus, the mechanisms for eliciting receptor potentials are individualized for each type of receptor.

Relationship of Amplitude of Receptor Potential to Nerve Impulse Rate. Referring once again to Figure 6–2, we see that the receptor potential generated in the core of the pacinian corpuscle causes a local circuit of current flow through the first node of Ranvier. When an action potential occurs at the node, this does not affect the receptor potential being emitted by the core of the pacinian corpuscle. Instead, the core continues to emit its current as long as an effective mechanical stimulus is applied. As a result, when the node of Ranvier repolarizes after its first action potential is over, it discharges once again, and action potentials continue as long as the receptor potential persists, which, in the case of the pacinian corpuscle, is only a few thousandths or hundredths of a second.

The frequency of action potentials in the nerve fiber (impulse rate) is almost directly proportional to the amplitude of the receptor potential. This relationship is illustrated in Figure 6–4, which shows the impulse rate corresponding to different voltages of receptor ("generator") potential recorded from a muscle spindle; there is an almost exact proportional relationship. This same relationship between receptor potential and impulse rate is approximately true for most sensory receptors.

ADAPTATION OF RECEPTORS

A special characteristic of all sensory receptors is that they *adapt* either partially or completely to their stimuli after a period of time. That is, when a continuous sensory stimulus is first applied, the receptors respond at a very high impulse rate at first, then progressively less rapidly until finally many of them no longer respond at all.

Figure 6–5 illustrates typical adaptation of certain types of receptors. Note that the pacinian corpuscle and the receptor at the hair bases adapt extremely rapidly, while joint capsule and muscle spindle receptors adapt very slowly.

Furthermore some sensory receptors adapt to a far greater extent than others. For example,

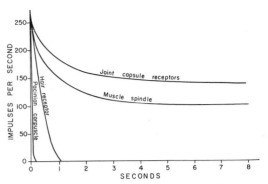

Figure 6–5. Adaptation of different types of receptors, showing rapid adaptation of some receptors and slow adaptation of others.

the pacinian corpuscles adapt to "extinction" within a few thousandths to a few hundredths of a second, and the hair base receptors adapt to extinction within a second or more.

Mechanisms by which Receptors Adapt. Adaptation of receptors is an individual property of each type of receptor in much the same way that development of a receptor potential is an individual property. For instance, in the eye, the rods and cones adapt by changing their chemical compositions (which will be discussed in Chapter 17). In the case of the mechanoreceptors, the receptor that has been studied in greatest detail is the pacinian corpuscle. Adaptation occurs in this receptor in two ways. First, the corpuscular structure itself very rapidly adapts to the deformation of the tissue. This can be explained as follows: The pacinian corpuscle is a viscoelastic structure so that when a distorting force is suddenly applied to one side of the corpuscle it is transmitted by the viscous component of the corpuscle directly to the same side of the central core, thus eliciting a receptor potential. However, within a few thousandths to a few hundredths of a second the fluid within the corpuscle redistributes so that the pressure becomes essentially equal all through the corpuscle; this applies an even pressure on all sides of the central core fiber, so that the receptor potential is no longer elicited. Thus, a receptor potential appears at the onset of compression but then disappears within a small fraction of a second. Then, when the distorting force is removed from the corpuscle, essentially the reverse events occur. The sudden removal of the distortion from one side of the corpuscle allows rapid expansion on that side and a corresponding distortion of the central core occurs once more. Again, within milliseconds, the pressure becomes equalized all

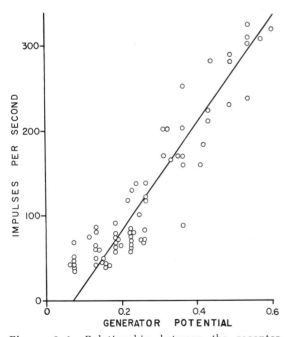

Figure 6–4. Relationship between the receptor (generator) potential of a muscle spindle and the frequency of sensory impulses transmitted from the spindle. [From Katz: *J. Physiol. (Lond.)*, 111:161, 1950.]

through the corpuscle and the stimulus is lost. Thus, the pacinian corpuscle signals the onset of compression and again signals the offset of compression.

The second mechanism of adaptation of the pacinian corpuscle results from a process of accommodation that occurs in the nerve fiber itself. That is, even if by chance the central core fiber should continue to be excited, as can be achieved after the capsule has been removed and the core is compressed with a stylus, the tip of the nerve fiber itself gradually becomes "accommodated" to the stimulus. This perhaps results from redistribution of ions across the nerve fiber membrane.

Presumably, these same two general mechanisms of adaptation apply to other types of receptors. That is, part of the adaptation results from readjustments in the structure of the receptor itself, and part results from accommodation in the terminal nerve fibril.

Function of the Poorly Adapting Receptors—The "Tonic" Receptors. The poorly adapting receptors (receptors that adapt very slowly and do not adapt to extinction) continue to transmit impulses to the brain as long as the stimulus is present (or at least for many minutes or hours). Therefore, they keep the brain constantly appraised of the status of the body and its relation to its surroundings. For instance, impulses from the slowly adapting joint capsule receptors allow the person to "know" at all times the degree of bending of the joints and therefore the positions of the different parts of his body. And impulses from the muscle spindles and Golgi tendon apparatuses allow the central nervous system to know respectively the status of muscle contraction and the load on the muscle tendon at each instant.

Other types of poorly adapting receptors include the receptors of the macula in the vestibular apparatus, the sound receptors of the ear, the pain receptors, the pressoreceptors of the arterial tree, the chemoreceptors of the carotid and aortic bodies, and some of the tactile receptors, such as the Ruffini endings and the Merkel's discs.

Because the poorly adapting receptors can continue to transmit information for many hours, they are also called *tonic* receptors. It is probable that many of these poorly adapting receptors would adapt to extinction if the intensity of the stimulus should remain absolutely constant over many days. Fortunately, because of our continually changing bodily state, the tonic receptors could almost never reach a state of complete adaptation.

Function of the Rapidly Adapting Receptors—The Rate Receptors or Movement Receptors or Phasic Receptors. Obviously, receptors that adapt rapidly cannot be used to transmit a continuous signal because these receptors are stimulated only when the stimulus strength changes. Yet they react strongly *while a change is actually taking place*. Furthermore, the number of impulses transmitted is directly related to the *rate at which the change takes place*. Therefore, these receptors are called *rate* receptors, *movement* receptors, or *phasic* receptors. Thus, in the case of the pacinian corpuscle, sudden pressure applied to the skin excites this receptor for a few milliseconds, and then its excitation is over even though the pressure continues. But then it transmits a signal again when the pressure is released. In other words, the pacinian corpuscle is exceedingly important in transmitting information about rapid changes in pressure against the body, but it is useless in transmitting information about constant pressure applied to the body.

Importance of the Rate Receptors–Their Predictive Function. If one knows the rate at which some change in his bodily status is taking place, he can predict ahead to the state of the body a few seconds or even a few minutes later. For instance, the receptors of the semicircular canals in the vestibular apparatus of the ear detect the rate at which the head begins to turn when one runs around a curve. Using this information, a person can predict that he will turn 10, 30, or some other number of degrees within the next 10 seconds, and he can adjust the motion of his limbs *ahead of time* to keep from losing his balance. Likewise, pacinian corpuscles located in or near the joint capsules help to detect the rates of movement of the different parts of the body. Therefore, when one is running, information from these receptors allows the nervous system to predict ahead of time where the feet will be during any precise fraction of a second, and appropriate motor signals can be transmitted to the muscles of the legs to make any necessary anticipatory corrections in limb position so that the person will not fall. Loss of this predictive function makes it impossible for the person to run.

PSYCHIC INTERPRETATION OF STIMULUS STRENGTH

The ultimate goal of most sensory stimulation is to appraise the psyche of the state of the body and its surroundings. Therefore, it is important that we discuss briefly some of the principles related to the transmission of sensory stimulus strength to the higher levels of the nervous system.

The first question that comes to mind is, "How is it possible for the sensory system to transmit sensory experiences of tremendously varying intensities?" For instance, the auditory system can detect the weakest possible whisper but can also discern the meanings of an explosive sound only a few feet away, even though the sound intensities of these two experiences can vary as much as a trillion-fold; the eyes can see visual images with light intensities that vary as much as a million-fold; or the skin can detect pressure differences of ten thousand- to one hundred thousand-fold.

As a partial explanation of these effects, note in Figure 6–3 the relationship of the receptor potential ("generator" potential) produced by the pacinian corpuscle to the strength of stimulus. At low stimulus strength, very slight changes in stimulus strength increase the potential markedly; whereas at high levels of stimulus strength, further increases in receptor potential are very slight. Thus, the pacinian corpuscle is capable of accurately measuring extremely minute changes in stimulus strength at low intensity levels and is also capable of detecting much larger changes in stimulus strength at high intensity levels.

The transduction mechanism for detecting sound by the cochlea of the ear illustrates still another method for separating gradations of stimulus intensity. When sound causes vibration at a specific point on the basilar membrane, weak vibration stimulates only those hair cells in the very center of the vibratory point. But, as the vibration intensity increases, not only do the centralmost hair cells become more intensely stimulated, but hair cells in each direction farther away from the central point also become stimulated. Thus, signals transmitted over progressively increasing numbers of cochlear nerve fibers as well as increasing intensity of signal strength in each nerve fiber are two mechanisms by which stimulus strength is transmitted into the central nervous system. These two mechanisms, which multiply each other, make it possible for the ear to operate reasonably faithfully at stimulus intensity levels changing as much as a trillion-fold.

Importance of the Tremendous Intensity Range of Sensory Reception. Were it not for the tremendous intensity range of sensory reception that we can experience, the various sensory systems would more often than not operate in the wrong range. This is illustrated by the attempt of most persons to adjust the light exposure on a camera without using a light meter. Left to intuitive judgment of light intensity, a person almost always overexposes the film on very bright days and greatly underexposes the film at twilight. Yet, his eyes are perfectly capable of discriminating with great detail the objects around him in both very bright sunlight and at twilight; the camera cannot do this because of the narrow critical range of light intensity required for proper exposure of film.

JUDGMENT OF STIMULUS STRENGTH

Physiopsychologists have evolved numerous methods for testing one's judgment of sensory stimulus strength, but only rarely do the results from the different methods agree with each other. For instance, one testing method requires a person to select a weight that is exactly 100 per cent heavier than another. But he usually selects a weight that is about 50 per cent heavier instead of 100 per cent heavier. Thus, the weak stimulus is underestimated and the strong stimulus is overestimated. In still another test procedure, a person is given a weight to hold and is then required to select the minimum amount of additional weight that must be added for him to detect a difference. In this case he might be holding a 50 gram weight and find out that an additional 5 grams are necessary to detect a difference. Then he holds a 500 gram weight and finds that 50 grams of additional weight are required. In this instance the discriminatory ability is far greater at the low intensity level than at the high intensity level. Thus, the results of these two different types of tests are exactly opposite to each other, which means that the real argument lies in the meaning of the tests themselves. Therefore, at present no real agreement exists as to a proper method for measuring one judgment of stimulus strength. Yet, two principles are widely discussed in the physiopsychology field of sensory interpretation: the *Weber-Fechner principle* and the *power principle*.

The Weber-Fechner Principle—Detection of "Ratio" of Stimulus Strength. In the mid–eighteen-hundreds, Weber first and Fechner later proposed the principle that *gradations of stimulus strength are discriminated approximately in proportion to the logarithm of stimulus strength*. This law is based primarily on one's ability to judge minimal changes in stimulus strength that can be detected, utilizing the second test described in the previous section; that is, in this example just given, a person can barely detect a 5 gram increase in weight when holding 50 grams, or a 50 gram increase when holding 500 grams. Thus, the *ratio* of the change in stimulus strength required for perception of a change remains essentially constant, which is what the logarithmic principle means.

Because the Weber-Fechner principle offers a ready explanation for the tremendous range of stimulus strength that our nervous system can discern, it unfortunately became widely accepted for all types of sensory experience and for all levels of background sensory intensity. More recently it has become evident that this principle applies mainly to higher levels of visual, auditory, and cutaneous sensory experience and that it applies only poorly to most other types of sensory experience.

Yet, the Weber-Fechner principle is still a good one to remember because it emphasizes that the greater the background sensory stimulus, the greater also must be the additional change in stimulus strength in order for the psyche to detect the change.

Figure 6–6. Graphical demonstration of the "power law" relationship between actual stimulus strength and strength that the psyche interprets it to be. Note that the power law does not hold at either very weak or very strong stimulus strengths.

The Power Law. Another attempt by physio-psychologists to find a good mathematical relationship between actual stimulus strength and interpretation of stimulus strength is the following formula, known as the power law:

Interpreted strength = K · (Stimulus strength)^y

In this formula K is a constant, and y is the power to which the stimulus strength is raised. The exponent y and the constant K are different for each type of sensation.

When this power law relationship is plotted on a graph using double logarithmic coordinates, as illustrated in Figure 6–6, a linear curve can be attained between interpreted stimulus strength and actual stimulus strength over a large range. However, as illustrated in the figure, even this power law relationship fails to hold satisfactorily at both low and high stimulus strengths.

Unfortunately, the power law is not of great philosophical importance for a very simple mathematical reason. Almost any curve (even the curve of a hill) that has a progressive change in slope in the same direction can be fitted over most of its range to the power law equation, provided one simply finds proper values for the exponent y and constant K. Therefore, use of the power law is more an exercise in mathematical curve fitting than it is a valuable tool in understanding sensory experience.

PHYSIOLOGICAL CLASSIFICATION OF NERVE FIBERS

Unfortunately, two separate classifications of nerve fibers are in general use. The first of these is a general classification given in Table 6–2. The fibers are divided into types A, B, and C; and the type A fibers are further subdivided into α, β, γ, and δ fibers.

Type A fibers are the typical myelinated fibers of spinal nerves. The type B fibers differ from very small type A fibers only in the fact that they do not display a negative after-potential following stimulation. However, they also are myelinated like type A fibers. They are the preganglionic autonomic nerve fibers.

Type C fibers are the very small unmyelinated nerve fibers that conduct impulses at low velocities. These constitute more than half the sensory fibers in

TABLE 6–2.   Properties of Different Mammalian Nerve Fibers

Type of Fiber	Diameter of Fiber (μ)	Velocity of Conduction (meters/sec.)	Duration of Spike (msec.)	Duration of Negative After-potential (msec.)	Duration of Positive After-potential (msec.)	Function
A (α)	13–22	70–120	0.4–0.5	12–20	40–60	Motor, muscle proprioceptors
A (β)	8–13	40–70	0.4–0.6	(?)	(?)	Touch, pressure, kinesthesia
A (γ)	4–8	15–40	0.5–0.7	(?)	(?)	Touch, motor excitation of muscle spindles
A (δ)	1–4	5–15	0.6–1.0	(?)	(?)	Pain. heat, cold, pressure
B	1–3	3–14	1.2	None	100–300	Preganglionic autonomic
C	0.2–1.0	0.2–2	2.0	50–80	300–1000	Pain, itch, heat(?), cold(?), pressure(?), postganglionic autonomic, smell

Compiled from various sources but mainly from Grundfest.

most peripheral nerves and also all of the post-ganglionic autonomic fibers.

The sizes, velocities of conduction, and functions of the different nerve fibers are given in Table 6–2. Note that the very large fibers can transmit impulses at velocities as great as 120 meters per second, a distance in one second that is longer than a football field. On the other hand, the smallest fibers transmit impulses as slowly as 0.2 meter per second, requiring several seconds to go from the big toe to the spinal cord.

Over two-thirds of all the nerve fibers in peripheral nerves are type C fibers. Because of their great number, these can transmit tremendous amounts of information from the surface of the body, even though their velocities of transmission are very slow. Utilization of type C fibers for transmitting this great mass of information represents an important economy of space in the nerves, for use of type A fibers would require peripheral nerves the sizes of large ropes and a spinal cord almost as large as the body itself.

Alternate Classification Used by Sensory Physiologists. Certain recording techniques have made it possible to separate the type $A\alpha$ fibers into two subgroups; and, yet, these same recording techniques cannot distinguish easily between $A\beta$ and $A\gamma$ fibers. Therefore, the following classification is frequently used by sensory physiologists:

GROUP I A. Fibers from the annulospiral endings of muscle spindles. (About 17 microns in diameter. These are alpha type A fibers in the classification of Table 6–2.)

GROUP I B. Fibers from the Golgi tendon apparatuses. (About 16 microns in diameter; these also are alpha type A fibers.)

GROUP II. Fibers from the discrete cutaneous tactile receptors and also from the flower-spray endings of the muscle spindles. (Average about 8 microns in diameter; these are beta and gamma type A fibers in the other classification.)

GROUP III. Fibers carrying temperature, crude touch, and pain sensations. (Average about 3 microns in diameter; these are delta type A fibers in the other classification.)

GROUP IV. Unmyelinated fibers carrying pain, itch, crude temperature, and crude touch sensations. (0.2 to 1 micron in diameter; called type C fibers in the other classification.)

REFERENCES

Anderson, D. J., Hannam, A. G., and Matthews, B.: Sensory mechanisms in mammalian teeth and their supporting structures. *Physiol. Rev.*, 50:171, 1970.

Appelle, S.: Perception and discrimination as a function of stimulus orientation: the "oblique effect" in man and animals. *Psychol. Bull.*, 78:266, 1972.

Babel, J., Bischoff, A., and Spoendlin, H.: Ultrastructure of the Peripheral Nervous System and Sense Organs. New York, Churchill Livingstone, Div. of Longman, Inc., 1971.

Bullock, T. H.: Seeing the world through a new sense: electroreception in fish. *Amer. Sci.*, 61:316, 1973.

Catton, W. T.: Mechanoreceptor function. *Physiol. Rev.*, 50:297, 1970.

Galun, R. (ed.): Sensory Physiology and Behavior. New York, Plenum Publishing Corporation, 1975.

Goldberg, J. M., and Lavine, R. A.: Nervous system: afferent mechanisms. *Ann. Rev. Physiol.*, 30:319, 1968.

Granit, R.: Receptors and Sensory Perception. New Haven, Yale University Press, 1955.

Gray, J. A. B.: Initiation of impulses at receptors. *In* Magoun, H. W. (ed.): Handbook of Physiology. Sec. 1, Vol. 1. Baltimore, The Williams & Wilkins Company, 1959.

Halata, Z.: The Mechanoreceptors of the Mammalian Skin. New York, Springer-Verlag New York, Inc., 1975.

Hunt, C. C., and Takeuchi, A.: Responses of the nerve terminal of the pacinian corpuscle. *J. Physiol. (Lond.)*, 160:1, 1962.

Jacobson, M., and Hunt, R. K.: The origins of nerve-cell specificity. *Sci. Amer.*, 228:26, 1973.

Kruger, L., and Kenton, B.: Quantitative neural and psychophysical data for cutaneous mechanoreceptor function. *Brain Res.*, 49:1, 1973.

Leibowitz, H. W., and Harvey, L. O., Jr.: Perception. *Ann. Rev. Psychol.*, 24:207, 1973.

Loewenstein, W. R.: The generation of electric activity in a nerve ending. *Ann. N.Y. Acad. Sci.*, 81:367, 1959.

Loewenstein, W. R.: Biological transducers. *Sci. Amer.*, 203:98, 1960.

Loewenstein, W. R.: Excitation and inactivation in a receptor membrane. *Ann. N.Y. Acad. Sci.*, 94:510, 1961.

Lynn, B.: Somatosensory receptors and their CNS connections. *Ann. Rev. Physiol.*, 37:105, 1975.

Perl, E. R., and Boivie, J. G.: Neural substrates of somatic sensation. *In* Guyton, A. C. (ed.): MTP International Review of Science: Physiology. Vol. 3. Baltimore, University Park Press, 1974, p. 303.

Somjen, G.: Sensory Coding in the Mammalian Nervous System. New York, Appleton-Century-Crofts, 1972.

Tamar, H.: Principles of Sensory Physiology. Springfield, Ill., Charles C Thomas, Publisher, 1972.

Thompson, R. F., and Patterson, M. (eds.): Bioelectric Recording Techniques, Part C. Receptor and Effector Processes. New York, Academic Press, Inc., 1974.

Thorson, J., and Biederman-Thorson, M.: Distributed relaxation processes in sensory adaptation. *Science*, 183:161, 1974.

Winkelmann, R. K.: Nerve Endings in Normal and Pathologic Skin. Springfield, Illinois, Charles C Thomas, Publisher, 1960.

Zotterman, Y.: Sensory Mechanisms. Progress in Brain Research. Vol. 23. New York, American Elsevier Publishing Co., Inc., 1967.

| 7 |

Somatic Sensations: I. The Mechanoreceptive Sensations

The *somatic senses* are the nervous mechanisms that collect sensory information from the body. These senses are in contradistinction to the *special senses,* which mean specifically sight, hearing, smell, taste, and equilibrium.

CLASSIFICATION OF SOMATIC SENSATIONS

The somatic senses can be classified into three different physiological types: (1) the *mechanoreceptive somatic senses,* stimulated by mechanical displacement of some tissue of the body, (2) the *thermoreceptive senses,* which detect heat and cold, and (3) the *pain sense,* which is activated by any factor that damages the tissues. The present chapter deals with the mechanoreceptive somatic senses, and the following chapter deals with the thermoreceptive and pain senses.

The mechanoreceptive senses include *touch, pressure,* and *vibration* senses (which are frequently called the *tactile senses*) and the *kinesthetic sense,* which determines the relative positions and rates of movement of the different parts of the body.

Other Classifications of Somatic Sensations. Different physiological types of somatic sensations are grouped together in special classes that are not necessarily mutually exclusive, as follows:

Exteroceptive sensations are those from the surface of the body.

Proprioceptive sensations are those having to do with the physical state of the body, including kinesthetic sensations, possible tendon and muscle sensations, pressure sensations from the bottom of the feet, and even the sensation of equilibrium, which is generally considered to be a "special" sensation rather than a somatic sensation.

Visceral sensations are those from the viscera of the body; in using this term one usually refers specifically to sensations from the internal organs.

The *deep sensations* are those that come from the deep tissues, such as from the bone, fasciae, and so forth. These include mainly "deep" pressure, pain, and vibration.

DETECTION AND TRANSMISSION OF TACTILE SENSATIONS

Interrelationship Between the Tactile Sensations of Touch, Pressure, and Vibration. Though touch, pressure, and vibration are frequently classified as separate sensations, they are all detected by the same types of receptors. The only differences among these three types of sensations are (1) touch sensation generally results from stimulation of tactile receptors in the skin or in tissues immediately beneath the skin, (2) pressure sensation generally results from deformation of deeper tissues, and (3) vibration sensation results from rapidly repetitive sensory signals, but some of the same types of receptors as those for both touch and pressure are utilized—specifically the rapidly adapting types of receptors.

The Tactile Receptors. At least six entirely different types of tactile receptors are known, but many more similar to these probably also exist. Some of these receptors were illustrated in Figure 6–1 of Chapter 6, and their special characteristics are the following:

First, some *free nerve endings,* which are found everywhere in the skin and in many other tissues, can detect touch and pressure. For instance, even light contact with the cornea of the eye, which contains no other type of nerve ending besides free nerve endings, can nevertheless elicit touch and pressure sensations.

Second, a touch receptor of special sensitivity is *Meissner's corpuscle,* an encapsulated nerve ending that excites a large myelinated sensory nerve fiber. Inside the capsulation are many whorls of terminal nerve filaments. These receptors are particularly abundant in the fingertips, lips, and other areas of the skin where one's ability to discern spatial characteristics of touch sensations is highly developed. These receptors, along with the expanded tip receptors described subsequently, are probably responsible for the ability to recognize exactly what point of the body is touched and to recognize the texture of objects touched. Meissner's corpuscles probably adapt within a second or perhaps even less after they are stimulated, which means that they are particularly sensitive to movement of very light objects over the surface of the skin and also to low-frequency vibration.

Third, the fingertips and other areas that contain large numbers of Meissner's corpuscles also contain *expanded tip tactile receptors,* one type of which is *Merkel's discs.* These receptors differ from Meissner's corpuscles in that they transmit an initial strong but partially adapting signal and then a continuing weaker signal that adapts only slowly. Therefore, they are probably responsible for giving steady state signals that allow one to determine continuous touch of objects against the skin. The hairy parts of the body contain almost no Meissner's corpuscles but do contain a few expanded tip receptors.

Fourth, slight movement of any hair on the body stimulates the nerve fiber entwining its base. Thus, each hair and its basal nerve fiber, called the *hair end-organ,* is also a type of touch receptor. This receptor adapts readily and, therefore, like Meissner's corpuscles, detects mainly movement of objects on the surface of the body.

Fifth, located in the deeper layers of the skin and also in deeper tissues of the body are many *Ruffini's end-organs,* which are multibranched endings, as described and illustrated in the previous chapter. These endings adapt very little and, therefore, are important for signaling continuous states of deformation of the skin and deeper tissues, such as heavy and continuous touch signals and pressure signals. They are also found in joint capsules and signal the degree of joint rotation.

Sixth, many *pacinian corpuscles,* which were discussed in detail in Chapter 6, lie both beneath the skin and also deep in the tissues of the body. These are stimulated only by very rapid movement of the tissues because these receptors adapt in a small fraction of a second. Therefore, they are particularly important for detecting tissue vibration or other extremely rapid changes in the mechanical state of the tissues.

Transmission of Tactile Sensations in Peripheral Nerve Fibers. The specialized sensory receptors, such as Meissner's corpuscles, expanded tip endings, pacinian corpuscles, and Ruffini's endings, all transmit their signals in beta type A nerve fibers that have transmission velocities of 30 to 60 meters per second. On the other hand, free nerve ending tactile receptors and probably some of the hair end-organs transmit signals via the small delta type A nerve fibers that conduct at velocities of 6 to 15 meters per second. Some of the tactile free nerve endings transmit via type C fibers at velocities of about 1 meter per second; it has not yet been proved that these send signals to the brain that can be detected consciously. Thus, the more critical types of sensory signals—those that help to determine precise localization on the skin, minute gradations of intensity, or rapid changes in sensory signal intensity—are all transmitted in the rapidly conducting types of sensory nerve fibers. On the other hand, the cruder types of signals, such as crude pressure and poorly localized touch, are transmitted via much slower nerve fibers, fibers that also require much less space in the nerves.

DETECTION OF VIBRATION

All the different tactile receptors are involved in detection of vibration, though different receptors detect different frequencies of vibration. Pacinian corpuscles can discern vibrations up to as high as 400 to 500 cycles per second, because they respond extremely rapidly to minute and rapid deformations of the tissues, and they also transmit their signals over beta type A nerve fibers, which can transmit more than 1000 impulses per second.

Low frequency vibrations up to 80 cycles per

second, on the other hand, stimulate other tactile receptors—especially Meissner's corpuscles, which are less rapidly adapting in preference to pacinian corpuscles.

POSSIBILITY OF A "MUSCLE SENSE"

Special sensory receptors are found in both skeletal muscles and tendons, *muscle spindles* in muscles and *Golgi tendon apparatuses* in tendons. These receptors transmit their signals into the spinal cord and cerebellum to control reflex contraction of the muscles. But, from what is known at present, these signals operate entirely at a subconscious level. These specialized receptors and the reflexes that they subserve will be considered in detail in relation to spinal cord reflexes and control of muscle contraction in Chapter 9.

However, some psychological effects have pointed to the existence of a conscious "muscle sense." For instance, one is capable of determining how heavy an object is, and this has long been believed to be detected by the specialized muscle spindles or tendon organs; but critical experiments show this not to be true. Instead, this type of information is probably signaled in two ways: (1) by usual tactile signals in the deep tissues and (2) by signals from the motor portions of the brain indicating intensity of motor signals to the muscles required to lift an object.

KINESTHETIC SENSATIONS

The term "kinesthesia" means conscious recognition of the orientation of the different parts of the body with respect to each other as well as of the rates of movement of the different parts of the body. These functions are subserved principally by extensive sensory endings in the joint capsules and ligaments.

The Kinesthetic Receptors. Three major types of nerve endings have been described in the joint capsules and ligaments about the joints. (1) By far the most abundant of these are spray type *Ruffini endings,* one of which was illustrated in Figure 6–1 of Chapter 6. These endings are stimulated strongly when the joint is suddenly moved; they adapt slightly at first but then transmit a steady signal thereafter. (2) A second type of ending resembling the stretch receptors found in muscle tendons (called *Golgi tendon receptors*) is found particularly in the ligaments about the joints. Though far less numerous than the Ruffini endings they have essentially the same response properties. (3) A few *pacinian corpuscles* are also found in the tissues around the joints. These adapt extremely rapidly and presumably help to detect *rate of rotation* at the joint.

Detection of the Degree of Joint Rotation by the Joint Receptors. Figure 7–1 illustrates the excitation of seven different nerve fibers leading from separate joint receptors in the capsule of a cat's knee joint. Note that at 180 degrees of joint rotation one of the receptors is stimulated; then at 150 degrees still another is stimulated; at 140 degrees two are stimulated, and so forth. The information from these joint receptors continually apprises the central nervous system of the momentary rotation of the joint. That is, the rotation determines *which* receptor is stimulated and how much it is stimulated, and from this the brain knows how far the joint is bent.

Detection of Rate of Movement at the Joint. Because pacinian corpuscles are especially adapted for detecting movement of tissues, it is tempting to suggest that rate of movement at the joints is detected by the pacinian corpuscles. However, the number of pacinian corpuscles in the joint tissues is small, for which reason rate of movement at the joint is probably detected mainly in the following way: The Ruffini and Golgi endings in the joint tissues are stimulated very strongly at first by the process of joint movement, but within a fraction of a second this strong level of stimulation fades to a lower, steady state rate of firing. Nevertheless, this early overshoot in receptor stimulation is directly proportional to the rate of joint movement and is believed to be the signal used by the brain to discern the rate of movement. However, it is likely that the few pacinian corpuscles also play at least some role in this process.

Transmission of Kinesthetic Signals in the Peripheral Nerves. Kinesthetic signals, like those from the critical tactile sensory receptors, are transmitted almost entirely in the beta type

Figure 7–1. Responses of seven different nerve fibers from knee joint receptors in a cat at different degrees of rotation. (Modified from Skogland: *Acta Physiol. Scand.,* Suppl. 124, 36:1, 1956.)

A sensory nerve fibers, which carry signals very rapidly to the cord and, thence, to the brain. This rapid transmission of kinesthetic signals is particularly important when parts of the body are moving rapidly, because it is essential for the central nervous system to "know" at each small fraction of a second the exact locations of the different parts of the body; otherwise one would not be capable of controlling further movements.

THE DUAL SYSTEM FOR TRANSMISSION OF MECHANORECEPTIVE SOMATIC SENSATIONS IN THE CENTRAL NERVOUS SYSTEM

All sensory information from the somatic segments of the body enters the spinal cord through the posterior roots. On entering the cord, most large sensory nerve fibers (mainly the beta type A fibers) immediately enter the *dorsal columns* of the cord and ascend the entire length of the cord. The smaller sensory fibers (type C and delta type A) as well as lateral collaterals from the larger fibers travel upward for one to six segments and downward for one to four segments, and then synapse with dorsal horn cells that give rise to the *ventral and lateral spinothalamic tracts*. These tracts ascend to the brain in the *anterior* and *lateral columns* of the spinal cord. This separation of the fibers at the dorsal roots represents a separation of the pathways for transmission of sensory impulses: the dorsal column pathway gives rise to the *dorsal column system,* and the spinothalamic tracts give rise to the *spinothalamic system.*

Comparison of the Dorsal Column System With the Spinothalamic System. The dorsal column system is composed of large, heavily myelinated nerve fibers that transmit signals to the brain at velocities of 35 to 70 meters per second. Also, there is a high degree of spatial orientation of the nerve fibers with respect to their origin on the surface of the body. On the other hand, the spinothalamic system is composed mainly of small fibers, some of which are not myelinated at all, or are poorly myelinated, and which transmit impulses at velocities perhaps as low as one meter per second but not over 15 meters per second. Some of these fibers are spatially oriented but only poorly so.

These differences in the two systems immediately characterize the types of sensory information that can be transmitted by the two pathways. First, sensory information that must be transmitted rapidly and with temporal fidelity is transmitted in the dorsal column system, while that which does not need to be transmitted rapidly is transmitted mainly in the spinothalamic system. Second, those sensations that detect fine gradations of intensity are transmitted in the dorsal column system, while those that lack the fine gradations are transmitted in the spinothalamic system. And, third, sensations that are discretely localized to exact points in the body are transmitted in the dorsal column system, while those transmitted in the spinothalamic system can be localized much less exactly. On the other hand, the spinothalamic system has a special capability that the dorsal column system does not have: the ability to transmit a broad spectrum of sensory modalities—pain, warmth, cold, and crude tactile sensations; the dorsal column system is limited to mechanoreceptive sensations alone. With this differentiation in mind we can now list the types of sensations transmitted in the two systems.

The Dorsal Column System

1. Touch sensations requiring a high degree of localization of the stimulus.
2. Touch sensations requiring transmission of fine gradations of intensity.
3. Phasic sensations, such as vibratory sensations.
4. Sensations that signal movement against the skin.
5. Kinesthetic sensations.
6. Pressure sensations having to do with fine degrees of judgment of pressure intensity.

The Spinothalamic System

1. Pain.
2. Thermal sensations, including both warm and cold sensations.
3. Crude touch and pressure sensations capable of very little localizing ability on the surface of the body and having very little capability for intensity discrimination.
4. Tickle and itch sensations.
5. Sexual sensations.

TRANSMISSION IN THE DORSAL COLUMN SYSTEM

Because the dorsal column system is large and its fibers numerous, we know much about transmission of sensory signals in this system in comparison with very little about transmission of signals in the spinothalamic system. Therefore, the dorsal column system will be discussed at length and then the known differences between this and the spinothalamic system will be pointed out.

ANATOMY OF THE DORSAL COLUMN PATHWAY

The dorsal column system is illustrated in Figure 7–2. The nerve fibers entering the *dorsal columns* pass all the way up these columns to the medulla, where they synapse in the *dorsal column nuclei* (the *cuneate* and *gracile nuclei*). From here, *second order neurons* decussate immediately to the opposite side and then pass upward to the thalamus through bilateral pathways called the *medial lemnisci*. Each medial lemniscus terminates in a *ventrobasal complex of nuclei* located in the ventral posterolateral nucleus of the *thalamus*. In its pathway through the hindbrain, the medial lemniscus is joined by additional fibers from the *main sensory nucleus of the trigeminal*

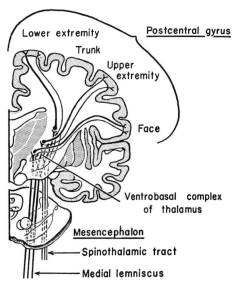

Figure 7–3. Projection of the dorsal column system from the thalamus to the somesthetic cortex. (Modified from Brodal: Neurological Anatomy in Relation to Clinical Medicine. Oxford University Press, 1969.)

nerve and from the upper portion of its descending nuclei; these fibers subserve the same sensory functions for the head that the dorsal column fibers subserve for the body.

From the ventrobasal complex, *third order neurons* project, as shown in Figure 7–3, mainly to the *postcentral gyrus* of the *cerebral cortex* called *somatic sensory area I*. But, in addition, neurons also project to closely associated regions of the cortex behind and in front of the postcentral gyrus. Finally, a few fibers project to the lowermost lateral portion of each parietal lobe, an area called *somatic sensory area II*.

Spatial Orientation of the Nerve Fibers in the Dorsal Column Pathway. All the way from the origin of the dorsal columns to the cerebral cortex, a distinct spatial orientation of the fibers from individual parts of the body is maintained. The fibers from the lower parts of the body lie toward the center of the dorsal columns, while those that enter the dorsal columns at progressively higher and higher levels form successive layers on the lateral sides of the dorsal columns.

In the thalamus, the distinct spatial orientation is still maintained, with the tail end of the body represented by the most lateral portions of the ventrobasal complex and the head and face represented in the medial component of the complex. However, because of the crossing of the medial lemnisci in the medulla, the left side of the body is represented in the right side of the

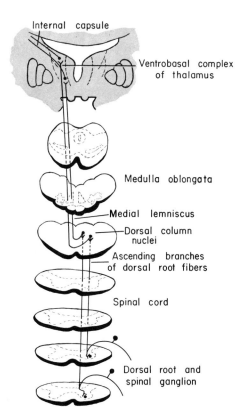

Figure 7–2. The dorsal column pathway for transmitting critical types of mechanoreceptive signals. (Modified from Ransom and Clark: Anatomy of the Nervous System, 1959.)

thalamus and the right side of the body is represented in the left side of the thalamus. In a similar manner, the fibers passing to the cerebral cortex also are spatially oriented so that a single part of the cortex receives signals from a discrete area of the body, as is described below.

THE SOMESTHETIC CORTEX

The area of the cerebral cortex to which the primary sensory impulses are projected is called the *somesthetic cortex*. In the human being, this area lies mainly in the anterior portions of the parietal lobes. Two distinct and separate areas are known to receive direct afferent nerve fibers from the relay nuclei of the thalamus; these, called *somatic sensory area I* and *somatic sensory area II*, are illustrated in Figure 7–4. However, somatic sensory area I is so much more important to the sensory functions of the body than is somatic sensory area II that in popular usage the term somesthetic cortex is almost always used to designate area I exclusive of area II. Yet, to keep these two areas separated, we will henceforth refer to them separately as somatic sensory area I and somatic sensory area II.

Projection of the Body in Somatic Sensory Area I. Somatic sensory area I lies in the postcentral gyrus of the human cerebral cortex. A distinct spatial orientation exists in this area for reception of nerve signals from the different areas of the body. Figure 7–5 illustrates a cross-section through the brain at the level of the postcentral gyrus, showing the representations of the different parts of the body in separate regions of somatic sensory area I. Note, however, that each side of the cortex receives sensory information exclusively from the oppo-

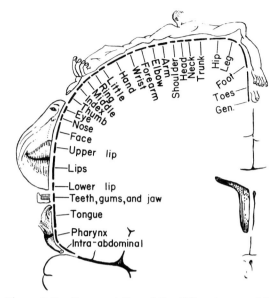

Figure 7–5. Representation of the different areas of the body in the somatic sensory area I of the cortex. (From Penfield and Rasmussen: Cerebral Cortex of Man: A Clinical Study of Localization of Function. The Macmillan Co., 1968.)

site side of the body (with the possible exception of a small amount of sensory information from the same side of the face).

Some areas of the body are represented by large areas in the somatic cortex—the lips by far the greatest area of all, followed by the face and thumb—while the entire trunk and lower part of the body are represented by relatively small areas. The sizes of these areas are directly proportional to the number of specialized sensory receptors in each respective peripheral area of the body. For instance, a great number of specialized nerve endings are found in the lips and thumb, while only a few are present in the skin of the trunk.

Note also that the head is represented in the lower or lateral portion of the postcentral gyrus, while the lower part of the body is represented in the medial or upper portion of the postcentral gyrus.

Modality Differentiation in Somatic Sensory Area I. Not only is there spatial projection of the body in somatic sensory area I, but there is also a moderate degree of modality separation between tactile signals and kinesthetic signals. Tactile signals stimulate neurons mainly in the anteriormost portion of the postcentral gyrus where it dips into the central sulcus. On the other hand, kinesthetic signals stimulate neurons mainly in the posteriormost portion of

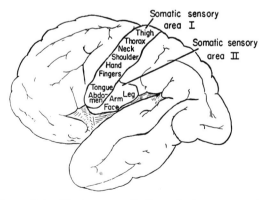

Figure 7–4. The two somesthetic cortical areas, somatic sensory areas I and II.

the postcentral gyrus. This separation of modalities is important because it helps us to understand how the brain dissects different types of information from incoming sensory signals, a subject that will be discussed in more detail later in the chapter.

Somatic Sensory Area II. The second cortical area to which somatic afferent fibers project, somatic sensory area II, lies posterior and inferior to the lower end of the postcentral gyrus and on the upper wall of the lateral fissure, as shown in Figure 7–4. The degree of localization of the different parts of the body is far less acute in this area than in somatic sensory area I. The face is represented anteriorly, the arms centrally, and the legs posteriorly.

So little is known about the function of somatic sensory area II that it cannot be discussed intelligently. It is known that signals enter this area from both the dorsal column system and the spinothalamic system, though much more from the latter. In fact, it has been suggested that somatic sensory area II might be the cortical terminus of pain information. Also, stimulation of somatic sensory area II in some instances causes complex body movements, for which reason it possibly plays a role in sensory control of motor functions.

Excitation of Vertical Columns of Neurons in the Somesthetic Cortex. The cerebral cortex contains *six* separate layers of neurons, and, as would be expected, the neurons in each layer perform functions different from those in other layers. Also, the neurons are arranged in vertical columns extending all the way through the six layers of the cortex, each column having a diameter of about one-half to one millimeter and containing hundreds of neuronal cell bodies in each layer. Unfortunately, we still know relatively little about the functions of these columns of cells but we are certain about the following facts:

1. The incoming sensory signal excites mainly neuronal layer IV first; then the signal spreads toward the surface of the cortex and also toward the deeper layers.

2. Layers I and II receive a diffuse, nonspecific input from the reticular activating system. This input perhaps controls the overall level of excitability of the cortex.

3. The neurons in layers V and VI send axons to other parts of the nervous system— some to other areas of the cortex, some to deeper structures of the brain, such as the thalamus or brain stem, and some even to the spinal cord.

Similar vertical columns of neurons exist in all other areas of the cortex as well as in the somesthetic cortex. In particular, they have been shown to be very important for function of the visual cortex and the motor cortex.

Each vertical column of neurons seems to be able to decipher a specific quality of information from the sensory signal. For instance, in the visual cortex one specific column will detect a line oriented in a particular direction, whereas an adjacent column will detect a similar line oriented in a slightly different direction. Presumably, in the somesthetic cortex each column detects separate qualities of signals (angles of orientation of rough spots, lengths of rough spots, perhaps roundness of objects, perhaps sharpness of objects, and so forth) from specific surface areas of the body.

Functions of Somatic Sensory Area I. The functional capabilities of different areas of the somesthetic cortex have been determined by selective excision of the different portions. Widespread excision of somatic sensory area I causes loss of the following types of sensory judgment:

1. The person is unable to localize discretely the different sensations in the different parts of the body. However, he can localize these sensations very crudely, such as to a particular hand, which indicates that the thalamus or parts of the cerebral cortex not normally considered to be concerned with somatic sensations can perform some degree of localization.

2. He is unable to judge critical degrees of pressure against his body.

3. He is unable to judge exactly the weights of objects.

4. He is unable to judge shapes or forms of objects. This is called *astereognosis.*

5. He is unable to judge texture of materials, for this type of judgment depends on highly critical sensations caused by movement of the skin over the surface to be judged.

6. He is unable to judge fine gradations in temperature.

7. He is unable to recognize the relative orientation of the different parts of his body with respect to each other.

Note in the above list that nothing has been said about loss of pain. However, in the absence of somatic sensory area I, the appreciation of pain is often altered, sometimes even the intensification of the pain. But more important, the pain that does occur is poorly localized, indicating that pain localization is probably dependent mainly upon simultaneous stimulation of tactile stimuli that use the topographical map of the body in somatic sensory area I to localize the source of the pain.

SOMATIC ASSOCIATION AREAS

Brodmann areas V and VII of the cerebral cortex, which are located in the parietal cortex immediately behind somatic sensory area I and above somatic sensory area II, play especially important roles in deciphering the sensory information that enters the somatic sensory areas. Therefore, these areas are called the *somatic association areas*.

Electrical stimulation in the somatic association area can occasionally cause a person to experience a complex somatic sensation, sometimes even the "feeling" of an object such as a knife or a ball. Therefore, it seems clear that the somatic association area combines information from multiple points in the somatic sensory area to decipher its meaning. This also fits with the anatomical arrangement of the neuronal tracts that enter the somatic association area, for it receives signals from (a) the primary somatic areas, (b) the ventrobasal complex of the thalamus, and (c) adjacent areas of the thalamus which themselves receive input from the ventrobasal complex.

Effect of Removing the Somatic Association Area—Amorphosynthesis. When the somatic association area is removed, the person especially loses his ability to recognize complex objects and complex forms that he feels. In addition, he loses a great deal of the sense of form of his own body. An especially interesting fact is that loss of the somatic association area on one side of the brain causes the person sometimes to be oblivious of the opposite side of his body— that is, to forget that it is there. Likewise, when he is feeling objects he will tend to feel only one side of the object and to forget that the other side even exists. This complex sensory deficit is called *amorphosynthesis*.

CHARACTERISTICS OF TRANSMISSION IN THE DORSAL COLUMN PATHWAY

Faithfulness of Transmission. The most important functional characteristic of the dorsal column pathway is its *faithfulness* of transmission. That is, each time a point in the periphery is stimulated, a signal ordinarily is transmitted all the way to the somesthetic cortex. Also, if this peripheral stimulus increases in intensity, the intensity of the signal at the cerebral cortex

increases proportionately. And, finally, when a discrete area of the body is stimulated, the signal from this area is transmitted to a discrete area of the cerebral cortex. Thus, the dorsal column pathway is adequately organized for transmission of accurate information from the periphery to the sensorium. Furthermore, the responsiveness of this system can be altered only moderately by stimuli from other areas of the nervous system, and it cannot be depressed to a significant extent by extraneous agents, such as moderate degrees of anesthesia.

Basic Neuronal Circuit and Discharge Pattern in the Dorsal Column System. The lower part of Figure 7–6 illustrates the basic organization of the neuronal circuit of the dorsal column system, showing that at each synaptic stage divergence occurs; indeed, there is as much as a 10-fold divergence at the dorsal column nuclei alone. However, the upper part of Figure 7–6 shows that a single receptor stimulus on the skin does not cause all the cortical neurons with which that receptor connects

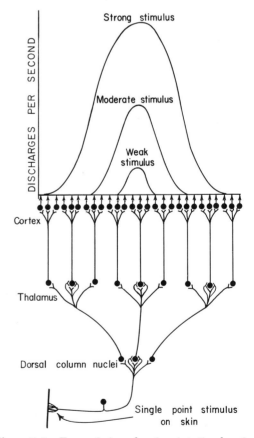

Figure 7–6. Transmission of a pinpoint stimulus signal to the cortex.

to discharge at the same rate. Instead, the cortical neurons that discharge to the greatest extent are those in a central part of the cortical "field" for each respective receptor. Thus, a weak stimulus causes only the centralmost neurons to fire. A moderate stimulus causes still more neurons to fire, but those in the center still discharge at a considerably more rapid rate than do those farther away from the center. Finally, a strong stimulus causes widespread discharge in the cortex but again a much more rapid discharge of the centralmost neurons in comparison with the peripheral neurons.

Localization of Signals From the Body. Referring once again to Figure 7–6, it is evident that, when a single receptor is stimulated in the skin, a particular point in the somesthetic cortex is excited more intensively than are all the surrounding areas. This does not mean that adjacent areas of the somesthetic cortex are not also stimulated. However, these adjacent areas are stimulated *less* intensively than a central point in the cortical field of the stimulated receptor. Thus, by this means, the sensory cortex is capable of detecting the precise localization of signals from the body, despite the spread of excitation in the cortex.

Two-Point Discrimination. A method frequently used to test a person's tactile capabilities is to determine his so-called "two-point discriminatory ability." In this test, two needles are pressed against the skin, and the subject determines whether he feels two points of stimulus or one point. On the tips of the fingers a person can distinguish two separate points even when the needles are as close together as 2 mm. However, on the back, the needles must usually be as far apart as 20 to 50 mm. before one can detect two separate points. The reason for this is that there are many specialized tactile receptors in the tips of the fingers in comparison with a small number in the skin of the back. Referring back to Figure 7–5, we can see also that the portions of the body that have a high degree of two-point discrimination have a correspondingly large cortical representation in somatic sensory area I.

Figure 7–7 illustrates the probable mechanism by which the dorsal column pathway transmits two-point discriminatory information. This shows two adjacent points on the skin that are strongly stimulated, and it shows the small area of the somesthetic cortex (greated enlarged) that is excited by signals from the two stimulated points in the skin. The two dashed curves show the individually ex-

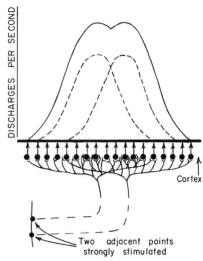

Figure 7–7. Transmission of signals to the cortex from two adjacent pinpoint stimuli.

cited cortical fields, and the solid curve shows the resultant cortical excitation when both the skin points are stimulated simultaneously. Note that the resultant zone of excitation has two separate peaks. It is believed to be these two peaks, separated by a valley, that allow the sensory cortex to detect the presence of two stimulatory points rather than a single stimulatory point.

Increase in Contrast in the Spatial Pattern Caused by Lateral Inhibition. In Chapter 5 it was pointed out that contrast in sensory patterns is increased by inhibitory signals transmitted laterally in the sensory pathway. This effect was illustrated in Figure 5–11 of that chapter.

In the case of the dorsal column system, an excited sensory receptor in the skin transmits not only excitatory signals to the somesthetic cortex but also inhibitory signals laterally to adjacent fiber pathways. These inhibitory signals help to block lateral spread of the excitatory signal, a process called *lateral inhibition* or *afferent inhibition*. As a result, the peak of excitation stands out, and much of the surrounding diffuse stimulation is blocked. Obviously, this mechanism accentuates the contrast between the areas of peak stimulation and the surrounding areas, thus greatly increasing the contrast or sharpness of the perceived spatial pattern.

Transmission of Rapidly Changing and Repetitive Sensations. The dorsal column system is of particular value for apprising the sensorium of rapidly changing peripheral conditions. This system can "follow" changing stimuli up to at least 100 cycles per second and can "detect" changes as high as 400 to 500 cycles. This rapid response allows one to direct his attention immediately to any point of contact, which, in turn, allows him to make necessary corrections before damage can be done.

Vibratory Sensation. Because vibratory signals are rapidly repetitive (can be detected up to 400 to 500 cycles per second), they can be transmitted only in the dorsal column system and not at all in the slowly transmitting spinothalamic system. For this reason, application of vibration with a tuning fork to different peripheral parts of the body is an important tool used by the neurologist for testing functional integrity of the dorsal column system.

PROCESSING OF INFORMATION IN THE DORSAL COLUMN SYSTEM

Despite the faithfulness of transmission of signals from the periphery to the sensory cortex through the dorsal column system, there is also some processing of sensory information at lower synaptic levels before it reaches the cerebral cortex. For instance, the signal pattern from kinesthetic receptors changes as it passes progressively up the dorsal column system. Figure 7–1 showed that individual joint receptors are stimulated maximally at specific degrees of rotation of the joint, with the intensity of stimulation decreasing on either side of the maximal point for each receptor. However, the kinesthetic signal is quite different at the level of the ventrobasal complex of the thalamus, as can be seen by referring to Figure 7–8. This

figure shows that the ventrobasal neurons are of two types: (1) those that are maximally stimulated when the joint is at full rotation and (2) those that are maximally stimulated when the joint is at minimal rotation. In each case, as the degree of rotation changes, the rate of stimulation of the neuron either decreases or increases depending on the direction in which the joint is being rotated. Furthermore, the intensity of neuronal excitation changes over angles of 40 to 60 degrees of angulation in contrast to 20 to 30 degrees for the individual receptors, as was illustrated in Figure 7–1. Thus, the signals from the individual joint receptors are integrated in the space domain by the thalamic neurons, giving a progressively stronger signal as the joint moves in only one direction rather than giving a peaked signal as occurs in stimulation of individual receptors.

Another instance of information processing in the dorsal column system is physical separation of signals of different modalities, with cutaneous sensibilities terminating anteriorly in somatic area I and kinesthetic sensibilities terminating posteriorly. It is presumably these types of changes in signal patterns and separation of modalities that allow the sensorium to separate out all the ingredients of sensory information.

TRANSMISSION IN THE SPINOTHALAMIC SYSTEM

It was pointed out earlier in the chapter that the spinothalamic system transmits sensory signals that do not require rapid transmission nor highly discrete localization in the body. These include pain, heat, cold, crude tactile sensations, and sexual sensations. In the following chapter, pain and temperature sensations are discussed specifically, but the present chapter is concerned principally with transmission of the crude tactile sensations in the spinothalamic system.

THE SPINOTHALAMIC PATHWAY

Most anatomists divide the spinothalamic pathway into three different tracts: (1) the ventral spinothalamic tract, (2) the lateral spinothalamic tract, and (3) the spinoreticular tract. In the following discussion we will follow this convention, though these tracts overlap each other greatly, and they course diffusely through the anterolateral quadrants of the white columns of the cord. For this reason, many physiologists simply speak of the anterolateral spinothalamic pathway.

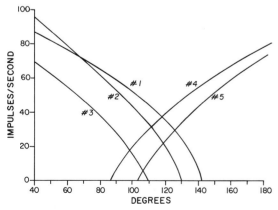

Figure 7–8. Typical responses of five different neurons in the knee joint receptor field of the ventrobasal complex when the knee joint is moved through its range of motion. (The curves were constructed from data in Mountcastle: *J. Neurophysiol., 26*:807, 1963.)

Ventral Spinothalamic Tract. Most of the spinothalamic fibers subserving the tactile sense (about 2500 of them) enter the dorsal columns along with the fibers of the dorsal column system, as shown in Figure 7–9, and then travel upward as much as six segments or downward as much as two segments before ending on second order neurons in the dorsal horns. Then fibers from these neurons cross through the anterior commissure to the opposite anterior column and form the *ventral spinothalamic tract* that passes all the way to the thalamus.

The ventral spinothalamic tract terminates, along with the terminations of the dorsal column system, in the ventrobasal nuclear complex of the thalamus, though many of the fibers also give off collaterals that terminate in the bulbar and mesencephalic reticular areas.

The fibers of the ventral spinothalamic tract are mainly larger size delta type A nerve fibers in contrast to smaller fibers found in the lateral spinothalamic tract. Furthermore, there is crude localization of touch and pressure sensations transmitted through this tract, indicating a moderate degree of *spatial orientation* of the fibers in the tract.

Lateral Spinothalamic Tract. On entering the cord through the posterior roots, the *pain* and *temperature* fibers travel upward in the *tract of Lissauer*

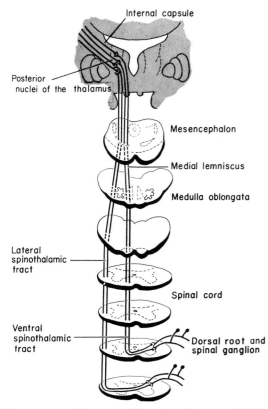

Figure 7–9. The spinothalamic pathways. (Modified from Ranson and Clark: Anatomy of the Nervous System, 1959.)

for one or two segments and then terminate in the gray matter of the dorsal horns. At this point, the signals probably pass through one or more local neurons, the last of which sends long fibers that cross through the anterior commissure of the cord gray matter, pass to the opposite lateral column of the spinal cord where they form the *lateral spinothalamic tract,* and eventually terminate mainly in the intralaminar nuclei of the thalamus, a different terminus from that of the ventral spinothalamic tract.

However, a few of the fibers (especially the delta pain fibers that will be discussed in the following chapter) terminate in the most caudal portion of the ventrobasal complex, an area that is the human analogue of the posterior nuclei of the thalamus of lower animals. Many of the fibers also give rise to collaterals that terminate in the reticular substance of the bulbar and mesencephalic areas.

The fibers of the lateral spinothalamic tract are mainly delta type A or type C fibers.

Spinoreticular Tract. In addition to the fibers of the ventral and lateral spinothalamic tracts, still other fibers originate in the dorsal horns of the spinal cord along with the fibers of these two tracts but never extend as far as the thalamus. Instead, these fibers terminate in the reticular substance of the bulbar and mesencephalic areas and therefore constitute the spinoreticular tract. Here they synapse with one or more successive neurons that eventually send fibers into the intralaminar nuclei of the thalamus, terminating in the same areas as many of the fibers from the lateral spinothalamic tract; from here signals are transmitted to other parts of the thalamus, the hypothalamus, and the cortex. The fibers of this tract are probably all of the type C variety, and they are concerned either entirely or almost entirely with the transmission of pain signals.

Fibers also enter the lateral and the ventral spinothalamic tracts and the spinoreticular tract from the spinal nucleus of the fifth nerve. These fibers transmit respective types of sensory information from the head.

Projection of Spinothalamic Signals from the Thalamus to the Cortex. Third order neurons from the ventrobasal complex of the thalamus, which carry tactile signals from the ventral spinothalamic tract, project primarily to somatic area I and, to a lesser extent, to somatic area II. However, on the basis of inadequate information, it has been suggested that the lateral spinothalamic system, which transmits pain and temperature signals, and which synapses in the intralaminar thalamic nuclei, probably projects to somatic area II, though even these projections are weak ones.

Separation of Modalities in the Spinothalamic Tracts. It has already been pointed out in the above description of the spinothalamic pathway that the nerve fibers that subserve the senses of touch and pressure are transmitted in the ventral spinothalamic tract, and those that subserve pain and temperature are transmitted in the lateral spinothalamic tract. In addition, the lateral spinothalamic tract is at least partially divided into *superficial* and *deep divisions,* the superficial division transmitting pain signals and the deep division transmitting temperature signals. Thus, the process of separating the different modalities of sensation actually begins in the spinal cord.

Characteristics of Transmission in the Spinothalamic Tracts.   The precise nature of transmission in the spinothalamic tracts is not nearly so well known as in the dorsal column system. In general, the same principles apply to transmission in this tract as in the dorsal column system, except for the following differences: (a) the velocities of transmission in the spinothalamic tracts are only one-fiftieth to one-quarter those in the dorsal column system; (b) the spatial localization of signals transmitted in the spinothalamic tracts is poor, especially in the lateral spinothalamic tract that transmits pain and temperature signals; (c) the gradations of intensities are also far less acute, most of the sensations being recognized in 10 to 20 gradations of strength rather than the 100 or more gradations for the dorsal column system; and (d) the ability to transmit rapidly repetitive sensations is almost nil in the spinothalamic system.

Thus, it is evident that the spinothalamic tracts are by far a cruder type of transmission system than is the dorsal column system. However, it must be realized that certain types of sensations are, nevertheless, transmitted only by the spinothalamic tracts, including pain, thermal sensations, and sexual sensations. Only the mechanoreceptive sensations are transmitted by both systems, the dorsal column system having to do with the critical types of mechanoreceptive sensations, and the ventral spinothalamic tract having to do with the cruder types of mechanoreceptive sensations.

SOME SPECIAL ASPECTS OF SENSORY FUNCTION

Function of the Thalamus in Somatic Sensations.   The major function of the thalamus in tactile sensation is probably to relay information to the cortex. However, since a person with his somesthetic cortex removed can redevelop a mild degree of tactile sensibility, it must be assumed that the thalamus can do much more than simply relay tactile information to the somesthetic cortex. The thalamus seems to be even more important in pain sensation, as pointed out in the following chapter.

Cortical Control of Sensory Sensitivity.   Almost all sensory information that enters the cerebrum, except that from the olfactory system, but including sensory information from the eyes, the ears, the taste receptors, and all the somatic receptors, is relayed through one or another of the thalamic nuclei. Furthermore, the conscious brain is capable of directing its attention to different segments of the sensory system. This function is believed to be mainly achieved through facilitation or inhibition of the cortical receptive areas.

But, in addition, ''corticofugal'' signals are transmitted from the cortex to the lower relay stations in the sensory pathways to *inhibit* transmission. For instance, corticofugal pathways control the sensitivity of the synapses in the thalamus as well as in the dorsal column nuclei and in the posterior horn relay station of the spinothalamic system. Also, similar systems are known for the visual, auditory, and olfactory systems, which are discussed in later chapters. Each corticofugal pathway begins in the cortex where the sensory pathway that it controls terminates. Thus, a feedback loop exists for each sensory pathway.

Obviously, corticofugal control of sensory input could allow the cerebral cortex to alter the threshold

Figure 7–10.   The dermatomes. (Modified from Grinker and Sahs: Neurology. Charles C Thomas, 1966.)

for different sensory signals. Also, it might help the brain focus its attention on specific types of information, which is an important and necessary quality of nervous system function.

Segmental Fields of Sensation—The Dermatomes. Each spinal nerve innervates a "segmental field" of the skin called a *dermatome*. The different dermatomes are illustrated in Figure 7–10. However, these are shown as if there were distinct borders between the adjacent dermatomes, which is far from true because much overlap exists from segment to segment. Indeed, because of the great overlap, the posterior roots from an entire segment of the spinal cord can be destroyed without causing significant loss of sensation in the skin.

Figure 7–10 shows that the anal region of the body lies in the dermatome of the most distal cord segment. In the embryo, this is the tail region and is the most distal portion of the body. The legs develop from the lumbar and upper sacral segments rather than from the distal sacral segments, which is evident from the dermatomal map. Obviously, one can use a dermatomal map such as that illustrated in Figure 7–10 to determine the level in the spinal cord at which various cord injuries may have occurred when the peripheral sensations are disturbed.

REFERENCES

Adrian, E. D.: The Physical Background of Perception. Oxford, Clarendon Press, 1947.

Albe-Fessard, D., and Iggo, A. (eds.): Somatosensory System. Berlin, New York, Springer-Verlag, 1973.

Asanuma, H.: Recent developments in the study of the columnar arrangement of neurons within the motor cortex. *Physiol. Rev.*, 55:143, 1975.

Bishop, P. O.: Central nervous system: afferent mechanisms and perception. *Ann. Rev. Physiol.*, 29:427, 1967.

Boudreau, J. C., and Tsuchitani, C.: Sensory Neurophysiology: with Special Reference to the Cat. New York, Van Nostrand Reinhold Company, 1973.

Darian-Smith, I.: Somatic sensation. *Ann. Rev. Physiol.*, 31:417, 1969.

Emmers, R., and Tasker, R. R.: The Human Somesthetic Thalamus. New York, Raven Press, 1975.

Frigyesi, T. L., Rinvik, E., and Yahr, M. D. (eds.): Corticothalamic Projections and Sensorimotor Activities. New York, Raven Press, 1972.

Lapresle, J., and Haguenau, M.: Anatomico-chemical correlation in focal thalamic lesions. *Z. Neurol.*, 205:29, 1973.

Lloyd, D. P.: Action in primary afferent fibers in the spinal cord. *Inter. J. Neurosci.*, 1:1, 1970.

Lynn, B.: Somatosensory receptors and their CNS connections. *Ann. Rev. Physiol.*, 37:105, 1975.

Mountcastle, V. B., Poggio, G. F., and Werner, G.: The relation of thalamic cell response to peripheral stimuli varied over an intensive continuum. *J. Neurophysiol.*, 26:807, 1963.

Omer, G. E., Jr.: Sensation and sensibility in the upper extremity. *Clin. Orthop.*, 104:30, 1974.

Perl, E. R., and Boivie, J. G.: Neural substrates of somatic sensation. In Guyton, A. C. (ed.): MTP International Review of Science: Physiology. Vol. 3. Baltimore, University Park Press, 1974, p. 303.

Persson, H. E.: Development of Somatosensory Cortical Functions; an Electrophysiological Study in Prenatal Sheep. Stockholm, Department of Physiology, Karolinska Institute, 1973.

Rodieck, R. W.: Central nervous system: afferent mechanisms. *Ann. Rev. Physiol.*, 33:203, 1971.

Sinclair, D. C.: Cutaneous Sensation. New York, Oxford University Press, 1967.

Wall, P. D., and Dubner, R.: Somatosensory pathways. *Ann. Rev. Physiol.*, 34:315, 1972.

Werner, G., and Mountcastle, V. B.: Neural activity in mechanoreceptive cutaneous afferents: stimulus-response relations, Weber functions, and information transmission. *J. Neurophysiol*, 28:359, 1965.

Whitsel, B. L., Petrucelli, L. M., and Werner, G.: Symmetry and connectivity in the map of the body surface in somatosensory area II of primates. *J. Neurophysiol.*, 32:170, 1969.

See also bibliographies at the ends of Chapters 6 and 8.

8

Somatic Sensations:
II. Pain, Visceral Pain, Headache,
and Thermal Sensations

Many, if not most, ailments of the body cause pain. Furthermore, one's ability to diagnose different diseases depends to a great extent on a knowledge of the different qualities of pain, a knowledge of how pain can be referred from one part of the body to another, how pain can spread from the painful site, and, finally, what the different causes of pain are. For these reasons, the present chapter is devoted mainly to pain and to the physiologic basis of some of the associated clinical phenomena.

The Purpose of Pain. Pain is a protective mechanism for the body; it occurs whenever any tissues are being damaged, and it causes the individual to react to remove the pain stimulus. Even such simple activities as sitting for a long time on the ischia can cause tissue destruction because of lack of blood flow to the skin where the skin is compressed by the weight of the body. When the skin becomes painful as a result of the ischemia, the person shifts his weight unconsciously. A person who has lost his pain sense, such as after spinal cord injury, fails to feel the pain and therefore fails to shift his weight. This eventually results in ulceration at the areas of pressure unless special measures are taken to move the person from time to time.

QUALITIES OF PAIN

Pain has been classified into three different major types: pricking, burning, and aching pain. Other terms used to describe different types of pain include throbbing pain, nauseous pain, cramping pain, sharp pain, electric pain, and others, most of which are well known to almost everyone.

Pricking pain is felt when a needle is stuck into the skin or when the skin is cut with a knife. It is also often felt when a widespread area of the skin is diffusely but strongly irritated.

Burning pain is, as its name implies, the type of pain felt when the skin is burned. It can be excruciating and is the most likely of the pain types to cause suffering.

Aching pain is not felt on the surface of the body, but, instead, is a deep pain with varying degrees of annoyance. Aching pain of low intensity in widespread areas of the body can summate into a very disagreeable sensation.

It is not necessary to describe these different qualities of pain in great detail because they are well known to all persons. The real problem, and one that is only partially solved, is what causes the differences in quality. Pricking pain results from stimulation of delta type A pain fibers, whereas burning and aching pain results from stimulation of the more primitive type C fibers, which will be discussed later in the chapter.

METHODS FOR MEASURING THE PERCEPTION OF PAIN

The intensity of a stimulus necessary to cause pain can be measured in many different ways, but the most used methods have been pricking the skin with a pin at measured pressures, pressing a solid object against a protruding bone with measured force, or heating the skin with measured amounts of heat. The latter methods has proved to be especially accurate from a quantitative point of view.

Figure 8–1 illustrates the basic principles of a heat apparatus used for measuring pain threshold. An intense light is focused by a large condenser lens onto a black spot painted on the forehead of the subject, and the heat intensity delivered by the light is controlled by a rheostat. In determining the subject's threshold for pain, the intensity of the heat is increased in progressive steps, and the length of time required for the forehead to heat sufficiently to elicit pain is recorded for each heat intensity. These data are then plotted in the form of a "strength-duration curve" to express pain threshold, as follows.

Strength-Duration Curve for Expressing Pain Threshold. Figure 8–2 illustrates a typical strength-duration curve obtained by using the above procedure for measuring pain threshold. This curve is almost identical with the strength-duration curves discussed in Chapter 1 for stimulation of nerve fibers by electrical currents of increasing intensities. Note that a very intense stimulus applied for only a second elicits a sensation of pain while a stimulus of much less intensity may require many seconds. The lowest intensity of stimulus that will excite the sensation of pain when the stimulus is applied for a prolonged period of time is called the *pain threshold*.

The Intensity of Pain—"JND's." The increase in stimulus intensity that will barely cause a detectable difference in degree of pain is called a *just noticeable difference* (JND). By applying all different stimulus intensities between the level of no pain at all and the most intense pain that a person can distinguish, it has been found that approximately 22 JND's can be discerned by the average person.

Figure 8–3 illustrates the relationship of stimulus intensity (applied by the apparatus of Fig. 8–1) to the intensity of pain expressed in JND's.

Uniformity of Pain Threshold in Different People. Figure 8–4 shows graphically the

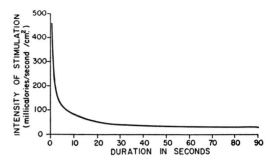

Figure 8–2. Strength-duration curve for depicting pain threshold. (From Hardy: *J. Chronic Dis.*, 4:20, 1956.)

skin temperature at which pain is first perceived by different persons. By far the greatest number of subjects perceive pain when the skin temperature reaches almost exactly 45° C., and almost everyone perceives pain before the temperature reaches 47° C. In other words, it is almost never true that some persons are unusually sensitive or insensitive to pain. Indeed, measurements in people as widely different as Eskimos, Indians, and whites have shown no significant differences in their *thresholds for pain*. However, different people do *react* very differently to pain, as is discussed below.

THE PAIN RECEPTORS AND THEIR STIMULATION

Free Nerve Endings as Pain Receptors. The pain receptors in the skin and other tissues are all free nerve endings. They are widespread in the superficial layers of the *skin* and also in certain internal tissues, such as the *periosteum*, the *arterial walls*, the *joint surfaces*, and the *falx* and *tentorium* of the cranial vault. Most of the other deep tissues are not extensively supplied with pain endings but are weakly supplied; nevertheless, any widespread tissue

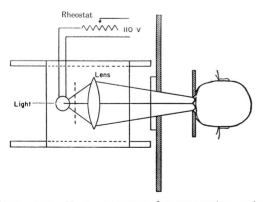

Figure 8–1. Heat apparatus for measuring pain threshold. (From Hardy, Wolff, and Goodell: *J. Clin. Invest*, 19:649, 1940.)

Figure 8–3. Pain intensity, expressed in JND's, at different intensities of stimulus. (From Hardy: *J. Chronic Dis.*, 4:22, 1956.)

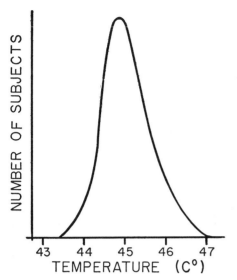

Figure 8–4. Distribution curve obtained from a large number of subjects of the minimal skin temperature that causes pain. (Modified from Hardy: *J. Chronic Dis.*, 4:22, 1956.)

damage can still summate to cause the aching type of pain in these areas.

Nonadapting Nature of Pain Receptors. In contrast to most other sensory receptors of the body the pain receptors adapt either not at all or almost not at all. In fact, under some conditions, the threshold for excitation of the pain fibers becomes progressively lower and lower as the pain stimulus continues, thus allowing these receptors to become progressively more activated with time. This increase in sensitivity of the pain receptors is called *hyperalgesia*.

One can readily understand the importance of this failure of pain receptors to adapt, for it allows them to keep the person apprised of a damaging stimulus that causes the pain as long as it persists.

RATE OF TISSUE DAMAGE AS THE CAUSE OF PAIN

The average critical temperature of 45° C. at which a person first begins to perceive pain is also the temperature at which the tissues begin to be damaged by heat; indeed, the tissues are eventually completely destroyed if the temperature remains at this level indefinitely. Therefore, it is immediately apparent that pain resulting from heat is closely correlated with the ability of heat to damage the tissues.

Furthermore, in studying soldiers who had been severely wounded in World War II, it was found that the majority of them felt little or no pain except for a short time after the severe wound had been sustained. This, too, indicates that *pain generally is not felt after damage has been done* but only *while damage is being done*.

Bradykinin and Similar Polypeptides as Possible Stimulators of Pain Endings. The precise mechanism by which tissue damage stimulates pain endings is not known. However, many research workers have shown that extracts from damaged tissues cause intense pain when injected beneath the normal skin. Therefore, it is almost certain that some chemical substance or substances released from damaged tissues excite the pain nerve endings.

There are many reasons to believe that the substance *bradykinin* or some similar polypeptide might be the principal substance that stimulates pain endings. For instance, when this substance is injected in extremely minute quantities underneath the skin, severe pain is felt. Furthermore, cell damage releases proteolytic enzymes that almost immediately split bradykinin and other similar substances from the globulins in the interstitial fluid. And, finally, bradykinin and similar substances can be found in the skin when painful stimuli are applied.

Thus, the postulated mechanism for eliciting pain: damage to cells releases proteolytic enzymes that then split bradykinin and associated substances from globulin, and these in turn stimulate the nerve endings.

Tissue Ischemia and Muscle Spasm as Causes of Pain. When blood flow to a tissue is blocked, the tissue becomes very painful within a few minutes. And the greater the rate of metabolism of the tissue, the more rapidly the pain appears. For instance, if a blood pressure cuff is placed around the upper arm and inflated until the arterial blood flow ceases, exercise of the forearm muscles can cause severe muscle pain within 15 to 20 seconds. In the absence of muscle exercise, the pain will not appear for three to four minutes. Cessation of blood flow to the skin, in which the metabolic rate is very low, usually does not cause pain for about 20 to 30 minutes.

Muscle spasm is also a frequent cause of pain. The reason for this is probably two-fold. First, the contracting muscle compresses the intramuscular blood vessels and either reduces or cuts off the blood flow. Second, muscle contraction increases the rate of metabolism of the muscle. Therefore, muscle spasm probably causes relative muscle ischemia so that typical ischemic pain results.

The cause of pain in ischemia is yet unknown; however, it is relieved by supplying oxygen to the ischemic tissue. Flow of unoxygenated blood to the tissue will not relieve the pain.

One of the suggested causes of pain in ischemia is accumulation of large amounts of lactic acid in the tissues, formed as a consequence of the anaerobic metabolism (metabolism without oxygen) that occurs during ischemia. However, it is also possible that other chemical agents, such as bradykinin and the polypeptides, are formed in the tissues because of muscle cell damage and that these, rather than lactic acid, stimulate the pain nerve endings.

TICKLING AND ITCH

The phenomenon of tickling and itch has often been stated to be caused by very mild stimulation of pain nerve endings, since whenever pain is blocked by anesthesia of a nerve or by compressing the nerve, the phenomenon of tickling and itch also disappears. However, recent neurophysiologic studies have demonstrated the existence of very sensitive free nerve endings that elicit only the itch sensation. Furthermore, these endings are found almost exclusively in the superficial layers of the skin, which is also the only tissue from which the itch sensation can usually be elicited. Furthermore, exciting itch receptors in animals initiates scratch reflexes, which contrasts with the effect of exciting pain nerve endings that always causes withdrawal reflexes instead.

Therefore, it seems clear that the itch and tickle sensations are transmitted by very small type C fibers similar to those that transmit the burning type of pain; these fibers, however, are distinctly separate from the pain fibers. Furthermore, the endings of these fibers are readily excited by light mechanoreceptive stimuli, indicating that they are mechanoreceptors in contradistinction to the probable chemoreceptor nature of pain fibers.

The purpose of the itch sensation is presumably to call attention to mild surface stimuli such as a flea crawling on the skin or a fly about to bite, and the elicited signals then lead to scratching or other maneuvers that rid the host of the irritant.

The relief of itch by the process of scratching occurs only when the irritant is removed or when the scratch is strong enough to elicit pain. The pain signals are believed to suppress the itch signals in the cord by a process of inhibition that will be described later in the chapter.

TRANSMISSION OF PAIN SIGNALS INTO THE CENTRAL NERVOUS SYSTEM

"Fast" Pain Fibers and "Slow" Pain Fibers. Pain signals are transmitted by small delta type A fibers at velocities of between 3 and 20 meters per second and also by type C fibers at velocities between 0.5 and 2 meters per second. When the delta type A fibers are blocked without blocking the C fibers by moderate compression of the nerve trunk, the pricking type of pain disappears. On the other hand, when the type C fibers are blocked without blocking the delta fibers by low concentrations of local anesthetic, the burning and aching types of pain disappear.

Therefore, a sudden onset of painful stimulus gives a "double" pain sensation: a fast pricking pain sensation followed a second or so later by a slow burning pain sensation. The pricking pain presumably apprises the person very rapidly of a damaging influence and, therefore, plays an important role in making the person react immediately to remove himself from the stimulus. On the other hand, the slow burning sensation tends to become more and more painful over a period of time. It is this sensation that gives one the intolerable suffering of pain.

Transmission in the Spinothalamic and Spinoreticular Tracts. Pain fibers enter the cord through the dorsal roots, ascend or descend one to two segments in the *tract of Lissauer,* and then terminate on neurons in the dorsal horns of the cord gray matter. Here the signals probably pass through one or more additional short-fibered neurons, the last of which gives rise to long fibers that cross immediately to the opposite side of the cord in the *anterior commissure* and pass upward to the brain via the spinothalamic and spinoreticular tracts. As discussed in the previous chapter, most of the pain fibers lie in the lateral portions of the spinothalamic and spinoreticular tracts; some pain fibers, however, are found in all areas of the entire anterolateral quadrant of the cord white columns.

We shall see later that the intensity of pain signals can be modified markedly as they pass through the neuronal synapses of the gray matter of the dorsal horns, especially in response to simultaneous signals transmitted by mechanoreceptor sensory nerve fibers and in response to signals entering the dorsal horns from the brain via corticofugal fibers.

As the pain pathways pass into the brain they separate into two separate pathways: *the pricking pain pathway* composed almost entirely of small type A delta fibers, and *the burning pain pathway* composed almost entirely of the slow type C fibers.

The Pricking Pain Pathway. Figure 8–5 illustrates that the pricking pain pathway terminates in the caudalmost portion of the ventrobasal complex, an area that is the human analogue of the posterior nuclear group in lower animals. From here signals are transmitted into other areas of the thalamus and to the somatic sensory cortex. Most of the fibers from this area probably go to somatic sensory area II, as was explained in the previous chapter. However, it is possible that a few pass also to somatic sensory area I.

The Burning Pain Pathway—Stimulation of the Reticular Activating System. Figure 8–5 shows that the burning and aching pain fibers terminate in the reticular area of the brain stem and in the intralaminar nuclei of the thalamus, the nonspecific nuclei located among the thalamic specific nuclei. Both the reticular area of the brain stem and the intralaminar nuclei are parts of the reticular activating system. In Chapter 54 we will discuss in detail the func-

tions of this system; briefly, however, it transmits activating signals into essentially all parts of the brain, especially upward through the thalamus to all areas of the cerebral cortex and also into the basal regions of the brain around the thalamus including very importantly the hypothalamus.

Thus, the burning and aching pain fibers, because they do excite the reticular activating system, have a very potent effect on activating essentially the entire nervous system, that is, to arouse one from sleep, to create a state of excitement, to create a sense of urgency, and to promote defense and aversion reactions designed to rid the person or animal of the painful stimulus.

The signals that are transmitted through the burning pain pathway can be localized only to very gross areas of the body, if they can be localized at all. Therefore, these signals are designed almost entirely for the single purpose of calling one's attention to injurious processes in the body. They create suffering that is sometimes intolerable. Their gradation of intensity is poor; instead, weak pain signals can summate over a period of time by a process of temporal summation to create an unbearable feeling even though the same pain for short periods of time may be relatively mild.

Function of the Thalamus and Cerebral Cortex in the Appreciation of Pain. Complete removal of the somatic sensory areas of the cerebral cortex does not destroy one's ability to perceive pain. Therefore, it is believed that pain impulses entering only the thalamus and lower centers cause at least some conscious perception of pain. However, this does not mean that the cerebral cortex has nothing to do with normal pain appreciation; indeed, electrical stimulation of the somesthetic cortical areas causes a person to perceive mild pain in approximately 3 per cent of the stimulations. Furthermore, lesions in these areas, particularly in somatic sensory area II, at times give rise to severe pain. Thus, there is reason to believe that somatic sensory area II may be more concerned with pain sensation than is somatic sensory area I.

Localization of Pain in the Body. Most localization of pain probably results from simultaneous stimulation of tactile receptors along with the pain stimulation. However, the pricking type of pain, transmitted through delta type A fibers, can be localized perhaps within 10 to 20 cm. of the stimulated area. On the other hand, the burning and aching types of pain,

Figure 8–5. Transmission of pain signals into the hindbrain, thalamus, and cortex.

transmitted through type C fibers, is localizable only very grossly, perhaps to a major part of the body such as a limb but certainly not to small areas. This is in keeping with the fact that these fibers terminate extremely diffusely in the hindbrain and thalamus.

Surgical Interruption of Pain Pathways. Often a person has such severe and intractable pain (this often results from rapidly spreading cancer), that it is necessary to relieve the pain. To do this the pain pathway can be destroyed at any one of several different points. If the pain is in the lower part of the body, a *cordotomy* in the upper thoracic region usually relieves the pain. To do this, the spinal cord on the side opposite to the pain is sectioned almost entirely through its anterolateral quadrant, which interrupts the spinothalamic tracts.

A cordotomy does not relieve pain in the upper part of the body because many pain fibers from the upper body do not cross to the opposite side of the spinal cord before reaching the medulla. In these patients, the lateral spinothalamic tract is sectioned in the brain stem where it passes over the inferior olive. This procedure is called a *bulbar tractotomy.*

Finally, if the pain originates in the neck or face, even a bulbar tractotomy is not satisfactory. Pain sometimes originates within the thalamus or elsewhere in the central pain pathways beyond the tractotomy site, as will be discussed later in the chapter. To relieve these types of pain, extirpation of either somatic sensory area I or somatic sensory area II has been attempted, but almost always without success—indeed, sometimes with exacerbation of the pain. Recently, however, it has been claimed that destruction of specific portions of the intralaminar nuclei in the thalamus can relieve the suffering elicited by pain while still leaving intact one's appreciation of the pricking quality of pain, which remains an important protective mechanism. Unfortunately, such operations are so difficult to perform without damaging other vital areas of the thalamus that they have been successful in only a few instances.

THE REACTION TO PAIN

Even though the threshold for recognition of pain remains approximately equal from one person to another, the degree to which each one reacts to pain varies tremendously. Stoical persons, such as members of the American Indian race, react to pain far less intensely than do more emotional persons. In the preceding chapter, it was pointed out that conditioning impulses entering the sensory areas of the central nervous system from various portions of the central and peripheral nervous systems can determine whether incoming sensory impulses will be transmitted extensively or weakly to other areas of the brain. It is probably some

such mechanism as this that determines how much one reacts to pain.

Pain causes both reflex motor reactions and psychic reactions. Some of the reflex actions occur directly from the spinal cord, for pain impulses entering the gray matter of the cord can directly initiate "withdrawal reflexes" that remove the body or a portion of the body from the noxious stimulus, as will be discussed in Chapter 9. These primitive spinal cord reflexes, though important in lower animals, are mainly suppressed in the human being by the higher centers of the central nervous system. Yet, in their place, much more complicated and more effective reflexes from the motor cortex are initiated by the pain stimuli to eliminate the painful stimulus.

The psychic reactions to pain are likely to be far more subtle; they include all the well-known aspects of pain such as anguish, anxiety, crying, depression, nausea, and excess muscular excitability throughout the body. These reactions vary tremendously from one person to another following comparable degrees of pain stimuli.

THE "GATING" THEORY FOR CONTROL OF THE REACTION TO PAIN

It is common experience that two types of nonpain signals from other parts of the nervous system can greatly alter the degree of transmission of pain through the spinal cord.

1. Stimulation of the large sensory fibers from peripheral mechanoreceptors greatly depresses the transmission of pain signals either from the same area of the body or from areas sometimes located many segments away.

2. Corticofugal signals from the brain can decrease pain sensitivity.

A special quality of the suppression caused both by the cutaneous mechanoreceptors and by the brain is that even after the signals are over the pain sometimes remains suppressed for an hour or more thereafter.

Mechanism of Pain Gating. Unfortunately, the detailed mechanism of pain gating is not known. However, the general mechanism is probably the following: After the pain fibers enter the spinal cord and pass into the tract of Lissauer, within one or two segments they terminate in the *substantia gelatinosa,* a group of small neurons located near the tip of the dorsal horn. The pain signals are then transmitted through one or more additional neurons before passing upward through the long pathways to the brain. However, there are other inputs to the substantia gelatinosa in addition to the pain fibers. For instance, collaterals from the mechanoreceptors terminate in the mid-portion of the dorsal horns, and from here second order neurons send short axons dorsally in the dorsal horns to terminate in the substantia gelatinosa. Most of these terminate on the pain fiber axons before they synapse with the neurons of the substantia gelatinosa, and they cause *presynaptic inhibition,* a mechanism explained in Chapter 4. In a similar manner, corticofugal pathways also terminate in the substantia gelatinosa where they, too, cause presynaptic inhibition.

Thus, signals either from the mechanoreceptors or from the corticofugal fibers can greatly depress the transmission of pain signals from the pain fibers into the successive levels of the pain pathway.

Treatment of Pain by Exciting the Dorsal Column Sensory Pathway. Experiments have shown that mild electrical excitation of the large sensory fibers of peripheral nerves or even electrical excitation of the large fibers of the dorsal columns in the spinal cord can often suppress pain. When the large peripheral fibers are stimulated, the suppression probably results from presynaptic inhibition in the substantia gelatinosa. When the dorsal columns are excited, a similar type of inhibition probably occurs at the brain stem level. It is possible that future advances in this area of "counter-stimulation" will allow relief from many types of presently unbearable pain.

A Possible Physiologic Basis for Acupuncture. One will recognize that the gating theory of pain control provides a partial physiologic basis for the claims of acupuncture. That is, stimulation of non-painful fibers, the mechanoreceptor sensory afferents, can suppress pain signals. In addition, strong conditioning signals from the brain can also suppress pain. A combination of these two could help to provide an explanation for the success of acupuncture in some people. Also, it can explain the efficacy of skin irritants or heat to relieve pain—for instance, the use of liniments on the skin to relieve pain of overly exercised muscles.

REFERRED PAIN

Often a person feels pain in a part of his body that is considerably removed from the tissues causing the pain. This pain is called *referred pain.* On occasion, pain can even be referred from one surface area of the body to another, but more frequently it is initiated in one of the visceral organs and referred to an area of the body surface. Also, pain may originate in a viscus and be referred to another deep area of the body not exactly coincident with the location of the viscus producing the pain. A knowledge of these different types of referred pain is extremely important because many visceral ailments cause no other signs except referred pain.

Mechanism of Referred Pain. Figure 8–6 illustrates the most generally accepted mech-

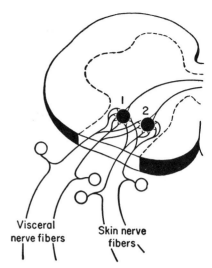

Figure 8–6. Mechanism of referred pain and referred hyperalgesia.

anism by which most pain is referred. In the figure, branches of visceral pain fibers are shown to synapse in the spinal cord with some of the same second order neurons that receive pain fibers from the skin. When the visceral pain fibers are stimulated intensely, pain sensations from the viscera spread into some of the neurons that normally conduct pain sensations only from the skin, and the person has the feeling that the sensations actually originate in the skin itself. It is also possible that some referred pain results from convergence of visceral and skin impulses at the level of the thalamus rather than in the spinal cord.

REFERRED PAIN CAUSED BY REFLEX MUSCULAR SPASM

Some types of referred pain are caused secondarily by reflex muscular spasm. For instance, pain in a ureter can cause reflex spasm of the lumbar muscles. Often the pain from the ureter itself is hardly felt at all, but instead almost all the pain results from spasm of the lumbar muscles.

Many back pains and some types of headache also appear to be caused by muscular spasm, the spasm originating reflexly from much weaker pain impulses originating elsewhere in the body.

VISCERAL PAIN

In clinical diagnosis, pain from the different viscera of the abdomen and chest is one of the few criteria that can be used for diagnosing visceral inflammation, disease, and other ailments.

In general, the viscera have sensory receptors for no other modalities of sensation besides pain, and visceral pain differs from surface pain in many important aspects.

One of the most important differences between surface pain and visceral pain is that highly localized types of damage to the viscera rarely cause severe pain. For instance, a surgeon can cut the gut entirely in two in a patient who is awake without causing significant pain. On the other hand, any stimulus that causes *diffuse stimulation of pain nerve endings* throughout a viscus causes pain that can be extremely severe. For instance, occluding the blood supply to a large area of gut stimulates many diffuse pain fibers at the same time and can result in extreme pain.

CAUSES OF TRUE VISCERAL PAIN

Any stimulus that excites pain nerve endings in diffuse areas of the viscera causes visceral pain. Such stimuli include ischemia of visceral tissue, chemical damage to the surfaces of the viscera, spasm of the smooth muscle in a hollow viscus, distention of a hollow viscus, or stretching of the ligaments. Essentially all of the true visceral pain originating in the thoracic and abdominal cavities is transmitted through sensory nerve fibers that run in the sympathetic nerves. These fibers are small type C fibers and, therefore, can transmit only burning and aching types of pain. The pathways for transmitting true visceral pain will be discussed in detail later in the chapter.

Ischemia. Ischemia causes visceral pain in exactly the same way that it does in other tissues, presumably because of the formation of acidic metabolic end-products or tissue degenerative products, such as bradykinin, that stimulate the pain nerve endings.

Chemical Stimuli. On occasion, damaging substances leak from the gastrointestinal tract into the peritoneal cavity. For instance, proteolytic acidic gastric juice often leaks through a ruptured gastric or duodenal ulcer. This juice causes widespread digestion of the visceral peritoneum, thus stimulating extremely broad areas of pain fibers. The pain is usually extremely severe.

Spasm of a Hollow Viscus. Spasm of the gut, the gallbladder, a bile duct, the ureter, or any other hollow viscus can cause pain in exactly the same way that spasm of the skeletal muscle causes pain. This presumably results from diminished blood flow to the muscle, combined with increased metabolic need of the muscle for nutrients. Thus, *relative* ischemia develops, which causes severe pain.

Often, pain from a spastic viscus occurs in the form of *cramps,* the pain increasing to a high degree of severity and then subsiding, this process continuing rhythmically once every few minutes. The rhythmic cycles result from rhythmic contraction of smooth muscle. For instance, each time a peristaltic wave travels along an overly excitable spastic gut, a cramp occurs. The cramping type pain frequently occurs in gastroenteritis, constipation, menstruation, parturition, gallbladder disease, or ureteral obstruction.

Overdistention of a Hollow Viscus. Extreme overfilling of a hollow viscus also results in pain, presumably because of overstretch of the tissues themselves. However, overdistention can also collapse the blood vessels that encircle the viscus, or that pass into its wall, thereby perhaps promoting ischemic pain.

"PARIETAL" PAIN CAUSED BY VISCERAL DAMAGE

In addition to true visceral pain, some pain sensations are also transmitted from the viscera through nerve fibers that innervate the parietal peritoneum, pleura, or pericardium. The parietal surfaces of the visceral cavities are supplied mainly by spinal nerve fibers that penetrate from the surface of the body inward.

Characteristics of Parietal Visceral Pain. When a disease affects a viscus, it often spreads to the parietal wall of the visceral cavity. This wall, like the skin, is supplied with extensive innervation including the "fast" delta fibers, which are different from the fibers in the true visceral pain pathways of the sympathetic nerves. Therefore, pain from the parietal wall of a visceral cavity is frequently very sharp and pricking in quality, though it can also have burning and aching qualities if the pain stimulus is diffuse. Thus, a knife incision through the *parietal* peritoneum is very painful, even though a similar cut through the visceral peritoneum or through a gut is not painful.

INSENSITIVE VISCERA

A few visceral areas are almost entirely insensitive to pain of any type. These include the parenchyma of the liver and the alveoli of the lungs. Yet the liver *capsule* is extremely sensitive to both direct trauma and stretch, and the *bile ducts* are also sensitive to pain. In the lungs, even though the aveoli are insensitive, the bronchi and the parietal pleura are both very sensitive to pain.

LOCALIZATION OF VISCERAL PAIN– REFERRED VISCERAL PAIN

Pain from the different viscera is frequently difficult to localize for a number of reasons. First, the brain does not know from firsthand experience that the different organs exist, and, therefore, any pain that is localized internally can be localized only generally. Second, sensations from the abdomen and thorax are transmitted by two separate pathways to the central nervous system—the *true visceral pathway* and the *parietal pathway*. The true visceral pain is transmitted via sensory fibers of the autonomic nervous system, and the sensations are *referred* to surface areas of the body often far from the painful organ. On the other hand, parietal sensations are conducted *directly* from the parietal peritoneum, pleura, or pericardium, and the sensations are usually *localized directly over the painful area*.

The Visceral Pathway for Transmission of Pain. Most of the internal organs of the body are supplied by type C pain fibers that pass along the visceral sympathetic nerves into the spinal cord and thence up the lateral spinothalamic tract along with the pain fibers from the body's surface. A few visceral pain fibers—those from the distal portion of the colon, from the rectum, and from the bladder—enter the spinal cord through the sacral parasympathetic nerves, and some enter the central nervous system through various cranial nerves. These include fibers in the glossopharyngeal and vagus nerves, which transmit pain from the pharynx, trachea, and upper esophagus. And fibers from the surfaces of the diaphragm as well as from the lower esophagus are carried in the phrenic nerves.

Localization of Referred Pain Transmitted by the Visceral Pathways. The position in the cord to which visceral afferent fibers pass from each organ depends on the segment of the body from which the organ developed embryologically. For instance, the heart originated in the neck and upper thorax. Consequently, the heart's visceral pain fibers enter the cord all the way from C-3 down to T-5. The stomach had its origin approximately from the seventh to the ninth thoracic segments of the embryo, and consequently the visceral afferents from the stomach

enter the spinal cord between these levels. The gallbladder had its origin almost entirely in the ninth thoracic segment, so that the visceral afferents from the gallbladder enter the spinal cord at T-9.

Because the visceral afferent pain fibers are responsible for transmitting referred pain from the viscera, the location of the referred pain on the surface of the body is in the dermatome of the segment from which the visceral organ was originally derived in the embryo. Some of the areas of referred pain on the surface of the body are shown in Figure 8–7.

The Parietal Pathway for Transmission of Abdominal and Thoracic Pain. Where spinal nerves overlie the abdomen or thorax, pain fibers penetrate inward to innervate the parietal peritoneum, parietal pleura, and parietal pericardium, Also, retroperitoneal visceral organs and perhaps portions of the mesentery are innervated to some extent by parietal pain fibers. The kidney, for instance, is supplied by both visceral and parietal fibers.

Pain from the viscera is frequently localized in two surface areas of the body because of the dual pathways for transmission of pain. Figure 8–8 illustrates dual transmission of pain from an inflamed appendix. Impulses pass from the appendix through the sympathetic visceral pain fibers into the sympathetic chain and then into the spinal cord at approximately T-10 or T-11; this pain is referred to an area around the um-

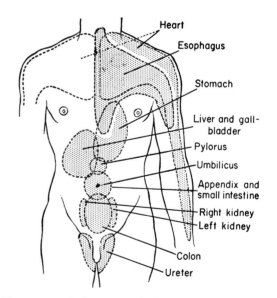

Figure 8–7. Surface areas of referred pain from different visceral organs.

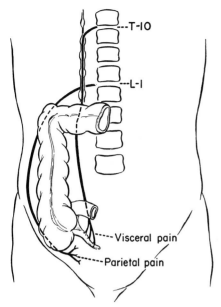

Figure 8–8. Visceral and parietal transmission of pain from the appendix.

bilicus and is of the aching, cramping type. On the other hand, pain impulses also often originate in the parietal peritoneum where the inflamed appendix touches the abdominal wall, and these impulses pass directly through the spinal nerves into the spinal cord at a level of approximately L-1 or L-2. This pain is localized directly over the irritated peritoneum in the right lower quadrant of the abdomen and is of the sharp type.

VISCERAL PAIN FROM VARIOUS ORGANS

Cardiac Pain.   Almost all pain that originates in the heart results from ischemia secondary to coronary sclerosis, which blocks the coronary arteries. This pain is referred mainly to the base of the neck, over the shoulders, over the pectoral muscles, and down the arms. Most frequently, the referred pain is on the left side rather than on the right—probably because the left side of the heart is much more frequently involved in coronary disease than is the right side—but occasionally mild referred pain occurs on the right side of the body as well as on the left.

The pain impulses are conducted through nerves passing to the middle cervical ganglia, to the stellate ganglia, and to the first four or five thoracic ganglia of the sympathetic chains. Then the impulses pass into the spinal cord through the second, third, fourth and fifth thoracic spinal nerves.

Direct Parietal Pain from the Heart.   When coronary ischemia is extremely severe, such as immediately after a coronary thrombosis, intense cardiac pain sometimes occurs directly underneath the sternum simultaneously with pain referred to other areas. This direct pain from underneath the sternum is difficult to explain on the basis of the visceral nerve connections. Therefore, it is highly probable that sensory nerve endings passing from the heart through the pericardial reflections around the great vessels conduct this direct pain.

In addition to pain from the heart, other sensations may accompany coronary thrombosis. One of these is a tight, oppressive sensation beneath the sternum. The exact cause of this is unknown, but a possible cause is reflex spasm of blood vessels, bronchioles, or muscles in the chest region.

Relief of Referred Cardiac Pain by Sympathectomy.   To interrupt pain impulses from the heart one can either cut the sympathetic nerves that pass from the heart to the sympathetic chains or, as is usually performed, cut nerve fibers as they pass through the sympathetic chains into the spinal cord. Relief of cardiac pain can frequently be accomplished simply by removing the sympathetic chain from T-2 through T-5 on only the left side, but sometimes it is necessary to remove the fibers on both sides in order to obtain satisfactory results.

Esophageal Pain.   Pain from the esophagus is usually referred to the pharynx, to the lower neck, to the arms, or to midline chest regions beginning at the upper portion of the sternum and ending approximately at the lower level of the heart. Irritation of the gastric end of the esophagus may cause pain directly over the heart, though the pain has nothing whatsoever to do with the heart. Such pain may be caused by spasm of the cardia, the area where the esophagus empties into the stomach, which causes excessive dilatation of the lower esophagus, or it may result from chemical, bacterial, or other types of inflammatory irritations.

Gastric Pain.   Pain arising in the fundus of the stomach—usually caused by gastritis—is referred to the anterior surface of the chest or upper abdomen from slightly below the heart to an inch or so below the xyphoid process. These pains are frequently characterized as burning pains; and they, or pains from the lower esophagus, cause the condition known as "heartburn."

Most peptic ulcers occur within 1 to 2 inches on either side of the pylorus in the stomach or in the duodenum, and pain from such ulcers is usually referred to a surface point approximately midway between the umbilicus and the xyphoid process. The origin of ulcer pain is almost undoubtedly chemical, because when the acid juices of the stomach are not allowed to reach the pain fibers in the ulcer crater the pain does not exist. This pain is characteristically intensely burning.

Biliary and Gallbladder Pain.   Pain from the bile ducts and gallbladder is localized in the midepigastrium almost coincident with pains caused by peptic ulcers. Also, biliary and gallbladder pain is often burning, like that from ulcers, though cramps often occur too.

Biliary disease, in addition to causing pain on the abdominal surface, frequently refers pain to a small area at the tip of the right scapula. This pain is transmitted through sympathetic afferent fibers that enter the ninth thoracic segment of the spinal cord.

Pancreatic Pain. Lesions of the pancreas, such as acute or chronic pancreatitis in which the pancreatic enzymes eat away the pancreas and surrounding structures, promote intense pain in areas both anterior to and behind the pancreas. It should be remembered that the pancreas is located beneath the parietal peritoneum and that it receives many sensory fibers from the posterior abdominal wall. Therefore, the pain is frequently localized directly behind the pancreas in the back and is severe and burning in character.

Renal Pain. The kidney, kidney pelvis, and ureters are all retroperitoneal structures and receive most of their pain fibers directly from skeletal nerves. Therefore, pain is usually felt directly behind the ailing structure. However, pain occasionally is referred via visceral afferents to the anterior abdominal wall below and about 2 inches to the side of the umbilicus.

Pain from the bladder is felt directly over the bladder, presumably because the bladder is well innervated by parietal pain fibers. However, pain is also frequently referred into the groin and testicles because some nerve fibers from the bladder apparently synapse in the cord in association with fibers from the genital areas.

Uterine Pain. Both parietal and visceral afferent pain may be transmitted from the uterus. The low abdominal cramping pains of dysmenorrhea are mediated through the sympathetic afferents, and an operation to cut the hypogastric nerves between the hypogastric plexus and the uterus will in many instances relieve this pain. On the other hand, lesions of the uterus that spread into the adnexa around the uterus, or lesions of the fallopian tubes and broad ligaments, usually cause pain in the lower back or side. This pain is conducted over parietal nerve fibers and is usually sharper in nature rather than resembling the diffuse cramping pain of true dysmenorrhea.

SOME CLINICAL ABNORMALITIES OF PAIN AND OTHER SENSATIONS

HYPERALGESIA

A pain pathway may become excessively excitable; this gives rise to hyperalgesia, which means hypersensitivity to pain. The basic causes of hyperalgesia are: (1) excessive sensitivity of the pain receptors themselves, which is called *primary hyperalgesia,* or facilitation of sensory transmission, which is called *secondary hyperalgesia.*

An example of primary hyperalgesia is the extreme sensitivity of sunburned skin. Secondary hyperalgesia frequently results from lesions in the spinal cord or in the thalmus. Several of these will be discussed in subsequent sections.

THE THALAMIC SYNDROME

Occasionally the posterolateral branch of the posterior cerebral artery, a small artery supplying the posteroventral portion of the thalamus, becomes blocked by thrombosis, so that the nuclei of this area of the thalamus degenerate, while the medial and anterior nuclei of the thalamus remain intact. The patient suffers a series of abnormalities, as follows: First, loss of almost all sensations from the opposite side of the body occurs because of destruction of the relay nuclei. Second, ataxia (inability to control movements precisely) may be evident because of loss of kinesthetic impulses normally relayed through the thalamus to the cortex. Third, after a few weeks to a few months some sensory perception in the opposite side of the body returns, but strong stimuli are usually necessary to elicit this. When the sensations do occur, they are poorly—if at all—localized, almost always very painful, sometimes lancinating, regardless of the type of stimulus applied to the body. Fourth, the person is likely to perceive many affective sensations of extreme unpleasantness or, rarely, extreme pleasantness; the unpleasant ones are often associated with emotional tirades.

The medial nuclei of the thalamus are not destroyed by thrombosis of the artery. Therefore, it is believed that these nuclei become facilitated and give rise to the enhanced sensitivity to pain transmitted through the reticular system as well as to the affective sensations.

HERPES ZOSTER

Occasionally a virus probably identical with that of chickenpox infects a dorsal root ganglion. This causes severe pain in the dermatomal segment normally subserved by the ganglion, thus eliciting a segmental type of pain that circles around the body. This pain is commonly called "shingles."

There are two possible causes of the pain of herpes zoster. One of these is that the disease destroys mainly the large mechanoreceptor afferent sensory fibers. This theoretically could reduce the normal inhibitory effect of these fibers on the pain pathway in the substantia gelatinosa of the dorsal horn. Therefore, pain signals could become exacerbated in the absence of this inhibition.

A second possibility is that the irritated neuronal cell bodies of the root ganglion are stimulated to excessive activity and thereby cause the pain.

TIC DOULOUREUX

Lancinating pains occur in some persons over one side of the face in part of the sensory distribution area of the fifth or ninth nerves; this phenomenon is called tic douloureux. The pains feel like sudden electric shocks, and they may appear for only a few seconds at a time or they may be almost continuous. Often, they are set off by exceedingly sensitive "trigger areas" on the surface of the head, in the mouth, or in the nose—almost always by a mechanoreceptive stimulus instead of a pain stimulus. For instance, when the patient swallows a bolus of food, as the food touches a tonsil it might set off a severe lancinating pain in the mandibular portion of the fifth nerve.

The pain of tic douloureux can usually be blocked by cutting the peripheral nerve from the hypersensitive area. The fifth nerve is often sectioned immediately inside the cranium, where the motor and sensory roots of the fifth nerve can be separated so that the motor portions, which are needed for many of the jaw movements, are spared while the sensory elements are destroyed. Obviously, this operation leaves the side of the face anesthetic, which in itself may be annoying. Furthermore, it is sometimes unsuccessful, indicating that the lesion might be more central than the nerves themselves. Therefore, still another operation is often performed in the medulla for relief of this pain, as follows:

The sensory nuclei of the fifth nerve divide into the main sensory nucleus, which is located in the pons, and the spinal sensory nucleus, which descends into the upper part of the spinal cord. It is the spinal nucleus that subserves the function of pain. Therefore, the spinal tract of the fifth nerve can be cut in the medulla as it passes to the spinal nucleus. This blocks pain sensations from the side of the face but does not block the sensations of touch and pressure.

THE BROWN-SÉQUARD SYNDROME

Obviously, if the spinal cord is transected entirely, all sensations and motor functions distal to the segments of transection are blocked, but if only one side of the spinal cord is transected, the socalled Brown-Séquard syndrome occurs. The following effects of such a transection occur, and these can be predicted from a knowledge of the cord fiber tracts illustrated in Figure 8–9: All motor functions are blocked on the side of the transection in all segments below the level of the transection; while only some of the modalities of sensation are lost on the transected side and others are lost on the opposite side. The sensations of pain, heat, and cold are lost on the opposite side of the body in all dermatomes two to six segments below the level of the transection. The sensations that are transmitted only in the dorsal columns—kinesthetic sensation, vibration sensation, discrete localization, and two-point discrimination—are lost entirely on the side of the transection in all dermatomes below the level of the transection. Touch is impaired on the side of the transection because the principal pathway for transmission of light touch, the dorsal columns, is transected. Yet, "crude touch," which is poorly localized, still persists be-

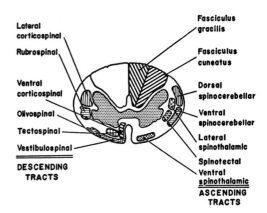

Figure 8–9. Cross-section of the spinal cord, showing principal ascending tracts on the right and principal descending tracts on the left.

cause of transmission in the opposite ventral spinothalamic tract.

HEADACHE

Headaches are actually referred pain to the surface of the head from the deep structures. Many headaches result from pain stimuli arising inside the cranium, but equally as many probably result from pain arising outside the cranium.

HEADACHE OF INTRACRANIAL ORIGIN

Pain-Sensitive Areas in the Cranial Vault. The brain itself is almost totally insensitive to pain. Even cutting or electrically stimulating the somesthetic centers of the cortex only occasionally causes pain; instead, it causes tactile paresthesias on the area of the body represented by the portion of the somesthetic cortex stimulated. Therefore, it is obvious from the outset that much or most of the pain of headache probably is not caused by damage within the brain itself.

On the other hand, *tugging on the venous sinuses, damaging the tentorium,* or *stretching the dura at the base of the brain* can all cause intense pain that is recognized as headache. Also, almost any type of traumatizing, crushing, or stretching stimulus to the *blood vessels of the dura* can cause headache. One of the most sensitive structures of the entire cranial vault is the middle meningeal artery, and neurosurgeons are careful to remain clear of this artery as much as possible when performing brain operations under local anesthesia.

Areas of the Head to which Intracranial Headache is Referred. Stimulation of pain receptors in the intracranial vault above the tentorium, including the upper surface of the tentorium itself, initiates impulses in the fifth nerve and, therefore, causes re-

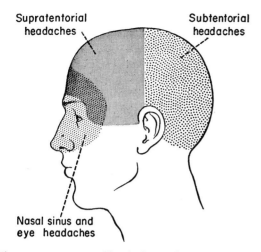

Figure 8–10.   Areas of headache resulting from different causes.

ferred headache on the outside of the head in the area supplied by the fifth cranial nerve. This area includes the upper part of the head anterior to the ear, as outlined by the dark shaded area of Figure 8–10. Thus, pain arising above the tentorium causes what is called "frontal headache."

On the other hand, pain impulses from beneath the tentorium enter the central nervous system mainly through the second cervical nerve, which also supplies the scalp behind the ear. Therefore, subtentorial pain stimuli cause "occipital headache" referred to the posterior part of the head shown in Figure 8–10.

Types of Intracranial Headache. *Headache of Meningitis.*   One of the most severe headaches of all is that resulting from meningitis, which causes inflammation of all the meninges, including the sensitive areas of the dura and the sensitive areas around the venous sinuses. Such intense damage as this can cause extreme headache pain referred over the entire head.

Headache Resulting from Direct Meningeal Trauma.   Following a brain operation one ordinarily has intense headache for several days to several weeks. Though part of this headache may result from the trauma of the brain itself, experiments indicate that most of it results from meningeal irritation.

Another type of meningeal trauma that almost invariably causes headache is the meningeal irritation resulting from brain tumor. Usually, tumor headache is referred to a localized area of the head, the exact area depending on the portion of the meninges affected by the tumor. Since any tumor above the tentorium refers its pain to the frontal areas and any tumor below the tentorium refers its pain to the occipital region of the skull, the general location of an intracranial tumor can often be predicted from the area of the headache.

Headache Caused by Low Cerebrospinal Fluid Pressure.   Removing as little as 20 ml. of fluid from the spinal canal, particularly if the person remains in the upright position, often causes intense intracranial headache. Removing this quantity of fluid removes the flotation for the brain that is normally provided by the cerebrospinal fluid. Therefore, the weight of the brain stretches the various dural surfaces and thereby elicits the pain which causes the headache.

Migraine Headache.   Migraine headache is a special type of headache that is thought to result from abnormal vascular phenomena, though the exact mechanism is unknown.

Migraine headaches often begin with various prodromal sensations, such as nausea, loss of vision in part of the fields of vision, visual aura, or other types of sensory hallucinations. Ordinarily, the prodromal symptoms begin half an hour to an hour prior to the beginning of the headache itself. Therefore, any theory that explains migraine headache must also explain these prodromal symptoms.

One of the theories of the cause of migraine headaches is that prolonged emotion or tension causes reflex vasospasm of some of the arteries of the head, including arteries that supply the brain itself. The vasospasm theoretically produces ischemia of portions of the brain, and this is responsible for the prodromal symptoms. Then, as a result of the intense ischemia, something happens to the vascular wall to allow it to become flaccid and incapable of maintaining vascular tone for 24 to 48 hours. The blood pressure in the vessels causes them to dilate and pulsate intensely, and it is supposedly the excessive stretching of the walls of the arteries—including the extracranial arteries such as the temporal artery—that causes the actual pain of migraine headaches. However, it is possible that diffuse after-effects of ischemia in the brain itself are responsible for this type of headache.

Alcoholic Headache.   As many people have experienced, a headache usually follows an alcoholic binge. It is most likely that alcohol, because it is toxic to tissues, directly irritates the meninges and causes the cerebral pain.

Headache Caused by Constipation.   Constipation causes headache in many persons. Because it has been shown that constipation headache can occur in persons whose spinal cords have been cut, we know that this headache is not caused by nervous impulses from the colon. Therefore, it possibly results from absorbed toxic products or from changes in the circulatory system. Indeed, constipation sometimes does cause temporary loss of plasma into the wall of the gut, and a resulting poor flow of blood to the head could be the cause of the headache.

EXTRACRANIAL TYPES OF HEADACHE

Headache Resulting from Muscular Spasm. Emotional tension often causes many of the muscles of the head, including especially those muscles attached to the scalp and the neck muscles attached to the occiput, to become moderately spastic, and it is postulated that this causes headache. The pain of the spastic head muscles supposedly is referred to the overlying areas of the head and gives one the same type of headache as do intracranial lesions.

Headache Caused by Irritation of the Nasal and Accessory Nasal Structures. The mucous membranes of the nose and also of all the nasal sinuses are sensitive to pain, but not intensely so. Nevertheless, infection or other irritative processes in widespread areas of the nasal structures usually cause headache that is referred behind the eyes or, in the case of frontal sinus infection, to the frontal surfaces of the forehead and scalp, as illustrated in Figure 8–10. Also, pain from the lower sinuses—such as the maxillary sinuses—can be felt in the face.

Headache Caused by Eye Disorders. Difficulty in focusing one's eyes clearly may cause excessive contraction of the ciliary muscles in an attempt to gain clear vision. Even though these muscles are extremely small, tonic contraction of them can be the cause of retroorbital headache. Also, excessive attempts to focus the eyes can result in reflex spasm in the various facial and extraocular muscles. Tonic spasm in these muscles is also a possible cause of headache.

A second type of headache originating in the eyes occurs when the eyes are exposed to excessive irradiation by ultraviolet light rays. Watching the sun or the arc of an arc-welder for even a few seconds may result in headache that lasts from 24 to 48 hours. The headache sometimes results from "actinic" irritation of the conjunctivae, and the pain is referred to the surface of the head or retroorbitally. However, focusing intense light from an arc or the sun on the retina can actually burn the retina, and this could result in headache.

THERMAL SENSATIONS

THERMAL RECEPTORS AND THEIR EXCITATION

The human being can perceive different gradations of cold and heat, progressing from *cold* to *cool* to *indifferent* to *warm* to *hot;* some persons perceive even freezing cold and burning hot.

The different thermal gradations in the body are discriminated by at least three different types of sensory end-organs, the *cold receptors,* the *warm receptors,* and the *pain receptors.* The pain receptors are stimulated only by extreme degrees of heat or cold and therefore will not be considered as thermal receptors but merely as pain receptors that become stimulated when either heat or cold becomes sufficiently severe to cause damage.

Both heat and cold can be perceived from areas of the body that contain only free nerve endings, such as the cornea. Therefore, it is known that free nerve endings can subserve these sensory functions. Thus far, no complex specialized receptors for either cold or warmth have been discovered.

Stimulation of Thermal Receptors— Sensations of Cold, Warmth, and Hot. Figure 8–11 illustrates the responses to different temperatures of three different types of nerve fibers: (1) a cold fiber, (2) a warm fiber, and (3) a pain fiber. Note especially that these fibers respond differently at different levels of temperature. For instance, in the *very* cold region only the pain fibers are stimulated (if the skin becomes even colder so that it nearly freezes or actually does freeze, even these fibers cannot be stimulated). As the temperature rises to 10 to 15° C., pain impulses cease, but the cold receptors begin to be stimulated. Then, above about 25° C. the warm end-organs become stimulated while the cold end-organs fade out at about 35° C. Finally, at around 45° C. the warm endings become nonresponsive once more; but the cold endings begin to respond again, and the pain endings also begin to be stimulated.

One can understand from Figure 8–11, therefore, that a person determines the different gradations of thermal sensations by the relative degrees of stimulation of the different types of endings. For instance, at 20° C. only cold endings are stimulated, whereas at 40° C. only warm endings are stimulated; at 33° C. both cold and warm endings are stimulated, and at 50° C. both cold and pain endings are stimulated. One can understand also from this figure why extreme degrees of cold or heat can be painful and why both these sensations, when intense enough, may give almost exactly the same quality of sensations—freezing cold and burning hot sensations feel almost alike to the person.

It is particularly interesting that a few areas of

Figure 8–11. Frequencies of discharge of a cold receptor, a warm receptor, and a pain nerve fiber at different temperatures. (The responses of the cold and warm receptors are modified from Zotterman: *Ann. Rev. Physiol.,* 15:357, 1953.)

the body, such as the tip of the penis, do not contain any warmth receptors; but these areas can experience the sensations of cold with ease and of "hot," which depends on stimulating cold and pain endings, but never the sensation of warmth.

Stimulatory Effects of Rising and Falling Temperature—Adaptation of Thermal Receptors. When a cold receptor is suddenly subjected to an abrupt fall in temperature, it becomes strongly stimulated at first, but this stimulation fades rapidly during the first minute and progressively more slowly during the next half hour or more. In other words, the receptor adapts to a great extent; this is illustrated in Figure 8–12, which shows that the frequency of discharge of a cold receptor rose approximately four-fold when the temperature fell suddenly from 32° to 30° C., but in less than a minute the frequency fell about five sixths of the way back to the original control value. Later, the temperature was suddenly raised from 30° to 32° C. At this point the cold receptor stopped firing entirely for a short time, but after adaptation returned to its original control level. The warm receptors, on the other hand, have not yet been shown to adapt, though psychological experience such as the entering of a hot tub of water indicates that the warmth signals do in some way adapt.

Thus, it is evident that the thermal senses respond markedly to *changes in temperature* in addition to being able to respond to steady states of temperature, as was depicted in Figure 8–11. This means, therefore, that when the temperature of the skin is actively falling, a person feels much colder than when the temperature remains at the same level. Conversely, if the temperature is actively rising the person feels much warmer than he would at the same temperature if it were constant.

The response to changes in temperature explains the extreme degree of heat that one feels when he first enters a hot tub of water and the extreme degree of cold he feels when he goes from a heated room to the out-of-doors on a cold day. The adaptation of the thermal senses explains the ability of the person to become gradually accustomed to his new temperature environmant.

Mechanism of Stimulation of the Thermal Receptors. It is believed that the thermal receptors are stimulated by changes in their metabolic rates, these changes resulting from the fact that temperature alters the rates of intracellular chemical reactions about 2.3 times for each 10° C. change. In other words, thermal detection probably results not from direct physical stimulation but instead from chemical stimulation of the endings as modified by the temperature.

Spatial Summation of Thermal Sensations. The number of cold or warmth endings in any small surface area of the body is very slight, so that it is difficult to judge gradations of temperature when small areas are stimulated. However, when a large area of the body is stimulated, the thermal signals from the entire area summate. Indeed, one reaches his maximum ability to discern minute temperature variations when his entire body is subjected to a temperature change all at once. For instance, rapid changes in temperature as little as 0.01° C. can be detected if this change affects the entire surface of the body simultaneously. On the other hand, temperature changes 100 times this great might not be detected when the skin surface affected is only a square centimeter or so in size.

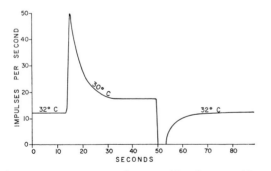

Figure 8–12. Response of a nerve fiber from a cold receptor following, first, instantaneous change in skin temperature from 32° to 30° C. and, second, instantaneous change back to 32° C. Note the adaptation of the receptor and also the higher steady state level of discharge at 30° than at 32°.

TRANSMISSION OF THERMAL SIGNALS IN THE NERVOUS SYSTEM

Thermal signals are transmitted by small myelinated fibers of the delta group with diameters of only 2 to 5 microns. It is also possible that some very crude thermal sensations, such as "burning hot" or "freezing cold," but with very poor differentiation of temperature gradations, are transmitted by type C fibers.

On entering the central nervous system, the thermal fibers travel in the lateral spinothalamic tract. The exact point in the thalamus at which the impulses synapse is not known, but since other delta spinothalamic fibers terminate mainly in the caudalmost portion of the ventrobasal complex of the thalamus, it is believed that the thermal tracts do too. Then, third order neurons travel to the somesthetic cortex, but the portion of the cerebral cortex to which the major share of thermal fibers radiate is also unknown.

Occasionally, a neuron in somatic sensory area I has been found by microelectrode studies to be directly responsive to either cold or warm stimuli in specific areas of the skin. Furthermore, it is known that removal of the postcentral gyrus in the human being reduces his ability to distinguish different gradations of temperature. Therefore, it is possible that somatic sensory area I, rather than area II, is the major somesthetic area concerned with thermal sensations.

REFERENCES

Bloedel, J. R.: The substrate for integration in the central pain pathways. *Clin. Neurosurg.*, 21:194, 1974.

Bonica, J. J. (ed.): International Symposium on Pain. New York, Raven Press, 1974.

Bonica, J. J., Procacci, P., and Pagni, C. A.: Recent Advances in Pain. Springfield, Ill., Charles C Thomas, Publisher, 1974.

Casey, K. L.: Pain: a current view of neural mechanisms. *Amer. Sci.*, 61:194, 1973.

Ciba Foundation Symposium: Touch, Heat and Pain. Boston, Little, Brown and Company, 1965.

Crue, B. L.: Pain: Research and Treatment. Further observations from City of Hope National Medical Center. New York, Academic Press, Inc., 1975.

Dalessio, D. J.: Wolff's Headache and Other Head Pain, 3rd Ed. New York, Oxford University Press, 1972.

Guyton, A. C., and Reeder, R. C.: Pain and contracture in poliomyelitis. *Arch. Neurol. Psychiatr.*, 63:954, 1950.

Hannington-Kiff, J. G.: Pain Relief. Philadelphia, J. B. Lippincott Company, 1974.

Hardy, J. D.: The nature of pain. *J. Chronic Dis.*, 4:22, 1956.

Hardy, J. D., Wolff, H. C., and Goodell, H.: Pain Sensations and Reactions. Baltimore, The Williams & Wilkins Company, 1952.

Johnson, R. H., and Spaulding, J. M.: Disorders of the autonomic nervous system. Chap 16: Pain. *Contemp. Neurol. Ser.*, 11:279, 1974.

Li, C. L.: Neurological basis of pain and its possible relationship to acupuncture-analgesia. *Amer. J. Chin. Med.*, 1:61, 1973.

Lim, R. K. S.: Pain. *Ann. Rev. Physiol.*, 32:269, 1970.

McMasters, R. E.: A clinical approach to pain. *South. Med. J.*, 67:173, 1974.

Merskey, H.: Assessment of pain. *Physiotherapy*, 60:96, 1974.

Nashold, B. S., Jr.: Central pain: its origins and treatment. *Clin. Neurosurg.*, 21:311, 1974.

Newman, P. O.: Visceral Afferent Functions of the Nervous System. Monograph of the Physiological Society, No. 25. Baltimore, The Williams & Wilkins Company, 1974.

Payne, J. P., and Burt, R. A. P. (eds.): Pain. New York, Churchill Livingstone, Div. of Longman, Inc., 1972.

Perl, E. R., and Boivie, J. G.: Neural substrates of somatic sensation. *In* Guyton, A. C. (ed.): MTP International Review of Science: Physiology. Vol. 3. Baltimore, University Park Press, 1974, p. 303.

Shepherd, J. A.: Concise Surgery of the Acute Abdomen. New York, Churchill Livingstone, Div. of Longman, Inc., 1974.

Swerdlow, M.: Relief of Intractable Pain. New York, American Elsevier Publishing Co., Inc., 1974.

Way, E. L.: New Concepts in Pain and Its Clinical Management. Philadelphia, F. A. Davis Company, 1967.

Wilkins, R. H.: Neurosurgical relief of pain: recent developments. *Tex. Med.*, 70:53, 1974.

Wilson, M. E.: The neurological mechanisms of pain. A review. *Anaesthesia*, 29:407, 1974.

Zotterman, Y.: Thermal sensations. *In* Magoun, H. W. (ed.): Handbook of Physiology. Sec. 1, Vol. 1. Baltimore, The Williams & Wilkins Co., 1959, p. 431.

See also bibliographies at the ends of Chapters 5, 6, and 7.

9

Motor Functions of the Spinal Cord and the Cord Reflexes

In the discussion of the nervous system thus far, we have considered principally the input of sensory information. In the following chapters we will discuss the origin and output of motor signals, the signals that cause muscle contraction and other motor effects throughout the body. Sensory information is integrated at all levels of the nervous system and causes appropriate motor responses, beginning in the spinal cord with relatively simple reflexes, extending into the brain stem with still more complicated responses, and, finally, extending to the cerebrum where the most complicated responses are controlled. The present chapter discusses the control of motor function especially in response to spinal cord reflexes.

Experimental Preparations for Studying Cord Reflexes. Normally the functions of the spinal cord are strongly controlled by signals from the brain. Therefore, to study the isolated cord reflexes it is necessary to separate the cord from the higher centers. This is usually done in one of two different types of preparations: (1) the *spinal animal* or (2) the *decerebrate animal*.

The spinal animal is prepared by cutting the spinal cord at any level above the region in which the cord reflexes are to be studied. For a variable period of time, depending upon the phylogenetic level of the animal, as will be discussed later in the chapter, the cord reflexes are deeply depressed immediately after removal of the signals from the brain. However, over a period of hours or days in animals and over a period of weeks or months in the human being, the cord reflexes become progressively more active and can then be studied independently of control by the upper levels of the nervous system. Sometimes the cord reflexes become even more excitable under these conditions than normally.

In the decerebrate preparation, the brain stem is usually transected between the superior and inferior colliculi. Transecting the brain at this level removes the voluntary control centers of the forebrain, and it also removes inhibitory influences from the basal ganglia that normally suppress the activities of the lower brain stem and spinal cord; this will be discussed in detail in the following chapter. Removal of this inhibition causes an immediate increase in the activity of many of the cord reflexes, especially the extensor reflexes that help the animal hold itself up against gravity. This preparation has an advantage over the spinal animal in that many of the cord reflexes are exacerbated even in the acute preparation and, therefore, can be studied without the long and tedious delay required to prepare the spinal animal.

ORGANIZATION OF THE SPINAL CORD FOR MOTOR FUNCTIONS

The cord gray matter is the integrative area for the cord reflexes and other motor functions. Figure 9–1 shows the typical organization of the cord gray matter in a single cord segment. Sensory signals enter the cord through the sensory roots. After entering the cord, every sensory signal travels to two separate destinations. First, either in the same segment of the cord or in nearby segments, the sensory nerve or its collaterals terminate in the gray matter of the cord and elicit local segmental responses—local excitatory effects, facilitatory effects, reflexes, and so forth. Second, the signals travel to higher levels of the nervous system—to higher levels in the cord itself, to the brain stem, or even to the cerebral cortex. It is these sensory

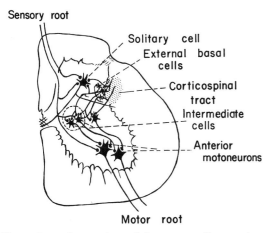

Figure 9–1. Connections of the sensory fibers and cortical fibers with the interneurons ("intermediate cells") and anterior motoneurons of the spinal cord. (Modified from Lloyd: *J. Neurophysiol.*, 4:525, 1941.)

signals that cause the conscious sensory experiences described in the past few chapters.

Each segment of the spinal cord has several hundred thousand neurons in its gray matter. Aside from the sensory relay neurons already discussed, these neurons are divided into two separate types, the *anterior motoneurons* and the *interneurons* (also called *internuncial cells* or *intermediate cells*).

The Anterior Motoneurons. Located in each segment of the anterior horns of the cord gray matter are several thousand neurons, 50 to 100 per cent larger than most of the others and called anterior motoneurons. These give rise to the nerve fibers that leave the cord via the anterior roots and then proceed to the muscles to innervate the skeletal muscle fibers. They can be divided into two major types, the *alpha motoneurons* and the *gamma motoneurons.*

The Alpha Motoneurons. The alpha motoneurons give rise to large type A alpha nerve fibers ranging from 9 to 16 microns in diameter and passing through the spinal nerves to innervate the skeletal muscle fibers. Stimulation of a single nerve fiber excites from 3 to 2000 skeletal muscle fibers (averaging about 180 fibers), which are collectively called the *motor unit.* Thus, it is the alpha motoneurons that control the contractile functions of the skeletal muscle fibers. Transmission of nerve impulses into skeletal muscles and their stimulation of the muscle fibers was discussed in Chapters 1 through 3.

The Gamma Motoneurons. In addition to the alpha motoneurons that excite contraction of the skeletal muscle fibers, about one-half as many much smaller motoneurons, located along with the alpha motoneurons also in the anterior horns, transmit impulses through type A gamma fibers, averaging 5 microns in diameter, to special skeletal muscle fibers called *intrafusal fibers*. These are part of the *muscle spindle,* which is discussed at length later in the chapter.

The Interneurons. The interneurons are present in all areas of the cord gray matter—in the dorsal horns, spread diffusely in the anterior horns, and also in the intermediate areas between these two. These cells are numerous—approximately 30 times as numerous as the anterior motoneurons. They are small and highly excitable, often exhibiting spontaneous activity and capable of firing as rapidly as 1500 times per second. They have many interconnections one with the other, and many of them directly innervate the anterior motoneurons as illustrated in Figure 9–1. The interconnections among the interneurons and anterior motoneurons are responsible for many of the integrative functions of the spinal cord that are discussed during the remainder of this chapter.

Essentially all the different types of neuronal circuits described in Chapter 5 are found in the interneuron pool of cells of the spinal cord, including the *diverging, converging,* and *repetitive-discharge* circuits. In the following sections of this chapter we will see the many applications of these different circuits to the performance of specific reflex acts by the spinal cord.

Only a few incoming sensory signals to the spinal cord or signals from the brain terminate directly on the anterior motoneurons. Instead, most of them are transmitted first through interneurons where they are appropriately processed before stimulating the anterior motoneurons. Thus, in Figure 9–1, it is shown that the corticospinal tract terminates almost entirely on interneurons, and it is through these that the cerebrum transmits most of its signals for control of muscular function.

The Renshaw Cell Inhibitory System. Located also in the ventral horns of the spinal cord in close association with the motoneurons are a large number of small interneurons called *Renshaw cells*. Almost immediately after the motor axon leaves a motoneuron, collateral branches pass to the Renshaw cells. These in turn are inhibitory cells that transmit inhibitory signals to the nearby motoneurons. Thus, stimulation of each motoneuron tends to inhibit the surrounding motoneurons. This effect is important for two major reasons:

1. It shows that the motor system utilizes the principle of lateral inhibition to focus, or sharpen, its

signals—that is, to allow unabated transmission of the primary signal while suppressing the tendency for signals to spread to adjacent neurons.

2. The peripheral axon of the anterior motoneuron is known to secrete acetylcholine at its nerve endings. Therefore, the ability of collateral nerve endings from the same axon to stimulate the Renshaw cells proves that acetylcholine is one of the central nervous system excitatory transmitters, acting in the same way that it acts as an excitatory transmitter at the neuromuscular junction.

Sensory Input to the Motoneurons and Interneurons

Most of the sensory fibrils entering each segment of the spinal cord terminate on interneurons, but a very small number of large sensory fibers from the muscle spindles terminate on the anterior motoneurons. Thus, there are two pathways in the spinal cord that cord reflexes can take: either directly to the anterior motoneuron itself, utilizing a monosynaptic pathway; or through one or more interneurons first, before passing to the anterior motoneuron. The monosynaptic pathway provides an extremely rapid reflex feedback system and is the basis of the very important muscle *stretch reflex* that will be discussed later in the chapter. All other cord reflexes utilize the interneuron pathway, a pathway that can modify the signals tremendously and that can cause complex reflex patterns. For instance, the very important protective reflex called the *withdrawal reflex* utilizes this pathway.

Multisegmental Connections in the Spinal Cord—the Propriospinal Fibers. About half of all the nerve fibers ascending and descending in the spinal cord are *propriospinal fibers*. These are fibers that run from one segment of the cord to another. In addition, the terminal fibrils of sensory fibers as they enter the cord branch both up and down the spinal cord, some of the branches transmitting signals only a segment or two in each direction, while others transmit signals many segments. These ascending and descending fibers of the cord provide pathways for the multisegmental reflexes that will be described later in this chapter, including many reflexes that coordinate movements in both the forelimbs and hindlimbs simultaneously.

ROLE OF THE MUSCLE SPINDLE IN MOTOR CONTROL

Muscles and tendons have an abundance of two special types of receptors: (1) *muscle spin-*

dles* that detect (a) change in length of muscle fibers and (b) rate of this change in length, and (2) *Golgi tendon organs* that detect the tension applied to the muscle tendon during muscle contraction or muscle stretch.

The signals from these two receptors operate entirely at a subconscious level, causing no sensory perception at all. But they do transmit tremendous amounts of information into the spinal cord and also to the cerebellum, thereby helping these two portions of the nervous system to perform their functions for controlling muscle contraction.

RECEPTOR FUNCTION OF THE MUSCLE SPINDLE

Structure and Innervation of the Muscle Spindle. The physiologic organization of the muscle spindle is illustrated in Figure 9–2. Each spindle is built around three to ten small *intrafusal muscle fibers* that are pointed at their ends and are attached to the sheaths of the surrounding *extrafusal* skeletal muscle fibers. The intrafusal fiber is a very small skeletal muscle fiber. However, the central region of each of these fibers has either no or few actin and myosin filaments. Therefore, this central portion does not contract when the ends do. The ends in turn are excited by small nerve fibers called *gamma efferent* motor nerve fibers. These average five microns in diameter and are much smaller than the sensory nerve fibers that also innervate the muscle spindle.

When the ends of the intrafusal fibers contract, this action stretches the central portion. Likewise, stretch of the entire muscle, which pulls on the ends of the intrafusal fibers where

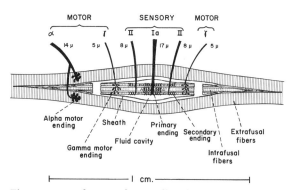

Figure 9–2. The muscle spindle, showing its relationship to the large extrafusal skeletal muscle fibers. Note also both the motor and the sensory innervation of the muscle spindle.

they attach to the muscle sheaths, also stretches the central portion of each intrafusal fiber. This central portion of the muscle spindle is the sensory receptor area of the muscle spindle.

The receptor portion of the muscle spindle is innervated by two different types of sensory nerves: one type Ia fiber and usually two type II fibers. The type Ia fiber averages 17 microns in diameter and transmits sensory signals from the muscle spindle to the spinal cord at a velocity approaching 100 meters per second, as rapidly as any sensory nerve fibers in the entire body. The type II nerve fibers average 8 microns in diameter and transmit signals to the central nervous system at a velocity of approximately 30 to 40 meters per second.

The Primary Ending. The type Ia fiber innervates the central portion of the spindle receptor. The tip of this fiber spirals around the intrafusal fibers, forming the so-called *primary ending,* also called the *annulospiral ending.*

The Secondary Endings. The two type II nerve fibers innervate the receptor region of the intrafusal fibers on either side of the primary ending. These fibers, like the Ia fiber, also spiral around the intrafusal fibers, and when the central portion of the intrafusal fibers is stretched, these nerve fibers are stimulated. These sensory endings are called *secondary endings.*

Division of the Intrafusal Fibers into Nuclear Bag and Nuclear Chain Fibers—Dynamic and Static Responses of the Muscle Spindle. There are also two different types of intrafusal fibers: (1) *nuclear bag fibers* (one to three), in which a large number of nuclei are congregated into a bag in the central portion of the receptor area, and (2) *nuclear chain fibers* (three to seven), which are about half as large in diameter and half as long as the nuclear bag fibers and have nuclei spread in a chain throughout the receptor area. The primary ending innervates both the nuclear bag intrafusal fibers *and* the nuclear chain fibers. On the other hand, the secondary endings are located almost entirely on the nuclear chain fibers. These relationships are illustrated in Figure 9–3.

Static Response of the Secondary Receptors. When the receptor portion of the muscle spindle is stretched, the number of impulses transmitted from the secondary endings increases almost directly in proportion to the degree of stretch, and the endings continue to transmit these impulses for many minutes. This effect is called the *static response* of the spindle receptor, meaning simply that the receptor transmits its signal for a prolonged period of time.

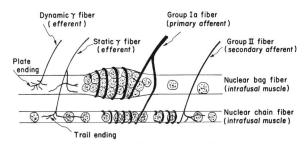

Figure 9–3. Details of nerve connections to the nuclear bag and nuclear chain muscle spindle fibers. (Modified from Stein: *Physiol. Rev.,* 54:225, 1974, and Boyd: *Philos. Trans. R. Soc. Lond.* [*Biol. Sci.*], 245:81, 1962.)

Dynamic Response of the Primary Endings. The primary ending also reacts with a static response, but it also exhibits a very strong *dynamic response,* which means that it responds extremely actively to a *change* in length. When the length of a spindle receptor area increases only a fraction of a micron, the primary receptor transmits tremendous numbers of impulses into the Ia fiber, but only *while the length is actually increasing.* As soon as the length has stopped increasing, the rate of impulse discharge returns almost back to its original level, except for the small static response that is still present in the signal.

Conversely, when the spindle receptor area shortens, this change momentarily decreases the impulse output from the primary ending; as soon as the receptor area has reached its new shortened length, the impulses reappear in the Ia fiber within a fraction of a second. Thus, the primary ending sends extremely strong signals to the central nervous system to apprise it of any change in length of the spindle receptor area.

Since both the primary and the secondary endings innervate the nuclear chain intrafusal fibers, it is assumed that it is these nuclear chain fibers that are responsible for the static response of both the primary and the secondary endings. On the other hand, only the primary endings innervate the nuclear bag fibers. Therefore, it is assumed that the nuclear bag fibers are responsible for the powerful dynamic response.

Control of the Static and Dynamic Responses by the Gamma Efferent Nerves. Some physiologists believe that the gamma efferent nerves to the muscle spindle can be divided into two different types: gamma-dynamic (gamma-d) and gamma-static (gamma-s). The first of these excites mainly the nuclear bag intrafusal fibers and the second excites mainly the nuclear chain intrafusal fibers. When the gamma-d fibers excite the nuclear bag fibers, the dynamic response of the muscle spindle becomes tremendously enhanced, whereas the static response remains very weak or even none at all. On the other hand, stimulation of the gamma-s fibers, which excite mainly the nuclear chain fibers, supposedly enhances the static response while having little influence on the dynamic response. We shall see in subsequent paragraphs that these two different types of responses of the muscle spindle are exceedingly important in different types of muscle control.

Function of the Muscle Spindle in Comparing Intrafusal and Extrafusal Muscle Lengths

From the foregoing description of the muscle spindle, one can see that there are two different ways in which the spindle can be stimulated:

1. By stretching the whole muscle. This lengthens the extrafusal fibers and therefore also stretches the spindle.

2. By contracting the intrafusal muscle fibers while the extrafusal fibers remain at their normal length. Since the intrafusal fibers contract only near their two ends, this stretches the central receptor portions of the intrafusal fibers, obviously exciting the spindles.

Therefore, in effect, the muscle spindle acts as a *comparator* of the lengths of the two types of muscle fibers, the extrafusal and the intrafusal. When the length of the extrafusal fibers is greater than that of the intrafusal fibers, the spindle becomes excited. On the other hand, when the length of the extrafusal fiber is shorter than that of the intrafusal fiber, the spindle becomes inhibited.

Continuous Discharge of the Muscle Spindles Under Normal Conditions. Normally, particularly when there is a slight amount of gamma efferent excitation, the muscle spindles emit sensory nerve impulses all of the time. Stretching the muscle spindles increases the rate of firing, whereas shortening the spindle decreases this rate of firing. Thus, the spindles can be either excited or inhibited.

THE MUSCLE SPINDLE REFLEX (ALSO CALLED STRETCH REFLEX OR MYOTATIC REFLEX)

From the above description of all the intricacies of the muscle spindle, one can readily see that the spindle is a very complex organ. Its function is manifested in the form of the muscle spindle reflex which, because of the static and the dynamic types of muscle spindle response, consists of a *static reflex* and a *dynamic reflex.*

Neuronal Circuitry of the Muscle Spindle Reflex. Figure 9–4 illustrates the basic circuit of the dynamic muscle spindle reflex, showing a type Ia nerve fiber originating in a muscle spindle and entering the dorsal root of the spinal cord. It then synapses directly with an anterior motoneuron whose motor nerve fiber transmits an appropriate reflex signal, with almost negligible delay, back to the same muscle containing the muscle spindle.

In addition to the direct synapse of the Ia muscle spindle nerve fiber with the anterior motoneuron, collaterals from this fiber, as well as the type II fibers from the secondary spindle endings, terminate on interneurons in the gray matter of the cord, and these in turn transmit more delayed signals to the anterior motoneuron.

The Stretch Reflex. The muscle spindle reflex is frequently called simply a *stretch reflex* because stretch of the muscle excites the muscle spindle and this in turn causes a muscle reflex contraction. This reflex has a dynamic component and a static component.

The Dynamic Stretch Reflex. The dynamic stretch reflex is caused by the potent dynamic signal believed to originate from the nuclear bag receptors and transmitted via the primary endings of the muscle spindles. That is, when the muscle fiber is suddenly stretched, a strong signal is transmitted to the spinal cord through the primary endings, but this signal is potent *only while the degree of stretch is increasing.* On entering the spinal cord, most of the signal goes directly to the anterior motoneurons without passing through interneurons, and it causes

STRETCH REFLEX

Figure 9–4. Neuronal circuit of the stretch reflex.

reflex contraction of the same muscle from which the muscle spindle signals originated. Thus, a sudden stretch of a muscle causes reflex contraction of the same muscle, and this returns the length of the muscle back toward its original length.

The Static Stretch Reflex. Though the dynamic stretch reflex is over within a fraction of a second after the muscle has been stretched to its new length, a much weaker static stretch reflex continues for a prolonged period of time thereafter. This reflex is elicited by continuous static receptor signals transmitted through both the primary and secondary endings of the muscle spindles and probably originating in the nuclear chain intrafusal fibers. The importance of the static stretch reflex is that it continues to cause muscle contraction as long as the muscle is maintained at an excessive length (for as long as several hours, but not for days). The muscle contraction in turn opposes the force that is causing the excess length.

The Negative Stretch Reflex. When a muscle is suddenly shortened, exactly opposite effects occur. If the muscle is already taut, any sudden release of the load on the muscle that allows it to shorten will elicit both dynamic and static inhibition rather than reflex excitation. Thus, *this negative stretch reflex* opposes the shortening of the muscle in the same way that the positive stretch reflex opposes lengthening of the muscle. Therefore, one can begin to see that the muscle spindle reflex tends to maintain the status quo for the length of a muscle.

FUNCTION OF THE STATIC MUSCLE SPINDLE REFLEX TO NULLIFY CHANGES IN LOAD DURING MUSCLE CONTRACTION

Let us assume that a person's biceps is contracted so that the forearm is horizontal to the earth. Then assume that a five-pound weight is put in the hand. The hand will immediately drop. However, the amount that the hand will drop is determined to a great extent by the degree of activity of the static muscle spindle reflex. If the gamma-s fibers to the muscle spindles are strongly stimulated so that the static reflex is very active, even slight lengthening of the biceps, and therefore also of the muscle spindles in the biceps, will cause a strong feedback contraction of the extrafusal skeletal muscle fibers of the biceps. This contraction in turn will limit the degree of fall of the hand, thus automatically maintaining the forearm in a nearly horizontal position. This response is called a *load reflex.*

Effect of Gamma Efferent Stimulation on Increasing the Effectiveness of the Load Reflex. If the gamma efferent nerves to the static portion of the muscle spindle (the gamma-s fibers) are not stimulated at all, then the spindle sensitivities are greatly depressed, and the effectiveness of the load reflex is almost zero. On the other hand, if these gama efferents are strongly stimulated so that the static muscle spindle reflex is an extremely potent one, then one would expect the length of the muscle to remain almost exactly constant regardless of the change in load. In many of our muscle activities a particular part of our body often is fixed in a given position, and any attempt to move that part of the body from the position is met by instantaneous reflex resistance. This probably results to a great extent from the load reflex. Furthermore, the fact that we can change the sensitivity of this load reflex by changing the intensity of gamma-s stimulation allows us to make a particular part of the body be either flail or tightly locked in place. To give an example, when a person is threading a needle he tends to fix both of his hands into precise positions, and any extra load applied to either of the two hands will hardly change its position.

The Damping Function of the Dynamic and Static Reflexes. Another extremely important function of the muscle spindle reflex—indeed, probably just as important as, if not more important than, the load reflex—is the ability of the muscle spindle reflex to prevent some types of oscillation and jerkiness of the body movements. This is a damping, or smoothing, function. An example is the following:

Use of the Damping Mechanism in Smoothing Muscle Contraction. Occasionally, signals from other parts of the nervous system are transmitted to a muscle in a very unsmooth form, first increasing in intensity for a few milliseconds, then decreasing in intensity, then changing to another intensity level, and so forth. When the muscle spindle apparatus is not functioning satisfactorily, the degree of muscle contraction changes jerkily during the course of such a signal. This effect is illustrated in Figure 9–5, which shows an experiment in which a sensory nerve signal entering one side of the cord is transmitted to a motor nerve from the other side of the cord to excite a muscle. In curve A the muscle spindle reflex of the excited muscle is intact. Note that the contraction is

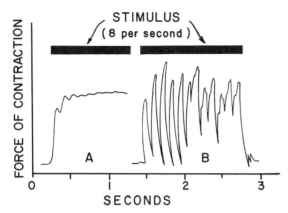

Figure 9–5. Muscle contraction caused by a central nervous system signal under two different conditions: (A) in a normal muscle, and (B) in a muscle whose muscle spindles had been denervated by section of the posterior roots of the cord 82 days previously. Note the smoothing effect of the muscle spindles in Part A. (Modified from Creed et al.: Reflex Activity of the Spinal Cord. Oxford University Press, 1932.)

relatively smooth even though the sensory nerve is excited at a frequency of 8 per second. Curve B, on the other hand, is the same experiment in an animal whose muscle spindle sensory nerves from the excited muscle had been sectioned three months earlier. Note the very unsmooth muscle contraction. Thus, curve A illustrates very graphically the ability of the damping mechanism of the muscle spindle to smooth muscle contractions even though the input signals to the muscle motor system may themselves be very jerky. This effect can also be called a *signal averaging* function of the muscle spindle.

Function of the Gamma Efferent System in Controlling the Degree of Damping. In the same way that the gamma efferent system can play a potent role in determining the effectiveness of the load reflex, so also can the gamma efferent system determine the degree of damping. For instance, there are times when a person wishes his limbs to move extremely rapidly in response to rapidly changing input signals. Under such conditions, one would wish less damping. On the other hand, there are other times when it is very important that the muscle contractions be very smooth. Under these conditions one would like a high degree of damping. Therefore, even though we are not completely sure how the nervous system can make such changes as this, psychophysiological tests do tell us that our motor system does have such capability to in-

crease or decrease the degree of damping in any given muscle response.

ROLE OF THE MUSCLE SPINDLE IN VOLUNTARY MOTOR ACTIVITY

To emphasize the importance of the gamma efferent system, one needs to recognize that 31 per cent of all the motor nerve fibers to the muscle are gamma efferent fibers rather than large type A alpha motor fibers. Whenever signals are transmitted from the motor cortex or from any other area of the brain to the alpha motoneurons, almost invariably the gamma motoneurons are stimulated simultaneously. This causes both the extrafusal and the intrafusal muscle fibers to contract at the same time.

The purpose of contracting the muscle spindle fibers at the same time that the large skeletal muscle fibers contract is probably two-fold: First, it keeps the muscle spindle from opposing the muscle contraction. Second, it also maintains proper damping and proper load responsiveness of the muscle spindle regardless of change in muscle length. For instance, if the muscle spindle should not contract and relax along with the large muscle fibers, the receptor portion of the spindle would sometimes be flail and at other times be overstretched, in neither instance operating under optimal conditions for spindle function.

Possible Servo Function of the Muscle Spindle Reflex. Several physiologists have suggested that the muscle spindle reflex can also operate as a servo controller of muscle contraction in the following way: Suppose that a gamma efferent nerve fiber to a muscle spindle were stimulated. This would contract the intrafusal fibers and excite the muscle spindle receptors. The signals from these receptors would then pass to the cord and thence back to the large skeletal muscle fibers to cause them to contract also. Thus, an initial contraction of the intrafusal fibers causes a similar contraction of the surrounding large skeletal muscle fibers.

If such a servo system as this did exist, signals transmitted from the brain downward through the gamma efferent system could cause secondary contractions of the muscles in accordance with the dictates of the muscle spindles. Unfortunately, most of the data indicate that a mechanism such as this does not occur to a significant extent. For a system of this type to function properly, it would be necessary to have a static response of the muscle spindles that is very potent and also unchanging. Unfortunately, the static response of the muscle spindles is usually very weak—that is, it has a low gain. Also, it decays very slowly over a period of a few minutes to an hour so that changes in length of a muscle spindle could cause only temporary changes in length of the surrounding large skeletal muscle fibers. Therefore, despite the attractiveness of this possible type of muscle control, it is doubtful that it does actually occur in normal function.

Probable Servo-Assist Function of the Muscle Spindle Reflex. It is much more likely that the muscle spindle reflex acts as a servo-assist device than as a pure servo controller. But, first, let us explain what is meant by a "servo-assist mechanism."

When both the alpha and gamma motoneurons are stimulated simultaneously, if the intra- and extrafusal fibers contract equal amounts, the degree of stimulation of the muscle spindles will not change at all—either to increase or to decrease. However, in case the extrafusal muscle fibers should contract less than the intrafusal fibers (as might occur when the muscle is contracting against a great load), this mismatch will stretch the receptor portions of the spindles and, therefore, elicit a stretch reflex that will further excite the extrafusal fibers. Thus, failure of the extrafusal fibers to contract to the same degree as the intrafusal fibers contract causes an accessory neuronal signal that increases the degree of stimulation of the extrafusal fibers. This is exactly the same mechanism as that employed by power steering in an automobile. That is, the steering wheel directly turns the front wheels and will do this even when the power steering is not effective. However, if the wheels fail to follow even the slightest extra force applied to the steering wheel, a servo-assist device is activated that applies additional power to turn the wheels.

The servo-assist type of motor function has several important advantages, as follows:

1. It allows the brain to cause a muscle contraction against a load without the brain having to expend much extra nervous energy.

2. It makes the muscle contract almost the desired amount even when the load is increased or decreased between successive contractions. In other words, it makes the degree of contraction less load-insensitive.

3. It compensates for fatigue or other abnormalities of the muscle itself because any failure of the muscle to provide the proper contraction elicits an additional muscle spindle reflex stimulus to make the contraction occur.

But, unfortunately, we still do not know how important this probable function of the muscle spindle reflex actually is.

Brain Areas for Control of the Gamma Efferent System

The gamma efferent system is excited primarily by the *bulboreticular facilitatory* region of the brain stem, and secondarily by impulses transmitted into this area from (a) the *cerebellum,* (b) the *basal ganglia,* and even (c) the *cerebral cortex.* Unfortunately, little is known about the precise mechanisms of control of the gamma efferent system. However, since the bulboreticular facilitatory area is particularly concerned with postural contractions, emphasis is given to the possible or probable important role of the gamma efferent mechanism in controlling muscle contraction for positioning the different parts of the body and for damping the movements of the different parts.

In addition to transmitting signals into the spinal cord, the muscle spindle also transmits signals up the cord to the cerebellum and thence into the bulboreticular areas, as will be discussed in greater detail in Chapter 11. However, both the signals that operate in the spinal cord and those that pass to the cerebellum are entirely subconscious, so that the conscious portion of the brain is never apprised of the immediate changes in length of the muscles. On the other hand, as has already been pointed out in Chapter 7, signals from the joint receptors constantly apprise the conscious brain of the positions of the different parts of the body, even though the muscle receptors do not.

CLINICAL APPLICATIONS OF THE STRETCH REFLEX

The Knee Jerk and Other Muscle Jerks. Clinically, a method used to determine the functional integrity of the stretch reflexes is to elicit the knee jerk and other muscle jerks. The knee jerk can be elicited by simply striking the patellar tendon with a reflex hammer; this stretches the quadriceps muscle and initiates a *dynamic stretch reflex* to cause the lower leg to jerk forward. The upper part of Figure 9–6 illustrates a myogram from the quadriceps muscle recorded during a knee jerk.

Similar reflexes can be obtained from almost any muscle of the body either by striking the tendon of the muscle or by striking the belly of the muscle itself. In other words, sudden stretch of muscle spindles is all that is required to elicit a stretch reflex.

The muscle jerks are used by neurologists to assess the degree of facilitation of spinal cord centers. When large numbers of facilitatory impulses are being transmitted from the upper regions of the central nervous system into the cord, the muscle jerks are greatly exacerbated. On the other hand, if the facilitatory impulses are depressed or abrogated, the muscle jerks are considerably weakened or completely absent. These reflexes are used most frequently to determine the presence or absence of muscle spasticity following lesions in the motor areas of the brain. Ordinarily, diffuse lesions in the contralateral motor areas of the cerebral cortex cause greatly exacerbated muscle jerks.

Clonus. Under appropriate conditions, the muscle jerks can oscillate, a phenomenon called clonus

Figure 9–6. Myograms recorded from the quadriceps muscle during elicitation of the knee jerk and from the gastrocnemius mucle during ankle clonus.

(see lower myogram, Fig. 9–6). Oscillation can be explained particularly well in relation to ankle clonus, as follows:

If a person is standing on his tiptoes and suddenly drops his body downward to stretch one of his gastrocnemius muscles, impulses are transmitted from the muscle spindles into the spinal cord. These reflexly excite the stretched muscle, which lifts the body back up again. After a fraction of a second, the reflex contraction of the muscle dies out and the body falls again, thus stretching the spindles a second time. Again a dynamic stretch reflex lifts the body, but this too dies out after a fraction of a second, and the body falls once more to elicit still a new cycle. In this way, the stretch reflex of the gastrocnemius muscle continues to oscillate, often for long periods of time; this is clonus.

Clonus ordinarily occurs only if the stretch reflex is highly sensitized by facilitatory impulses from the cerebrum. For instance, in the decerebrate animal, in which the stretch reflexes are highly facilitated, clonus develops readily. Therefore, to determine the degree of facilitation of the spinal cord, neurologists test patients for clonus by suddenly stretching a muscle and keeping a steady stretching force applied to the muscle. If clonus occurs, the degree of facilitation is certain to be very high.

THE TENDON REFLEX

The Golgi Tendon Organ and Its Excitation. Golgi tendon organs, illustrated in Figure 9–7, lie within muscle tendons immediately beyond their attachments to the muscle fibers. An average of 10 to 15 muscle fibers is usually connected in series with each Golgi tendon organ, and the organ is stimulated by the tension produced by this small bundle of muscle fibers. Thus, the major difference between the function

of the Golgi tendon apparatus and the muscle spindle is that the spindle detects relative muscle length, and the tendon organ detects muscle *tension.*

The tendon organ, like the primary receptor of the muscle spindle, responds with overexcitation to the onset of increased muscle tension, but within a small fraction of a second it settles down to a lower level of steady state firing that is almost directly proportional to the muscle tension. Thus, the Golgi tendon organs provide to the central nervous system instantaneous information of the degree of tension on each small segment of each muscle.

Transmission of Impulses from the Tendon Organ into the Central Nervous System. Signals from the tendon organ are transmitted through large, rapidly conducting type A alpha nerve fibers, fibers only slightly smaller than those from the primary receptors of the muscle spindle. These fibers, like those from the primary receptors, transmit signals both into local areas of the cord and through the spinocerebellar tracts into the cerebellum. The local signal is believed to excite a single inhibitory interneuron that in turn inhibits the anterior alpha motoneuron. Thus, this local circuit directly inhibits the individual muscle without affecting adjacent muscles. The signals to the cerebellum will be discussed in Chapter 11.

Inhibitory Nature of the Tendon Reflex. The Golgi tendon organ detects tension applied to the tendon by muscle contraction, as was discussed earlier in the chapter. Signals from the tendon organ are then transmitted into the spinal cord to cause reflex effects in the respective muscle. However, this reflex is entirely inhibitory, the exact opposite to the muscle spindle reflex. The signal from the tendon organ supposedly excites inhibitory interneurons, and these in turn inhibit the alpha motoneurons to the respective muscle.

When tension on the muscle and, therefore, on the tendon becomes extreme, the inhibitory effect from the tendon organ can be so great that it causes sudden relaxation of the entire muscle. This effect is called the *lengthening reaction;* it is probably a protective mechanism

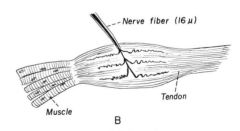

Figure 9–7. Golgi tendon organ.

to prevent tearing of the muscle or avulsion of the tendon from its attachments to the bone. We know, for instance, that direct electrical stimulation of muscles in the laboratory can frequently cause such destructive effects.

However, possibly as important as this protective reaction is function of the tendon reflex as a part of the overall servo control of muscle contraction in the following manner:

The Tendon Reflex as a Servo Control Mechanism for Muscle Tension. In the same way that the stretch reflex possibly operates as a feedback mechanism to control length of a muscle, the tendon reflex theoretically can operate as a servo feedback mechanism to control muscle tension. That is, if the tension on the muscle becomes too great, inhibition from the tendon organ decreases this tension back to a lower value. On the other hand, if the tension becomes too little, impulses from the tendon organ cease; and the resulting loss of inhibition allows the alpha motoneurons to become active again, thus increasing muscle tension back toward a higher level.

Very little is known at present about the function of or control of this tension servo feedback mechanism, but it is postulated to operate in the following basic manner: Signals from the brain are presumably transmitted to the cord centers to set the gain of the tendon feedback system. This can be done by changing the degree of facilitation of the neurons in the feedback loop. If the gain is high, then this system will be extremely sensitive to signals coming from the tendon organs; on the other hand, lack of excitatory signals from the brain could make the system very insensitive to the signals from the tendon organ. In this way, control signals from higher nervous centers could automatically set the level of tension at which the muscle would be maintained. If the required tension is high, then the muscle tension would be set by the servo feedback mechanism to this high level of tension. On the other hand, if the desired tension level is low, the muscle tension would automatically adjust to this low level.

This description of the tension servo system is obviously very incomplete and almost entirely theoretical at the present time, but it does depict some of the speculation on this effect. Yet, a word of caution: Despite the speculation, the measured feedback gains of the tendon-muscle feedback system have been far too little to prove that it can be useful as a tension servo controller.

Value of a Servo Mechanism for Control of Tension. An obvious value of a mechanism for setting the degree of muscle tension would be to allow the different muscles to apply a desired amount of force irrespective of how far the muscles contract. An example of this would be paddling a boat, during which a person sets the amount of force that he pulls backwards on the paddle and maintains that degree of force throughout the entire movement. Were it not for some type of tension feedback mechanism, the same amount of force would not be maintained

throughout the stroke because uncontrolled muscles change their force of contraction as their lengths change. One can imagine hundreds of different patterns of muscle function that might require maintenance of constant tension rather than maintenance of constant lengths of the muscles.

THE FLEXOR REFLEX

In the spinal or decerebrate animal, almost any type of sensory stimulus to a limb is likely to cause the flexor muscles of the limb to contract strongly, thereby withdrawing the limb from the stimulus. This is called the flexor reflex.

In its classical form the flexor reflex is elicited most frequently by stimulation of pain endings, such as by pinprick, heat, or some other painful stimulus, for which reason it is also frequently called a *nociceptive reflex.* However, even stimulation of the touch receptors can also occasionally elicit a weaker and less prolonged flexor reflex.

If some part of the body besides one of the limbs is painfully stimulated, this part, in a similar manner, will be withdrawn from the stimulus, but the reflex may not be confined entirely to flexor muscles even though it is basically the same type of reflex. Therefore, the reflex is frequently called a *withdrawal reflex,* too.

Neuronal Mechanism of the Flexor Reflex. The left-hand portion of Figure 9–8 il-

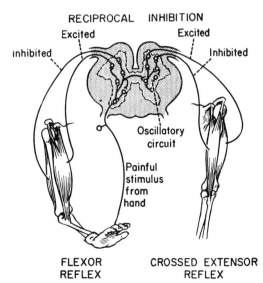

Figure 9–8. The flexor reflex, the crossed extensor reflex, and reciprocal inhibition.

lustrates the neuronal pathways for the flexor reflex. In this instance, a painful stimulus is applied to the hand; as a result, the flexor muscles of the upper arm become reflexly excited, thus withdrawing the hand from the painful stimulus.

The pathways for eliciting the flexor reflex do not pass directly to the anterior motoneurons but, instead, pass first into the interneuron pool of neurons and then to the motoneurons. The shortest possible circuit is a three- or four-neuron arc; however, most of the signals of the reflex traverse many more neurons than this and involve the following basic types of circuits: (1) diverging circuits to spread the reflex to the necessary muscles for withdrawal, (2) circuits to inhibit the antagonist muscles, called *reciprocal inhibition circuits,* and (3) circuits to cause a prolonged repetitive after-discharge even after the stimulus is over.

Figure 9–9 illustrates a typical myogram from a flexor muscle during a flexor reflex. Within a few milliseconds after a pain nerve is stimulated, the flexor response appears. Then, in the next few seconds the reflex begins to *fatigue,* which is characteristic of essentially all of the more complex integrative reflexes of the spinal cord. Then, soon after the stimulus is over, the contraction of the muscle begins to return toward the base line, but, because of *after-discharge,* will not return all the way for many milliseconds. The duration of the after-discharge depends on the intensity of the sensory stimulus that had elicited the reflex; a weak stimulus causes almost no after-discharge, in contrast to an after-discharge lasting for several seconds following a strong stimulus. Furthermore, a flexor reflex initiated by nonpainful stimuli and transmitted through the large sensory fibers causes essentially no after-discharge, whereas nociceptive impulses transmitted through the small type A fibers and type C fibers cause prolonged after-discharge.

The after-discharge that occurs in the flexor reflex almost certainly results from all three types of repetitive-discharge circuits that were discussed in Chapter 5. Electrophysiological studies indicate that the immediate after-discharge, lasting for about 6 to 8 milliseconds, results from the interneuron repetitive firing mechanism and from the parallel type of circuit, with impulses being transmitted from one interneuron to another to another and all these in turn transmitting their signals successively to the anterior motoneurons. However, the prolonged after-discharge that occurs following strong pain stimuli almost certainly involves reverberating circuits in the interneurons, these transmitting impulses to the anterior motoneurons sometimes for several seconds after the incoming sensory signal is completely over.

Thus, the flexor reflex is appropriately organized to withdraw a pained or otherwise irritated part of the body away from the stimulus. Furthermore, because of the after-discharge it will hold the irritated part away from the stimulus for as long as 1 to 3 seconds even after the irritation is over. During this time, other reflexes and actions of the central nervous system can move the entire body away from the painful stimulus.

The Pattern of Withdrawal.   The pattern of withdrawal that results when the flexor (or withdrawal) reflex is elicited depends on the sensory nerve that is stimulated. Thus, a painful stimulus on the inside of the arm not only elicits a flexor reflex in the arm but also contracts the abductor muscles to pull the arm outward. In other words, the integrative centers of the cord cause those muscles to contract that can most effectively remove the pained part of the body from the object that causes pain. This same principle applies for any part of the body but especially to the limbs, because they have highly developed flexor reflexes.

THE CROSSED EXTENSOR REFLEX

Approximately 0.2 to 0.5 second after a stimulus elicits a flexor reflex in one limb, the opposite limb begins to extend. This is called the *crossed extensor reflex.* Extension of the opposite limb obviously can push the entire body away from the object causing the painful stimulus.

Neuronal Mechanism of the Crossed Extensor Reflex.   The right-hand portion of Figure 9–8 illustrates the neuronal circuit responsible

Figure 9–9. Myogram of a flexor reflex, showing rapid onset of the reflex, an interval of fatigue, and finally after-discharge after the stimulus is over.

for the crossed extensor reflex, showing that signals from the sensory nerves cross to the opposite side of the cord to cause exactly opposite reactions to those that cause the flexor reflex. Because the crossed extensor reflex usually does not begin until 200 to 500 milliseconds following the initial pain stimulus, it is certain that many internuncial neurons are in the circuit between the incoming sensory neuron and the motoneurons of the opposite side of the cord responsible for the crossed extension. Furthermore, after the painful stimulus is removed, the crossed extensor reflex continues for an even longer period of after-discharge than that for the flexor reflex. Therefore, again, it is almost certain that this prolonged after-discharge results from reverberatory circuits among the internuncial cells.

Figure 9–10 illustrates a myogram recorded from a muscle involved in a crossed extensor reflex. This shows the relatively long latency before the reflex begins and also the very long after-discharge following the end of the stimulus. The prolonged after-discharge obviously would be of benefit in holding the entire body away from a painful object until other neurogenic reactions should cause the body to move away.

RECIPROCAL INNERVATION

In the foregoing paragraphs we have pointed out several times that excitation of one group of muscles is often associated with inhibition of another group. For instance, when a stretch reflex excites one muscle, it simultaneously inhibits the antagonist muscles. This is the phenomenon of *reciprocal inhibition,* and the neuronal mechanism that causes this reciprocal relationship is called *reciprocal innervation.* Likewise, reciprocal relationships exist between the two sides of the cord as exemplified

Figure 9–11. Myogram of a flexor reflex, illustrating crossed inhibition caused by a stronger flexor reflex in the opposite limb.

by the flexor and extensor reflexes as described above.

We will see below that the principle of reciprocal innervation is also important in most of the cord reflexes that subserve locomotion, for it helps to cause forward movement of one limb while causing backward movement of the opposite limb, and it also causes alternate movements between the forelimbs and the hindlimbs.

Figure 9–11 illustrates a typical example of reciprocal inhibition. In this instance, a moderate but prolonged flexor reflex is elicited from one limb of the body, and while this reflex is still being elicited a still stronger flexor reflex is elicited from the opposite limb, causing reciprocal inhibition of the first limb. Then removal of the strong flexor reflex allows the original reflex to reassume its previous intensity.

FATIGUE (DECREMENT) OF REFLEXES; REBOUND

Figure 9–9 illustrated that the flexor reflex begins to *fatigue* within a few seconds after its initiation. This is a common effect in most of the cord reflexes as well as many other reflexes of the central nervous system, and it presumably results from progressive fatigue of synaptic transmission in the reflex circuits, a subject that was discussed more fully in Chapter 4.

Another effect closely allied to fatigue is *rebound.* This means that, immediately after a reflex is over, a second reflex of the same type is much more difficult to elicit for a given time thereafter. However, because of reciprocal innervation, reflexes of the antagonist muscles become even more easily elicited during that same period of time. For instance, if a flexor reflex occurs in a left limb, a second flexor reflex is more difficult to establish for a few seconds thereafter, but a crossed extensor reflex in this same limb will be greatly exacerbated. Rebound is probably one of the important

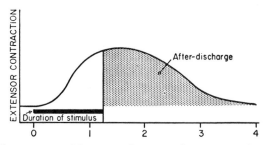

Figure 9–10. Myogram of a crossed extensor reflex, showing slow onset but prolonged after-discharge.

mechanisms by which the rhythmic to-and-fro movements required in locomotion are effected, which are described in more detail later in the chapter.

THE REFLEXES OF POSTURE AND LOCOMOTION

THE POSTURAL AND LOCOMOTIVE REFLEXES OF THE CORD

The Positive Supportive Reaction. Pressure on the footpad of a decerebrate animal causes the limb to extend against the pressure that is being applied to the foot. Indeed, this reflex is so strong an animal whose spinal cord has been transected for several months can often be placed on its feet, and the pressure on the footpads will reflexly stiffen the limbs sufficiently to support the weight of the body—the animal will stand in a rigid position. This reflex is called the *positive supportive reaction.*

The positive supportive reaction involves a complex circuit in the interneurons similar to those responsible for the flexor and the crossed-extensor reflexes. Furthermore, the locus of the pressure on the pad of the foot determines the position to which the limb is extended.

The Magnet Reaction. If pressure is applied on one side of the foot, the foot moves in that direction, or, if the pressure is applied forward, the foot moves forward, or, if it is applied backward, the foot moves backward. In this way, the bottom of the foot remains continuously extended toward the pressure that is being applied. This is called the magnet reaction, and it obviously could help in the maintenance of equilibrium, for, if an animal should tend to fall to one side, that side of the footpad would be stimulated, and the limb would automatically extend toward the falling side to push the body of the animal in the opposite direction.

The Cord "Righting" Reflexes. When a spinal cat or even a well-recovered young spinal dog is laid on its side, it will make incoordinate movements that indicate that it is trying to raise itself to the standing position. This is called a *cord righting reflex,* and it illustrates that relatively complicated reflexes associated with posture are at least partially integrated in the spinal cord. Indeed, a puppy with a well-healed transected thoracic cord caudal to the cord level for the forelegs can completely right itself from the lying position and can even walk on its hindlimbs. And, in the case of the opossum with a similar transection of the thoracic cord, the walking movements of the hindlimbs are hardly

different from those in the normal opossum—except that the hindlimb movements are not synchronized with those of the forelimbs as is normally the case.

The Rhythmic Stepping Reflex of a Single Limb. Rhythmic stepping movements are frequently observed in the limbs of spinal animals. Indeed, even when the lumbar portion of the spinal cord is separated from the remainder of the cord and a longitudinal section is made down the center of the cord to block neuronal connections between the two limbs, each hind limb can still perform stepping functions. Forward flexion of the limb is followed a second or so later by backward extension. Then flexion occurs again, and the cycle is repeated over and over.

This oscillation back and forth between the flexor and extensor muscles seems to result mainly from reciprocal inhibition and rebound. That is, the forward flexion of the limb causes reciprocal inhibition of extensor muscles, but shortly thereafter the flexion begins to die out; as it does so, *rebound* inhibition of the flexors and reciprocal excitation of the extensors cause the leg to move downward and backward. After extension has continued for a time, it, too, begins to die and is followed by reciprocal excitation of the flexor muscles.

Reciprocal Stepping of Opposite Limbs. If the lumbar spinal cord is not sectioned down its center as noted above, every time stepping occurs in the forward direction in one limb, the opposite limb ordinarily steps backward. This effect results from reciprocal innervation between the two limbs.

Diagonal Stepping of All Four Limbs—The "Mark Time" Reflex. If a well healed spinal animal is held up from the table and its legs are allowed to fall downward as illustrated in Figure 9–12, the stretch on the limbs occasionally elicits stepping reflexes that involve all four limbs. In general, stepping occurs diagonally between the fore- and hindlimbs. That is, the right hindlimb and the left forelimb move backward together while the right forelimb and left hindlimb move forward. This diagonal response is another manifestation of reciprocal innervation, this time occurring the entire distance up and down the cord between the fore- and hindlimbs. Such a walking pattern is often called a *mark time reflex.*

The Galloping Reflex. Another type of reflex that occasionally develops in the spinal animal is the galloping reflex, in which both forelimbs move backward in unison while both

Walking movement

Figure 9–12. Diagonal stepping movements exhibited by a spinal animal.

hindlimbs move forward. If stretch or pressure stimuli are applied almost exactly equally to opposite limbs at the same time, a galloping reflex will likely result, whereas unequal stimulation of one side versus the other elicits the diagonal walking reflex. This is in keeping with the normal patterns of walking and of galloping, for, in walking, only one limb at a time is stimulated, and this would predispose to continued walking. Conversely, when the animal strikes the ground during galloping, the limbs on both sides are stimulated approximately equally; this obviously would predispose to further galloping and, therefore, would continue this pattern of motion in contradistinction to the walking pattern.

THE SCRATCH REFLEX

An especially important cord reflex in lower animals is the scratch reflex, which is initiated by the *itch and tickle sensation*. It actually involves two different functions: (1) a *position sense* that allows the paw to find the exact point of irritation on the surface of the body and (2) a *to-and-fro scratching movement*.

Obviously, the scratch reflex, like the stepping movements of locomotion, involves reciprocal innervation circuits that cause oscillation. One of the important discoveries in relation to the to-and-fro movement of the scratch reflex is that it can still occur even when all the sensory roots from the oscillating limb are sectioned. In other words, feedback from the limb itself is not necessary to maintain the neuronal oscillation, which almost certainly means that the oscillation can occur intrinsically as a result of oscillating circuits within the spinal interneurons themselves.

The *position sense* of the scratch reflex is also a highly developed function, for even though a flea

might be crawling as far forward as the shoulder of a spinal animal, the hind paw can find its position. Furthermore, this can be accomplished even though 19 different muscles in the limb must be contracted simultaneously in a precise pattern to bring the paw to the exact position of the crawling flea. To make the reflex even more complicated, when the flea crosses the midline, the paw stops scratching, but the opposite paw suddenly begins the to-and-fro motion and finds the flea immediately.

THE SPINAL CORD REFLEXES THAT CAUSE MUSCLE SPASM

In human beings, local muscle spasm is often observed. The mechanism of this has not been elucidated to complete satisfaction even in experimental animals, but it is known that pain stimuli can cause reflex spasm of local muscles, which presumably is the cause of much if not most of the muscle spasm observed at localized regions of the human body.

Muscle Spasm Resulting from a Broken Bone. One type of clinically important spasm occurs in muscles surrounding a broken bone. This seems to result from the pain impulses initiated from the broken edges of the bone, which cause the muscles surrounding the area to contract powerfully and tonically. Relief of the pain by injection of a local anesthetic relieves the spasm; a general anesthetic also relieves the spasm. One of these procedures is often necessary before the spasm can be overcome sufficiently for the two ends of the bone to be set back into appropriate positions.

Abdominal Spasm in Peritonitis. Another type of local spasm caused by a cord reflex is the abdominal spasm resulting from irritation of the parietal peritoneum by peritonitis. Here, again, relief of the pain caused by the peritonitis allows the spastic muscles to relax. Almost the same type of spasm often occurs during surgical operations; pain impulses from the parietal peritoneum cause the abdominal muscles to contract extensively and sometimes actually to extrude the gut through the surgical wound. For this reason deep surgical anesthesia is usually required for intraabdominal operations.

Muscle Cramps. Still another type of local spasm is the typical muscle cramp. In the past this has been ascribed to local contraction of the muscle in response to abnormal metabolic end-products in the muscle itself. However, electromyographic studies indicate that the cause of at least some muscle cramps is the following:

Any local irritating factor or metabolic abnormality of a muscle—such as severe cold, lack of blood flow to the muscle, or overexercise of the muscle—can elicit pain or other types of sensory impulses that are transmitted from the muscle to the spinal cord, thus causing reflex muscle contraction. The contraction in turn stimulates the same sensory receptors still more, which causes the spinal cord to increase the intensity of contraction still further. Thus, a positive feedback mechanism occurs so that a small amount of initial irritation causes more and more contraction until a full-blown muscle cramp ensues. Reciprocal inhibition of the muscle can sometimes completely relieve the cramp. That is, if a person purposefully contracts the muscle on the opposite side of the joint from the cramped muscle while at the same time using another hand or leg to prevent movement of the joint, the reciprocal inhibition that occurs in the cramped muscle can at times relieve the cramp immediately.

THE AUTONOMIC REFLEXES IN THE SPINAL CORD

Many different types of segmental autonomic reflexes occur in the spinal cord, most of which are discussed in other chapters. Briefly, these include: (1) changes in vascular tone resulting from heat and cold, (2) sweating, which results from localized heat at the surface of the body, (3) intestino-intestinal reflexes that control some motor functions of the gut, (4) peritoneo-intestinal reflexes that inhibit gastric motility in response to peritoneal irritation, and (5) evacuation reflexes for emptying the bladder and the colon. In addition, all the segmental reflexes can at times be elicited simultaneously in the form of the so-called mass reflex as follows:

The Mass Reflex. In a spinal animal or human being, the spinal cord sometimes suddenly becomes excessively active, causing massive discharge of large portions of the cord. The usual stimulus that causes this is a strong nociceptive stimulus to the skin or excessive filling of a viscus, such as overdistention of the bladder or of the gut. Regardless of the type of stimulus, the resulting reflex, called the mass reflex, involves large portions or even all of the cord, and its pattern of reaction is the same. The effects are: (1) a major portion of the body goes into strong flexor spasm, (2) the colon and bladder are likely to evacuate, (3) the arterial pressure often rises to maximal values—sometimes to a mean pressure well over 200 mm. Hg, and (4) large areas of the body break out into profuse sweating. The mass reflex might be likened to the epileptic attacks that involve the central nervous system in which large portions of the brain become massively activated.

The precise neuronal mechanism of the mass reflex is unknown. However, since its duration is prolonged, it presumably results from activation of great masses of reverberating circuits that excite large areas of the cord at once.

SPINAL CORD TRANSECTION AND SPINAL SHOCK

When the spinal cord is suddenly transected, essentially all cord functions, including the cord re-

flexes, immediately become depressed to the point of oblivion, a reaction called *spinal shock*. The reason for this is that normal activity of the cord neurons depends to a great extent on continual tonic discharges from higher centers, particularly discharges transmitted through the vestibulospinal tract, the excitatory portions of the reticulospinal tracts, and the corticospinal tracts.

After a few days to a few months of spinal shock, the spinal neurons gradually regain their excitability. This seems to be a natural characteristic of neurons everywhere in the nervous system—that is, after they lose their source of facilitatory impulses, they increase their own natural degree of excitability to make up for the loss. In most nonprimates, the excitability of the cord centers returns essentially to normal within a few hours to a few weeks, but in man the return is often delayed for several months and occasionally is never complete; or, on the other hand, recovery is sometimes excessive, with resultant hyperexcitability of all or most cord functions.

Some of the spinal functions specifically affected during or following spinal shock are: (1) The arterial blood pressure falls immediately—sometimes to as low as 40 mm. Hg—thus illustrating that sympathetic activity becomes blocked almost to extinction. However, the pressure ordinarily returns to normal within a few days. (2) All skeletal muscle reflexes integrated in the spinal cord are completely blocked during the initial stages of shock. In lower animals, a few hours to three weeks are required for these reflexes to return to normal, and in man several months are often required. Sometimes, both in animals and man, some reflexes eventually become hyperexcitable, particularly if a few facilitatory pathways remain intact between the brain and the cord while the remainder of the spinal cord is transected. The first reflexes to return are the stretch reflex, followed in order by the progressively more complex reflexes, the flexor reflexes, the postural antigravity reflexes, and remnants of stepping reflexes. (3) The sacral reflexes for control of bladder and colon evacuation are completely suppressed in man for the first few weeks following cord transection, but they eventually return.

REFERENCES

Adams, E. B., Laurence, D. R., and Smith, J. W. G.: Tetanus. Philadelphia, J. B. Lippincott Company, 1969.

Banker, B. Q. (ed.): Research in Muscle Development and the Muscle Spindle. New York, American Elsevier Publishing Co., Inc., 1972.

Creed, R. S., Denny-Brown, D., Eccles, J. C., Liddell, E. G. T., and Sherrington, C. S.: Reflex Activity of the Spinal Cord. New York, Oxford University Press, Inc., 1932.

Easton, T. A.: On the normal use of reflexes. Amer. Sci., 60:591, 1972.

Gawronski, R. (ed.): Bionics: The Nervous System as a Control System. New York, American Elsevier Publishing Co., Inc., 1972.

Granit, R., Pompeiano, O., and Waltman, B.: First supraspinal control of mammalian muscle spindles: extra- and intrafusal co-activation. *J. Physiol. (Lond.)*, 147:385, 1959.

Granit, R.: Muscular tone, *J. Sport Med.*, 2:46, 1962.

Guttman, L.: Spinal Cord Injuries. Philadelphia, J. B. Lippincott Company, 1973.

Houk, J., and Henneman, E.: Responses of Golgi tendon organs to active contractions of the soleus muscle of the cat. *J. Neurophysiol.*, 30:466, 1967.

Hunt, C. C., and Perl, E. R.: Spinal reflex mechanisms concerned with skeletal muscle. *Physiol. Rev.*, 40:538, 1960.

Liddell, E. G. T.: The Discovery of Reflexes. New York, Oxford University Press, Inc., 1960.

Lippold, O.: Physiological tremor. *Sci. Amer.*, 224:65, 1971.

Lloyd, D. P.: Action in primary afferent fibers in the spinal cord. *Inter. J. Neurosci.*, 1:1, 1970.

Matthews, P. B. C.: Mammalian Muscle Receptors and Their Central Actions. Baltimore, The Williams & Wilkins Company, 1972.

Merton, P. A.: How we control the contraction of our muscles. *Sci. Amer.*, 226:30, 1972.

Porter, R.: The neurophysiology of movement performance. *In* Guyton, A. C. (ed.): MTP International Review of Science: Physiology. Vol. 3. Baltimore, University Park Press, 1974, p. 151.

Roberts, T. D. M.: Neurophysiology of Postural Mechanisms. New York, Plenum Publishing Corporation, 1967.

Sherrington, C. S.: The Integrative Action of the Nervous System. New Haven, Yale University Press, 1911.

Stein, R. B.: Peripheral control of movement. *Physiol. Rev.*, 54:215, 1974.

Wilson, D. M.: Genetic and sensory mechanisms for locomotion and orientation in animals. *Amer. Sci.*, 60:358, 1972.

See also bibliographies at the ends of Chapters 6 and 7.

10

Motor Functions of the Brain Stem and Basal Ganglia—Reticular Formation, Vestibular Apparatus, Equilibrium, and Brain Stem Reflexes

The brain stem is a complex extension of the spinal cord. Collected in it are numerous neuronal circuits to control respiration, cardiovascular function, gastrointestinal function, eye movement, equilibrium, support of the body against gravity, and many special stereotyped movements of the body. Some of these functions—such as control of respiration and cardiovascular functions—are described in special sections of this text. The present chapter deals primarily with the control of whole body movement and equilibrium.

THE RETICULAR FORMATION, AND SUPPORT OF THE BODY AGAINST GRAVITY

Throughout the entire extent of the brain stem—in the medulla, pons, mesencephalon, and even in portions of the diencephalon—are areas of diffuse neurons collectively known as the *reticular formation*. Figure 10–1 illustrates the extent of the reticular formation, showing it to begin at the upper end of the spinal cord and to extend (a) upward through the central portions of the thalamus, (b) into the hypothalamus, and (c) into other areas adjacent to the thalamus. The lower end of the reticular formation is continuous with the interneurons

of the spinal cord, and, indeed, the reticular formation of the brain stem functions in a manner quite analogous to many of the functions of the interneurons in the intermediolateral portions of the cord gray matter.

Interspersed throughout the reticular formation are both motor and sensory neurons; these vary in size from very small to very large. The small neurons, which constitute the greater number, have short axons that make multiple connections within the reticular formation itself. The large neurons are mainly motor in function, and their axons usually bifurcate almost immediately, with one division extending downward to the spinal cord and the other extending upward to the thalamus or other basal regions of the diencephalon or cerebrum. In general, the medial portions of the reticular formation tend to be more motor in function, whereas the more lateral portions tend to be either sensory or associative in function.

The sensory input to the reticular formation is from multiple sources, including: (1) the spinoreticular tracts and collaterals from the spinothalamic tracts, (2) the vestibular tracts, (3) the cerebellum, (4) the basal ganglia, (5) the cerebral cortex, especially the motor regions, and (6) the hypothalamus and other nearby associated areas.

Though most of the neurons in the reticular

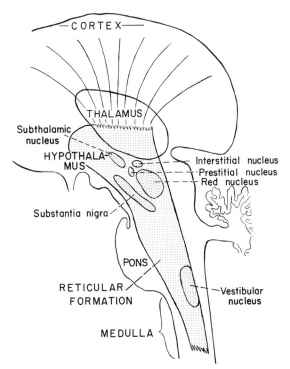

Figure 10–1. The reticular formation and associated nuclei.

formation are evenly dispersed, some of them are collected into *specific nuclei,* which are labeled in Figure 10–1. In general, these specific nuclei are not considered to be part of the reticular formation per se even though they do operate in association with it. In most instances they are the loci of "preprogrammed" control of stereotyped movements. As an example, the vestibular nuclei provide preprogrammed attitudinal contractions of the muscles for maintenance of equilibrium, as will be discussed later in the chapter.

EXCITATORY FUNCTION OF THE RETICULAR FORMATION—THE BULBORETICULAR FACILITATORY AREA

By far the majority of the reticular formation is excitatory, including especially the reticular formation in the uppermost and lateral parts of the medulla and all of that in the pons, mesencephalon, and diencephalon. These areas are known collectively as the *bulboreticular facilitatory area.* Diffuse stimulation in this facilitatory area causes a general increase in muscle tone either throughout the body or in localized areas.

The bulboreticular facilitatory area and also the vestibular nuclei, which are really also part of the facilitatory system, are intrinsically excitable. That is, if they are not inhibited by signals from other parts of the nervous system, they have a natural tendency to transmit continuous nerve impulses both downward to the motor areas of the cord and upward to the cerebrum. But, in the normal animal, inhibitory signals are continually available from the basal ganglia, the cerebellum, and the cerebral cortex to keep the facilitatory system from becoming overactive. As will be noted later in the chapter in the discussion of the decerebrate animal, removal of the higher portions of the nervous system removes this inhibition and allows the reticular facilitatory area to become tonically active, which causes rigidity of the extensor, anti-gravity skeletal muscles throughout the body.

On the other hand, when the brain stem is sectioned at a level slightly lower than the vestibular nuclei, most of the motor functions of the reticular facilitatory area are then blocked, which causes almost all the musculature throughout the body to become totally flaccid.

INHIBITORY FUNCTION OF THE LOWER RETICULAR FORMATION—THE BULBORETICULAR INHIBITORY AREA

A small portion of the reticular formation located in the ventral medial region of the lower three-fourths of the medulla has potent inhibitory functions and is known as the *bulboreticular inhibitory area.* Diffuse stimulation in this area causes decreased tone in most musculature of the body. The bulboreticular inhibitory area is not itself intrinsically excitable. However, signals arrive in this area almost all the time from the basal ganglia, the cerebral cortex, and the cerebellum to keep it excited.

The inhibitory effect of the bulboreticular inhibitory area is continually pitted against the excitatory effect of the bulboreticular facilitatory area. Consequently, when the two areas are both functioning normally, the motor functions of the spinal cord are neither excited nor inhibited. But if the excitation of the inhibitory area from the basal ganglia, cerebral cortex, and cerebellum is removed or even partially removed, then the inhibitory area becomes less active and facilitation predominates. Indeed, this is one of the usual causes of spasticity of the muscles throughout the body after a major part of the brain has been destroyed by a cerebral infarct.

SUPPORT OF THE BODY AGAINST GRAVITY

When a person or an animal is in a standing position, continuous impulses are transmitted from the reticular formation and from closely allied nuclei, particularly from the vestibular nuclei, into the spinal cord and thence to the extensor muscles to stiffen the limbs. This allows the limbs to support the body against gravity. These impulses are transmitted mainly by way of the reticulospinal and vestibulospinal tracts.

The normal excitatory nature of the vestibular nuclei and of the bulboreticular facilitatory area provides much of the intrinsic excitation required to maintain tone in the extensor muscles. However, the degree of activity in the individual extensor muscles is determined by the equilibrium mechanisms. Thus, if an animal begins to fall to one side, the extensor muscles on that side stiffen while those on the opposite side relax. And analogous effects occur when it tends to fall forward or backward.

In essence, then, the reticular facilitatory system provides the nervous energy to support the body against gravity. But other factors, particularly the vestibular apparatuses, control the relative degree of extensor contraction in the different parts of the body, which provides the function of equilibrium.

VESTIBULAR SENSATIONS AND THE MAINTENANCE OF EQUILIBRIUM

THE VESTIBULAR APPARATUS

The vestibular apparatus is the sensory organ that detects sensations concerned with equilibrium. It is composed of a *bony labyrinth* containing the *membranous labyrinth,* the functional part of the apparatus. The top of Figure 10–2 illustrates the membranous labyrinth; it is composed mainly of the *cochlear duct,* the three *semicircular canals,* and the two large chambers known as the *utricle* and the *saccule.* The cochlear duct is concerned with hearing and has nothing to do with equilibrium. However, the *utricle,* the *saccule,* and the *semicircular canals* are especially important for maintaining equilibrium.

MEMBRANOUS LABYRINTH

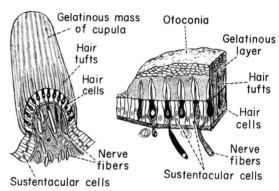

CRISTA AMPULLARIS AND MACULA

Figure 10–2. The membranous labyrinth, and organization of the crista ampullaris and the macula. (From Goss: Gray's Anatomy of the Human Body. Lea & Febiger; modified from Kolmer by Buchanan: Functional Neuroanatomy. Lea & Febiger.)

The Utricle and the Saccule. Located on the wall of both the utricle and the saccule is a small area slightly over 2 mm. in diameter called a *macula.* Each of these maculae is a sensory area for detecting the orientation of the head with respect to the direction of gravitational pull or of other acceleratory forces, as will be explained in subsequent sections of this chapter. Each macula is covered by a gelatinous layer in which many small calcium carbonate crystals called *otoconia* are imbedded. Also, in the macula are thousands of *hair cells,* which project *cilia* up into the gelatinous layer. Around the bases of the hair cells are entwined sensory axons of the vestibular nerve.

Even under resting conditions, most of the

nerve fibers surrounding the hair cells transmit a continuous series of nerve impulses. Bending the cilia of a hair cell to one side causes the impulse traffic in its nerve fibers to increase markedly; bending the cilia to the opposite side decreases the impulse traffic, often turning it off completely. Therefore, as the orientation of the head in space changes and the weight of the otoconia (whose specific gravity is about three times that of the surrounding tissues) bends the cilia, appropriate signals are transmitted to the brain to control equilibrium.

In each macula the different hair cells are oriented in different directions so that some of them are stimulated when the head bends forward, some when it bends backward, others when it bends to one side, and so forth. Therefore, a different pattern of excitation occurs in the macula for each position of the head; it is this "pattern" that apprises the brain of the head's orientation.

The Semicircular Canals. The three semicircular canals in each vestibular apparatus, known respectively as the *superior, posterior,* and *external* (or *horizontal*) *semicircular canals,* are arranged at right angles to each other so that they represent all three planes in space. When the head is bent forward approximately 30 degrees, the two external semicircular canals are located approximately horizontal with respect to the surface of the earth. The superior canals are then located in vertical planes that project *forward and 45 degrees outward,* and the posterior canals are also in vertical planes but project *backward and 45 degrees outward.* Thus, the superior canal on each side of the head is in a plane parallel to that of the posterior canal on the opposite side of the head, whereas the two external canals on the two sides are located in approximately the same plane.

In the *ampullae* of the semicircular canals, as illustrated in Figure 10–2, are small crests, each called a *crista ampullaris,* and on top of the crista is a gelatinous mass similar to that in the utricle and known as the *cupula.* Into the cupula are projected hairs from hair cells located along the ampullary crest, and these hair cells in turn are connected to sensory nerve fibers that pass into the *vestibular nerve.* Bending the cupula to one side, caused by flow of fluid in the canal, stimulates the hair cells, while bending in the opposite direction inhibits them. Thus, appropriate signals are sent through the vestibular nerve to apprise the central nervous system of fluid movement in the respective canal.

Recent experiments indicate that the upper end of the cupula is either attached or semi-attached to the opposite side of the ampulla and therefore might not bend as a whole unit as illustrated in Figure 10–2. Instead, the fluid accumulating on one side of the cupula simply bulges the structure in the opposite direction as if it were a diaphragm. Because of this, the hair cells in the center of the cupula will be stimulated much more powerfully at first, whereas the more lateral hair cells will be stimulated progressively more powerfully as the cupula bulges still more. This effect may account for the tremendous range of acceleration that can be detected accurately by the semicircular canal system.

Directional Sensitivity of the Hair Cells— The Kinocilium. Each hair cell has a large number of very small cilia plus one very large cilium called the *kinocilium.* This kinocilium is located to one side of the hair cell, always on the same side of the cell with respect to its orientation on the ampullary crest. This presumably is the cause of the directional sensitivity of the hair cells: namely, stimulation when the hairs are bent in one direction and inhibition when bent in the opposite direction.

Neuronal Connections of the Vestibular Apparatus with the Central Nervous System. Figure 10–3 illustrates the central connections of the vestibular nerve. Most of the vestibular nerve fibers end in the vestibular nuclei, which are located approximately at the junction of the medulla and the pons, but some fibers pass without synapsing to the fastigial nuclei, uvula, and flocculonodular lobes of the cerebellum. The fibers that end in the vestibular nuclei synapse with second order neurons that in turn send fibers into the flocculonodular lobe of the cerebellum, to the cortex of other portions of the cerebellum, into the vestibulospinal tract, into the medial

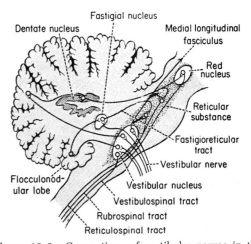

Figure 10–3. Connections of vestibular nerves in the central nervous system.

longitudinal fasciculus, and to other areas of the brain stem, particularly the reticular nuclei.

Note especially the very close association between the vestibular apparatus, the vestibular nuclei, and the cerebellum. The primary pathway for the reflexes of equilibrium begins in the vestibular nerves and passes next to both the vestibular nuclei and the cerebellum. Then, after much two-way traffic of impulses between these two, signals are sent into the reticular nuclei of the brain stem as well as down the spinal cord via vestibulospinal and reticulospinal tracts. In turn, the signals to the cord control the interplay between facilitation and inhibition of the extensor muscles, thus automatically controlling equilibrium.

The *flocculonodular lobes* of the cerebellum seem to be especially concerned with equilibrium functions of the semicircular canals because destruction of these lobes gives almost exactly the same clinical symptoms as destruction of the semicircular canals themselves. That is, severe injury to either of these structures causes loss of equilibrium during *rapid changes in direction of motion* but does not disturb equilibrium under static conditions, as will be discussed in subsequent sections. It is also believed that the uvula of the cerebellum plays an important role in static equilibrium.

Signals transmitted upward in the brain stem from both the vestibular nuclei and the cerebellum via the *medial longitudinal fasciculus* cause corrective movements of the eyes every time the head rotates so that the eyes can remain fixed on a specific visual object. Signals also pass upward (either through this same tract or through reticular tracts) to the cerebral cortex, probably terminating in a primary cortical center for equilibrium located near the auditory area of the superior temporal gyrus. These signals apprise the psyche of the equilibrium status of the body.

FUNCTION OF THE UTRICLE AND THE SACCULE IN THE MAINTENANCE OF STATIC EQUILIBRIUM

It is especially important that the different hair cells be oriented in all different directions in the maculae of the utricles and saccules so that at different positions of the head, different hair cells become stimulated. The "patterns" of stimulation of the different hair cells apprise the nervous system of the position of the head with respect to the pull of gravity. In turn, the vestibular, cerebellar, and reticular motor systems reflexly excite the appropriate muscles to maintain proper equilibrium.

The maculae in the utricle and saccule are especially attuned to detecting the precise position of the head with respect to the pull of gravity when the head is in the near-vertical position. That is, a person can determine as little as ½ degree mal-equilibrium when the head leans from the precise upright position. On the other hand, as the head is leaned further and further from the upright, the determination of head orientation by the vestibular sense becomes poorer and poorer. Obviously, extreme sensitivity in the upright position is of major importance for maintenance of precise vertical static equilibrium, which is the most essential function of the vestibular apparatus.

Detection of Linear Acceleration by the Utricle. When the body is suddenly thrust forward, the otoconia, which have greater inertia than the surrounding fluids, fall backward on the hair cilia, and information of mal-equilibrium is sent into the nervous centers causing the individual to feel as if he were falling backward. This automatically causes him to lean his body forward until the anterior shift of the otoconia exactly equals the tendency for the otoconia to fall backward because of the linear acceleration. At this point, the nervous system detects a state of proper equilibrium and therefore shifts the body no farther forward. As long as the degree of linear acceleration remains constant and the body is maintained in this forward leaning position, the person falls neither forward nor backward. Thus, the otoconia operate to maintain equilibrium during linear acceleration in exactly the same manner as they operate in static equilibrium.

The otoconia *do not* operate for the detection of linear *motion*. When a runner first begins to run, he must lean far forward to keep from falling over backward because of acceleration, but once he has achieved running speed, he would not have to lean forward at all if he were running in a vacuum. When running in air he leans forward to maintain equilibrium only because of the air resistance against his body, and in this instance it is not the otoconia that make him lean but the pressure of the air acting on pressure end-organs in the skin, which initiate the appropriate equilibrium adjustments to prevent falling.

THE SEMICIRCULAR CANALS AND THEIR DETECTION OF ANGULAR ACCELERATION AND ANGULAR VELOCITY

When the head suddenly *begins* to rotate in any direction, the endolymph in the membranous semicircular canals, because of its inertia, tends to remain stationary while the semicircular canals themselves turn. This causes relative fluid flow in the canals in a direction opposite to the rotation of the head.

Figure 10–4 illustrates an *ampulla* of one of the semicircular canals, showing the *capula* and its embedded hairs bending in the direction of fluid movement. And Figure 10–5 illustrates the discharge signal from a single hair cell in the crista ampullaris when an animal is rotated for 40 seconds, showing that (1) even when the cupula is in its resting position the hair cell emits a tonic discharge of approximately 15 impulses per second; (2) when the animal is rotated, the hairs bend to one side and the rate of discharge increases greatly; and (3) with continued rotation, the excess discharge of the hair cell gradually subsides back to the resting level in about 20 seconds.

The reason for this adaptation of the receptor is that within a second or more of rotation, friction in the semicircular canal causes the endolymph to rotate as rapidly as the semicircular canal itself; then in an additional 15 to 20 seconds the cupula slowly returns to its resting position in the middle of the ampulla.

When the rotation suddenly stops, exactly the opposite effects take place: the endolymph continues to rotate while the semicircular canal stops. This time the cupula is bent in the opposite direction, causing the hair cell to stop discharging entirely. After another few seconds, the endolymph stops moving, and the cupula returns gradually to its resting position in about 20 seconds, thus allowing the discharge of the hair cell to return to its normal tonic level as shown to the right in Figure 10–5.

Thus, the semicircular canal transmits a signal when the head *begins* to rotate and a negative signal when it *stops* rotating. Furthermore,

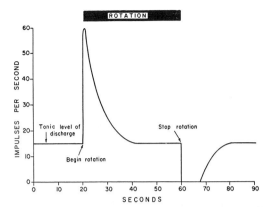

Figure 10–5. Response of a hair cell when a semicircular canal is stimulated first by rotation and then by stopping rotation.

at least some hair cells will always respond to rotation in any plane—horizontal, sagittal, or coronal—for fluid movement always occurs in at least one semicircular canal.

Detection of Angular Acceleration and Angular Velocity. Angular velocity means the rate of rotation; that is, it is the number of revolutions about an axis in a given period of time. Angular acceleration means the rate at which the angular velocity is changing.

The semicircular canals always give a person a feeling of increasing rotation when he begins to rotate or a feeling of decreasing rotation when he stops rotating—that is, they give a signal for angular acceleration. Therefore, it is commonly stated that the semicircular canals are primarily a detector of angular acceleration. However, a person also continues to feel that he is rotating for 15 to 30 seconds after he has begun to rotate. That is, he feels angular velocity during this period of time. Therefore, the semicircular canals actually detect a combination of angular acceleration and angular velocity, although the angular velocity effect may last only for 15 to 30 seconds.

To explain these effects, let us refer again to Figure 10–5. This shows that the hair cell of the semicircular canal detects neither pure angular velocity nor pure angular acceleration but, instead, detects a combination of these two. Angular acceleration occurs at the onset of the rotation, and negative angular acceleration occurs when the rotation stops. Therefore, if the signal depicted only angular acceleration, there would be a positive spike at the onset and a negative spike at the offset, but the signal would be at baseline level at all other times. On the other hand, if the hair cell detected only angular velocity, there would be a positive signal of the same intensity during the entire period of rotation. Note that the actual record of Figure 10–5 is a combination of these two types of records.

Rate of Angular Acceleration Required to Stimulate the Semicircular Canals. The angular

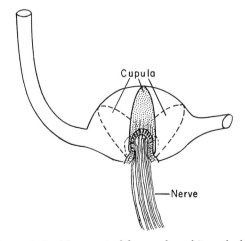

Figure 10–4. Movement of the cupula and its embedded hairs during rotation first in one direction and then in the opposite direction.

acceleration required to stimulate the semicircular canals in the human being averages about 1 degree per second per second. In other words, when one begins to rotate, his velocity of rotation must be as much as 1 degree per second by the end of the first second, 2 degrees per second by the end of the second second, 3 degrees per second by the end of the third second, and so forth, in order for him barely to detect that his rate of rotation is increasing.

"Predictive" Function of the Semicircular Canals in the Maintenance of Equilibrium. Since the semicircular canals do not detect that the body is off balance in the forward direction, in the side direction, or in the backward direction, one might at first ask: What is the function of the semicircular canals in the maintenance of equilibrium? All they detect is that the person's head is beginning to rotate or is stopping rotation in one direction or another. Therefore, the function of the semicircular canals is not likely to be to maintain static equilibrium or to maintain equilibrium during linear acceleration or when the person is exposed to steady centrifugal forces. Yet loss of function of the semicircular canals causes a person to have poor equilibrium, especially when he attempts to perform *rapid* and *intricate* body movements.

We can explain the function of the semicircular canals best by the following illustration. If a person is running forward rapidly, and then suddenly begins to turn to one side, he falls off balance a second or so later unless appropriate corrections are made *ahead of time*. But, unfortunately, the utricle cannot detect that he is off balance until *after* this has occurred. On the other hand, the semicircular canals will have already detected that the person is beginning to turn, and this information can easily apprise the central nervous system of the fact that the person *will* fall off balance within the next second or so unless some correction is made. In other words, the semicircular canal mechanism *predicts ahead of time* that mal-equilibrium is going to occur even before it occurs and thereby causes the equilibrium centers to make appropriate preventive adjustments. In this way, the person need not fall off balance before he begins to correct the situation.

Removal of the flocculonodular lobes of the cerebellum prevents normal function of the semicircular canals but does not prevent normal function of the macular receptors. It is especially interesting in this connection that the cerebellum serves as a "predictive" organ for most of the other rapid movements of the body as well as those having to do with equilibrium.

These other functions of the cerebellum are discussed in the following chapter.

VESTIBULAR REFLEXES

The Vestibular Phasic Postural Reflexes. Sudden changes in the orientation of an animal in space elicits reflexes that help to maintain equilibrium and posture. For instance, if an animal is suddenly pushed to the right, even before he can fall more than a few degrees his right legs extend instantaneously. In other words, this mechanism *anticipates* that the animal will be off balance in a few seconds and makes appropriate adjustments to prevent this.

Another type of vestibular phasic postural reflex occurs when the animal's head suddenly falls downward. When this occurs, the forepaws extend forward, the extensor muscles tighten, and the muscles in the back of the neck stiffen to prevent the animal's head from striking the ground. This reflex is probably also of importance in locomotion, for, in the case of the galloping horse, the downward thrust of the head could automatically provide reflex thrust of the forelimbs to move the animal forward for the next gallop.

The Vestibular "Righting" Reflex and Equilibrium. In the previous chapter it was pointed out that some of the crude motions required to move an animal from a lying to a standing position can be elicited by circuits in the spinal cord. However, these *cord* "righting" reflexes cannot perform the full function of righting an animal to the upright position without signals from the brain stem. The static equilibrium organs, the maculae of the utricle and saccule, transmit impulses into the brain stem to apprise the nervous system of the status of the animal with respect to the pull of gravity, and, if the animal is in a lying position, these can elicit appropriate reflexes from the vestibular and reticular nuclei to cause the animal to climb to his feet. This is called the vestibular righting reflex.

This vestibular righting reflex requires neuronal centers in all parts of the brain stem up to as high as and including the mesencephalon.

VESTIBULAR MECHANISM FOR STABILIZING THE EYES AND FOR NYSTAGMUS

When a person changes his direction of movement rapidly, or even leans his head sideways, forward, or backward, it would be impossible for him to maintain a stable image on the retinae of his eyes unless he had some automatic control mechanism to stabilize the direction of gaze of the eyes. In addition, the eyes would be of little use in detecting an image unless they remained "fixed" on each object long enough to gain a clear image. Fortunately, each time the head is angulated, signals from the semicircular canals cause the eyes to angulate in an equal and opposite direction to the angulation of the head. This results from reflexes transmitted through the *vestibular nuclei,* the *cerebellum,* and the *medial longitudinal fasciculus* to the *ocular nuclei.*

A special example of this stabilization of the eyes occurs when a person begins to rotate. At first the eyes remain glued to the object. But after the head has rotated far to one side, they jump suddenly in the direction of rotation of the head and "fix" on a new object; then they deviate slowly backward again as the rotation proceeds. This sudden jumping motion forward and then slow backward motion is known as *nystagmus.* The jumping motion is called the *fast component* of the nystagmus, and the slow movement is called the *slow component.*

Nystagmus always occurs automatically when the semicircular canals are stimulated. For instance, if a person's head begins to rotate to the right, backward movement of fluid in the left horizontal canal and forward movement in the right horizontal canal cause the eyes to move slowly to the left; thus, the slow component of nystagmus is initiated by the vestibular apparatuses. But, when the eyes have moved as far to the left as they reasonably can, centers located in the brain stem in close approximation with the nuclei of the abducens nerves cause the eyes to jump suddenly to the right; then the vestibular apparatuses take over once more to move the eyes again slowly to the left.

CLINICAL TESTS FOR INTEGRITY OF VESTIBULAR FUNCTION

Balancing Test. One of the simplest clinical tests for integrity of the equilibrium mechanism is to have the individual stand perfectly still with his eyes closed. If he no longer has a functioning static equilibrium system of the utricles, he will waiver to one side or the other and possibly even fall. However, as noted below, some of the proprioceptive mechanisms of equilibrium are occasionally sufficiently well developed to maintain balance even with the eyes closed.

Barany Test. A second test that is frequently performed determines the integrity of the semicircular canals. In this instance the individual is placed in a "Barany chair" and rotated rapidly while he places his head respectively in various planes—first forward, then angulated to one side or the other. By such positioning, each pair of semicircular canals is successively placed in the horizontal plane of rotation. When the rotation of the chair is stopped suddenly, the endolymph, because of its momentum, continues to rotate in the pair of semicircular canals that has been placed in the horizontal plane, this flow of endolymph causing the cupula to bend in the direction of rotation. As a result, nystagmus occurs, with the slow component in the direction of rotation and the fast component in the opposite direction. Also, as long as the nystagmus lasts (about 15 to 20 seconds) the individual has the sensation that he is rotating in

the direction *opposite* to that in which he was actually rotated in the chair. Obviously, this test checks the semicircular canals on both sides of the head at the same time.

Ice Water Test. A clinical test for testing one vestibular apparatus separately from the other depends on placing ice water in one ear. The external semicircular canal lies adjacent to the ear, and cooling the ear can transfer a sufficient amount of heat from this canal to cool the endolymph. This increases the density of the endolymph, thereby causing it to sink downward and resulting in slight movement of fluid around the semicircular canal. This stimulates the canal, giving the individual a sensation of rotating and also initiating nystagmus. From these two findings one can determine whether the respective semicircular canals are functioning properly. When the semicircular canals are normal, the utricles and saccules are usually normal also, for disease usually destroys the function of all of these components at the same time.

OTHER FACTORS CONCERNED WITH EQUILIBRIUM

The Neck Proprioceptors. The vestibular apparatus detects the orientation and movements *only of the head.* Therefore, it is essential that the nervous centers also receive appropriate information depicting the orientation of the head with respect to the body as well as the orientation of the different parts of the body with respect to each other. This information is transmitted from the proprioceptors of the neck and body both directly into the reticular nuclei of the brain stem and indirectly by way of the cerebellum and thence into the reticular nuclei.

By far the most important proprioceptive information needed for the maintenance of equilibrium is that derived from the *joint receptors of the neck,* for this apprises the nervous system of the orientation of the head with respect to the body. When the head is bent in one direction or the other, impulses from the neck proprioceptors keep the vestibular apparatuses from giving the person a sense of mal-equilibrium. They do this by transmitting signals that exactly oppose the signals transmitted from the vestibular apparatuses. However, *when the entire body* is changed to a new position with respect to gravity, the impulses from the vestibular apparatuses *are not opposed* by the neck proprioceptors; therefore, the person in this instance does perceive a change in equilibrium status.

The Neck Reflexes. In an animal *whose vestibular apparatuses have been destroyed,* bending the neck causes immediate muscular reflexes called *neck reflexes* occurring especially in the forelimbs. For instance, bending the head forward causes both forelimbs to relax. However, when the vestibular apparatuses are *intact,* this effect does *not* occur because the vestibular reflexes function almost exactly oppositely to the neck reflexes. Thus, if the head is flexed downward, the vestibular reflex tends to extend the forelimbs, while the neck reflexes tend to relax them. Since the equilibrium of the entire body and not of the head alone must be maintained, it is easy to understand that the vestibular and neck reflexes must function oppositely. Otherwise, each time the neck should bend, the animal would immediately fall off balance.

Proprioceptive and Exteroceptive Information from Other Parts of the Body. Proprioceptive information from other parts of the body besides the neck is also necessary for maintenance of equilibrium because appropriate equilibrium adjustments must be made whenever the body is angulated in the chest or abdomen region or elsewhere. Presumably, all this information is algebraically added in the cerebellum and reticular substance of the brain stem, thus causing appropriate adjustments in the postural muscles.

Also important in the maintenance of equilibrium are several types of exteroceptive sensations. For instance, pressure sensations from the footpads can tell one (a) whether his weight is distributed equally between his two feet and (b) whether his weight is more forward or backward on his feet.

Another instance in which exteroceptive information is necessary for maintenance of equilibrium occurs when a person is running. The air pressure against the front of his body signals that a force is opposing the body in a direction different from that caused by gravitational pull; as a result, the person leans forward to oppose this.

Importance of Visual Information in the Maintenance of Equilibrium. After complete destruction of the vestibular apparatuses, and even after loss of most proprioceptive information from the body, a person can still use his visual mechanisms effectively for maintaining equilibrium. Visual images help the person maintain equilibrium simply by visual detection of the upright stance. Also, slight linear or angular movement of the body instantaneously shifts the visual images on the retina, and this information is relayed to the equilibrium centers. In this respect the optic information is similar to that from the semicircular canals and can help the equilibrium centers predict that the person will fall off balance before this actually occurs if appropriate adjustments are not immediately made. Many persons with complete destruction of the vestibular apparatus have almost normal equilibrium as long as their eyes are open and as long as they perform all motions slowly. But, when moving rapidly or when the eyes are closed, equilibrium is immediately lost.

Conscious Perception of Equilibrium. A cortical center for conscious perception of the state of equilibrium is believed to lie in the upper portion of the temporal lobe in close association with the primary cortical area for hearing. The sensations from the vestibular apparatuses, from the neck proprioceptors, and from most of the other proprioceptors are probably first integrated in the equilibrium centers of the brain stem before being transmitted to the cerebral cortex. Various pathologic processes in the vestibular apparatuses or in the vestibular

neuronal circuits often affect the equilibrium sensations. Thus, loss of one or both flocculonodular lobes or one of both fastigial nuclei of the cerebellum gives the person a sensation of constant mal-equilibrium, or at least this feeling lingers for the first few weeks or months after the loss. This probably results because impulses from these cerebellar areas are normally integrated into the subconscious sense of equilibrium by the reticular nuclei even before equilibrium information is sent to the cerebral cortex.

FUNCTIONS OF THE RETICULAR FORMATION AND SPECIFIC BRAIN STEM NUCLEI IN CONTROLLING SUBCONSCIOUS, STEREOTYPED MOVEMENTS

Rarely, a child called an anencephalic monster is born without brain structures above the mesencephalic region, and some of these children have been kept alive for many months. Such a child is able to perform essentially all the functions of feeding, such as suckling, extrusion of unpleasant food from the mouth, and moving his hands to his mouth to suck his fingers. In addition, he can yawn and stretch. He can cry and follow objects with his eyes and by movements of his head. Also, placing pressure on the upper anterior parts of his legs will cause him to pull to the sitting position.

Therefore, it is obvious that many of the stereotyped motor functions of the human being are integrated in the brain stem. Unfortunately, the loci of most of these different motor control systems have not been found except for the following:

Stereotyped Body Movements. Most movements of the trunk and head can be classified into several simple movements, such as forward flexion, extension, rotation, and turning movements of the entire body. These types of movements are controlled by special nuclei located mainly in the mesencephalic and lower diencephalic region. For instance, *rotational movements* of the head and eyes are controlled by the *interstitial nucleus,* which is illustrated in Figure 10–1. This nucleus lies in close approximation to the *medial longitudinal fasciculus,* through which it transmits a major portion of its control impulses. The *raising movements* of the head and body are controlled by the *prestitial nucleus,* which is located approximately at the juncture of the diencephalon and mesencephalon. On the other hand, the *flexing movements* of the head and body are controlled by the *nucleus precommissuralis* located at the level of the posterior commissure. Finally, the *turning movements* of the entire body, which are much more complicated, involve both the pontile and mesencephalic reticular formation. However, for full expression of the turning movements, the caudate nucleus and the cingulate gyrus of the cerebral cortex are also required. The turning movements can cause an animal or person to continue circling around and around in one direction or the other.

Function of the Red Nucleus. The red nucleus is composed of two distinct parts, the *magnocellular portion* and a *small cellular portion*.

As illustrated in Figure 10–6, the magnocellular nuclei receive impulses both from the *caudate nucleus* and the *putamen* as well as from the *prestitial nucleus* and the *nucleus commissuralis*. In turn it transmits signals by way of the *rubrospinal tract* into the spinal cord and by way of collaterals from the rubrospinal tract into the *reticular nuclei* of the brain stem. Stimulation of this portion of the red nucleus causes the head and upper trunk to extend backward. Thus, this portion of the red nucleus enters into a particular type of gross body movement concerned with forward and backward deviation of the body axis.

The small cells of the red nucleus are excited principally by impulses from the *cerebellum* through the *cerebellorubral tracts*. In turn, they send impulses mainly into the reticular formation of the brain stem. These tracts are part of the overall cerebellar mechanism for control of motor function, which will be discussed in the following chapter.

Function of the Subthalamic Areas—Forward Progression. Much less is known about function of higher brain stem centers in posture and locomotion than of the lower centers, principally because of the complexity of the neuronal connections. However, it is known that stimulation of centers in or around the subthalamic nuclei can cause rhythmic motions, including crude forward walking reflexes. This does not mean that the individual muscles of walking are necessarily controlled from this region but simply that excitation of this region excites the appropriate patterns of action in the brain stem and cord to cause the walking movements.

A cat with its brain transected beneath the thalamus but above the subthalamus can walk in an almost completely normal fashion—so much so that the observer cannot tell the difference. However, when the animal comes to an obstruction it simply butts its head against the obstruction and tries to keep on walking. Thus, it lacks *purposefulness of locomotion.*

The function of the subthalamic region in walking is frequently described as that of controlling *forward progression.* In the foregoing discussions we have already noted that a decerebrate animal can stand perfectly well and that it can make attempts to right itself from the lying position. Unfortunately, though, the decerebrate animal, with the brain stem sectioned below the subthalamus cannot force itself to move forward in a normal walking pattern. This seems to be the function of areas either in or somewhere close to the subthalamic nuclei.

MOTOR FUNCTIONS OF THE BASAL GANGLIA

Physiologic Anatomy of the Basal Ganglia. The anatomy of the basal ganglia is so complex and is so poorly known in its details that it would be pointless to attempt a complete description at this time. However, Figure 10–6 illustrates the principal structures of the basal ganglia and their neural connections with other parts of the nervous system. Anatomically, the basal ganglia are the *caudate nucleus, putamen, globus pallidus, amygdaloid nucleus,* and *claustrum.* The amygdaloid nucleus, which will be discussed in Chapter 57, and the claustrum are not concerned directly with motor functions of the central nervous system. On the other hand, the *thalamus, subthalamus, substantia nigra,* and *red nucleus* all operate in close association with the caudate nucleus, putamen, and globus pallidus and are considered to be part of the basal ganglia system for motor control.

Some important features of the different pathways illustrated in Figure 10–6 are the following:

1. Numerous nerve pathways pass from the motor portions of the cerebral cortex, particularly the so-called premotor areas, to the caudate nucleus and putamen, which together are called the *striate body.* In turn, the caudate nucleus and putamen send numerous fibers to the globus pallidus, the globus pallidus to the ventroanterior nucleus of the thalamus, and this nucleus back to the motor areas of the cerebral cortex. Thus, circular pathways are established from the motor cortical regions to the basal ganglia, the thalamus, and back to the same motor regions from which the pathways begin. These circuits obviously could operate as a feedback system of the servo control type, as will be discussed later.

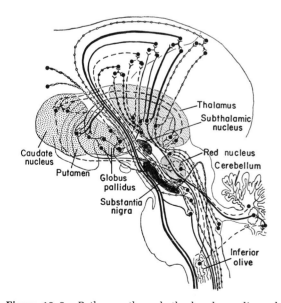

Figure 10–6. Pathways through the basal ganglia and related structures of brain stem, the thalamus, and cerebral cortex. (From Jung and Hassler: Handbook of Physiology, Sec. I, Vol. II, The Williams & Wilkins Co., 1960.)

2. In the following chapter it will be noted that signals also pass from the motor regions of the cerebral cortex to the pons and then into the cerebellum. In turn, signals from the cerebellum are transmitted back to the motor cortex by way of the ventrolateral nucleus of the thalamus, a nucleus closely associated with the ventroanterior thalamic nucleus through which the basal ganglial signals are transmitted. This circuit could allow integration between the basal ganglial feedback signals and the feedback signals from the cerebellum.

3. The basal ganglia have numerous short neuronal connections among themselves. Also, the lower basal ganglia, such as the globus pallidus, send tremendous numbers of nerve fibers into the lower brain stem, projecting especially onto the reticular nuclei, the red nucleus, and the inferior olive. It is presumably through these pathways that many of the so-called extrapyramidal signals for motor control are transmitted.

4. Large numbers of nerve fibers pass directly from the motor cortex to the reticular nuclei and other nuclei of the brain stem. These by-pass the basal ganglia but converge on the same brain stem nuclei that are innervated by the basal ganglia.

FUNCTIONS OF THE DIFFERENT BASAL GANGLIA

Before attempting to discuss the functions of the basal ganglia in man, we should speak briefly of the better known functions of these ganglia in lower animals. In birds, for instance, the cerebral cortex is poorly developed while the basal ganglia are highly developed. These ganglia perform essentially all the motor functions, even controlling the voluntary movements in much the same manner that the motor cortex of the human being controls voluntary movements. Furthermore, in the cat, and to a lesser extent in the dog, decortication removes only the discrete types of motor functions and does not interfere with the animal's ability to walk, eat, fight, develop rage, have periodic sleep and wakefulness, and even participate naturally in sexual activities. However, if a major portion of the basal ganglia is destroyed, only gross stereotyped movements remain, which were discussed above in relation to the mesencephalic animal.

Finally, in the human being, decortication of very young individuals destroys the discrete movements of the body, particularly of the hands and distal portions of the lower limbs, but does not destroy the person's ability to walk crudely, to control his equilibrium, or to perform many other subconscious types of movements. However, simultaneous destruction of a major portion of the caudate nuclei almost totally paralyzes the opposite side of the body except for a few stereotyped reflexes integrated in the cord or brain stem.

With this brief background of the overall function of the basal ganglia, we can attempt to dissect the functions of the individual portions of the basal ganglia system, realizing that the system actually operates as a total unit and that individual functions cannot be ascribed completely to the different parts of the basal ganglia.

Inhibition of Motor Tone by the Basal Ganglia. Though it is wrong to ascribe a single function to all the basal ganglia, nevertheless, one of the general effects of diffuse basal ganglia excitation is to inhibit muscle tone throughout the body. This effect results from inhibitory signals transmitted from the basal ganglia to the bulboreticular facilitatory area and excitatory signals to the bulboreticular inhibitory area. Therefore, whenever widespread destruction of the basal ganglia occurs, the facilitatory area becomes overactive and the inhibitory area underactive, and this causes muscle rigidity throughout the body. For instance, when the brain stem is transected at the mesencephalic level, which removes the inhibitory effects of the basal ganglia, the phenomenon of decerebrate rigidity occurs.

Yet, despite this general inhibitory effect of the basal ganglia, stimulation of specific areas within the basal ganglia can at times elicit positive muscle contractions and at times even complex patterns of movements.

Function of the Caudate Nucleus and Putamen—The Striate Body. The caudate nucleus and putamen, because of their gross appearance on sections of the brain, are together called the *striate body*. They seem to function together to initiate and regulate gross intentional movements of the body. To perform this function they transmit impulses through two different pathways: (1) into the *globus pallidus,* thence by way of the *thalamus* to the *cerebral cortex,* and finally downward into the spinal cord through the *corticospinal* and *extracorticospinal pathways;* (2) downward through the *globus pallidus* and the *substantia nigra* by way of short axons into the *reticular formation* and finally into the spinal cord mainly through the *reticulospinal tracts.*

In summary, the striate body helps to control gross intentional movements that we normally perform unconsciously. However, this control also involves the motor cortex, with which the striate body is very closely connected.

Function of the Globus Pallidus. It has been suggested that the principal function of the globus pallidus is to provide background muscle tone for intended movements, whether these be initiated by impulses from the cerebral cortex or from the striate body. That is, if a person wishes to perform an exact function with one hand, he positions his body and limbs appropriately and also tenses the muscles of the upper arm. These associated tonic contractions are supposedly initiated by a circuit that strongly involves the globus pallidus. Destruction of the globus pallidus removes these associated movements and, therefore, makes it difficult or impossible for the distal portions of the limbs to perform their more discrete activities.

The globus pallidus is believed to function through two pathways: first, through feedback circuits to the thalamus, to the cerebral cortex, and thence by way of corticospinal and extracorticospinal tracts to the spinal cord; and, second, by way of short axons to the reticular formation of the brain stem and thence mainly by way of the reticulospinal tracts into the spinal cord.

Electrical stimulation of the globus pallidus while an animal is performing a gross body movement will often stop the movement in a static position, the animal holding that position for many seconds while the stimulation continues. This fits with the concept that the globus pallidus is involved in some type of servo feedback motor control system that is capable of locking the different parts of the body into specific positions. Obviously, such a circuit could be extremely important in providing the background body movements and upper limb movements when a person performs delicate tasks with his hands.

CLINICAL SYNDROMES RESULTING FROM DAMAGE TO THE BASAL GANGLIA

Much of what we know about the function of the basal ganglia comes from study of patients with basal ganglia lesions whose brains have undergone pathologic studies after death. Among the different clinical syndromes are:

Chorea. Chorea is a disease in which random uncontrolled contractions of different muscle groups of the body occur continuously. Normal progression of movements cannot occur; instead, the person may perform a normal pattern of movements for a few seconds and then suddenly begin another pattern of movements; then still another pattern begins after a few seconds. Because of this peculiar progression of movements, one type of chorea is frequently called *St. Vitus' dance*.

Pathologically, chorea results from *diffuse and widespread damage of the striate body,* but the manner in which this causes the choreiform movements is not known.

Athetosis. In this disease, slow, writhing movements of the peripheral parts of one or more limbs— usually upper—occur continually. The movements are likely to be wormlike, first with overextension of the hands and fingers, then flexion, then rotary twisting to the side—all these continuing in a slow, rhythmic, writhing pattern. The contracting muscles exhibit a high degree of spasm, and the movements are enhanced by emotions or by excessive signals from the sensory organs. Furthermore, voluntary movements in the affected area are greatly impaired or sometimes even impossible.

The damage in athetosis is usually found in the *outer portion of the globus pallidus* or in this area and the striate body. Athetosis is usually attributed to the interruption of feedback circuits among the basal ganglia, thalamus, and cerebral cortex. The normal feedback circuits presumably allow a constant and rapid interplay between antagonistic muscle groups so that finely controlled movements can take place. However, if the feedback circuits are blocked, it is supposed that the detouring impulses may take devious routes through the basal ganglia, thalamus, and motor cortex, causing a succession of abnormal movements.

Hemiballismus. Hemiballismus is an uncontrollable succession of violent movements of large areas of the body. These may occur once every few seconds or sometimes only once in many minutes. For instance, an entire leg might suddenly jerk uncontrollably to full flexion, or the entire trunk might go through an extreme, sudden torsion movement, or an arm might be pulled upward suddenly with great force. Hemiballismus of the legs or trunk causes the person to fall to the ground if he is walking, and even when the person is in bed, he tosses violently when affected by these powerful and strong intermittent movements. Furthermore, attempts to perform voluntary movements frequently invoke ballistic movements in place of the normal movements.

Hemiballismus of one side of the body results from a *large lesion in the opposite subthalamus*. The smooth, rhythmic movements of the limbs or other parts of the body normally integrated in this area can no longer occur, but excitatory impulses attempting to evoke such movements elicit instead uncontrollable ballistic movements.

Parkinson's Disease. Parkinson's disease, which is also known as *paralysis agitans,* results almost invariably from *widespread destruction of the substantia nigra,* often associated with lesions of the *globus pallidus* and other related areas. It is characterized by (1) *rigidity* of the musculature in either widespread areas of the body or in isolated areas, (2) *tremor at rest* of the involved areas in most but not all instances, and (3) *loss of involuntary and associated* *movements, called "akinesia."* Also, there may be enhancement of salivation, sweating, and seborrheic secretion.

The rigidity in this disease is quite different from that which occurs in decerebrate rigidity, for decerebrate rigidity results from hyperactivity of the muscle spindle system, and even slight movement of a muscle is met with rather extreme reflex resistance resulting from feedback through the stretch reflex mechanism. Parkinsonian rigidity, on the other hand, is of a "plastic" type. That is, sudden movement is not met by intense resistance from the stretch reflexes as in the decerebrate type of rigidity, but instead both protagonist and antagonist muscles remain tightly contracted throughout the movement. Furthermore, the rigidity of Parkinson's disease seems to result from excess impulses transmitted in the corticospinal system, thus activating the alpha motor fibers to the muscles, whereas decerebrate rigidity results from excess activation of the gamma efferents to the muscle spindles.

Tremor usually, though not always, occurs in Parkinson's disease. Its frequency normally is 4 to 6 cycles per second. When the person performs voluntary movements, weak tremors become temporarily blocked, possibly because cortical signals to the spinal cord excite the gamma efferent fibers to the muscle spindles at the same time that they excite the alpha fibers; the gamma stimulation sensitizes the muscle spindles which theoretically could then damp out the tremor.

The mechanism of the tremor in Parkinson's disease is not known, but at least two different theories must be considered: (1) Loss of inhibitory influences from the substantia nigra or globus pallidus allows the control nuclei of antagonistic muscles in the *reticular substance of the brain stem* to oscillate. (2) Lack of inhibitory impulses in the lower basal ganglia enhances feedback in the globus pallidus-thalamus-cortical circuit, causing it to oscillate.

Another abnormality of Parkinson's disease is a high degree of "motor stiffness" and loss of automatisms (akinesia). When a person begins to perform a discrete voluntary movement with his hands, the automatic "associated" adjustments of the trunk of his body and the upper arm segments do not occur. Instead, he must voluntarily adjust these segments before he can use his hands. Furthermore, a tremendous amount of nervous effort must be made by the voluntary motor control system to overcome the motor stiffness of his musculature. Thus, the person with Parkinson's disease has a masklike face, showing almost no automatic, emotional facial expressions; he is usually bent forward because of his muscle rigidity, and all his movements of necessity are highly deliberate rather than the many casual subconscious movements that are normally a part of our everyday life. This loss of automatisms is believed to result from diminished transmission of signals into the globus pallidus and other basal ganglia from the substantia nigra. Most of the pathways from the substantia nigra to these areas are inhibitory, and

when they are absent the globus pallidus and other basal ganglia become excessively active, leading to rigidity of the muscles that are usually responsible for the automatisms. Thus, as the automatisms are lost they are replaced by rigidity.

Treatment with L-Dopa and Anticholinergic Drugs. Administration of L-dopa to patients with Parkinson's disease ameliorates most of the symptoms, especially the rigidity and the akinesia, in about two-thirds of the patients. The reason for this seems to be the following: The neurons that originate in the substantia nigra and then project to the globus pallidus and striate body are inhibitory neurons whose terminals probably secrete *dopamine,* a derivative of L-dopa. When the substantia nigra is destroyed and the person develops Parkinson's disease, the administered L-dopa is believed to substitute for the dopamine no longer secreted by the destroyed neurons. This causes more or less normal inhibition of the basal ganglia and relieves much or most of the akinesia and rigidity.

The same basal ganglia that are inhibited by dopamine seem to be excited by other nerve terminals derived elsewhere; these terminals probably secrete acetylcholine. Therefore, as would be expected, administration of anticholinergic drugs such as scopolamine can also benefit the parkinsonian patient.

Coagulation of the Ventrolateral Nucleus of the Thalamus for Treatment of Parkinson's Disease. In recent years neurosurgeons have treated Parkinson's disease patients, with varying success, by destroying portions of the basal ganglia or of the thalamus. The most prevalent treatment at present is widespread destruction of the ventrolateral nucleus of the thalamus usually by electrocoagulation. Most fiber pathways from the basal ganglia and cerebellum to the cerebral cortex pass through this nucleus so that its destruction blocks many or most of the feedback functions of the basal ganglia and cerebellum. It is presumed that blockage of some of these feedbacks limits the functions of at least certain basal ganglia and thereby removes the factors that cause the rigidity and tremor of Parkinson's disease.

FUNCTIONS OF THE CEREBRAL CORTEX IN POSTURE AND LOCOMOTION— PURPOSEFULNESS OF LOCOMOTION

The principal function of the cerebral cortex in locomotion is to add *purposefulness* to the locomotion, as illustrated above by the subthalamic cat that would not go around an obstruction but would simply butt its head against the obstruction and continue its attempts to move forward. Such an effect obviously would not occur in an animal with a cerebral cortex. However, in addition to the purposefulness added by cortical function, several postural and righting reflexes are also integrated in the cortex. These include the *visual righting reflex,* certain aspects of *exteroceptive righting reflexes,* the *placing reaction,* and the *hopping reaction.*

The Visual and Exteroceptive Righting Reflexes. The visual righting reflexes depend on function of the visual cortex. That is, an animal can tell by images from the periphery whether his body is in the appropriate position with respect to its surroundings. From this information, he can raise himself from the lying position to the standing position even in the absence of the vestibular righting reflexes.

Similarly, the animal's sensory and motor cortex causes righting in response to exteroceptive information that is transmitted into the cerebrum. It has been pointed out that sensations from the skin can cause crude righting responses even in the spinal animal and even much better responses in the decerebrate animal. However, for full expression of the exteroceptive righting reflexes, the cerebral cortex is also required.

The Placing Reaction. A blindfolded animal held in the air and then brought in contact with a surface so that almost any part of his body makes contact with the surface immediately brings his paws toward the point of contact, thus placing his feet in an advantageous position to gain support. This is called the placing reaction. Though a weak expression of the placing reaction can occur even in animals without the cerebral cortex, here again the complete reaction can occur only when the cortex is available to provide stereognostic orientation of the different parts of the body in relation to each other, thus allowing the animal to "know" where his feet need to be moved in order to make appropriate contact.

The Hopping Reaction. The hopping reaction is another reaction that requires the cerebral cortex for full attainment. This reaction probably results mainly from direct transmission of proprioceptive and vestibular information to the motor cortex to cause the hopping.

SUMMARY OF THE DIFFERENT FUNCTIONS OF THE CENTRAL NERVOUS SYSTEM IN POSTURE AND LOCOMOTION

From the discussions in the previous chapter, we could see that almost all of the discrete "patterns" of muscle movement required for posture and locomotion can be elicited by the spinal cord alone. However, coordination of these patterns to provide equilibrium, progression, and purposefulness of movement requires neuronal function at progressively higher levels of the central nervous system. Centers in the brain stem provide most of the nervous energy required to maintain postural tone and therefore to support the body against gravity. But, in ad-

dition, the brain stem centers provide especially the equilibrium reflexes. Then moving still higher we find a control center for "progression" in the subthalamic region, a center that makes the animal move forward in a normal rhythmic pattern of walking and also in a straight line. Even so, this animal still does not have purposefulness in his motion. For this the basal ganglia, the thalamus, and the cerebral cortex are required.

With this background, we can now describe the characteristics of animals with transections through their nervous systems at the different levels shown in Figure 10–7.

The Spinal Animal. In the spinal animal, the flexor reflex, the crossed extensor reflex, the stretch reflex, and the reflexes that control the basic rhythm and pattern of locomotion are intact after the stage of spinal shock is over. Furthermore, under the most favorable conditions the animal can even stand for a few seconds because of the positive supportive reaction.

Transection of the Medulla Below the Vestibular Nuclei. If the medulla is cut below the vestibular nuclei, the lower portion of the reticular substance of the brain stem will be intact; this, if anything, transmits *inhibitory* impulses into the spinal cord. Therefore, few cord reflexes can be elicited, and the animal certainly cannot stand.

Transection of the Brain Stem Above the Vestibular Nuclei. If the brain stem is transected above the vestibular nuclei, the vestibular nuclei and the upper reticular substance of the brain stem transmit *facilitatory* impulses into the spinal cord and actually provide far more facilitation than normal. If

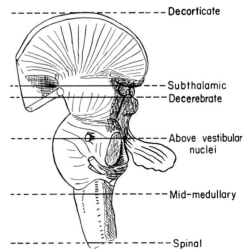

Figure 10–7. Levels of transection in the brain, the descriptions of which are given in the text.

the transection is well above the vestibular nuclei, sufficient postural tone can be attained for the animal to stand for minutes at a time.

The Classical Decerebrate Animal—Decerebrate Rigidity. The classical decerebrate animal has a transection between the superior and the inferior colliculi. In this animal the inhibitory signals from the basal ganglia and cerebral cortex to the reticular facilitatory area are removed, which allows the bulboreticular facilitatory area to become intrinsically very active, as explained earlier in the chapter. Impulses are transmitted downward to cause muscle rigidity called *decerebrate rigidity.* Especially the extensor muscles, but to some extent the flexor muscles as well, are maintained in a state of strong tonic contraction. The animal can occasionally stand, supporting its body against gravity. It also can make crude equilibrium adjustments; but for full expression of equilibrium, it needs a completely intact mesencephalon.

A major part of the increased postural tone in decerebrate rigidity results from stimulation of the *gamma activating system of the muscle spindles* and not from direct activation of the alpha motor neurons.

The Subthalamic Animal. With the transection above the superior colliculi, preserving the subthalamus as well as adjacent regions of the brain stem, the animal has less rigidity and is capable of walking with normal progression.

The Decorticate Animal. In a decorticate animal the cortex has been removed but the thalamus and basal ganglia are still intact. The capabilities of this type of animal depend on its degree of cerebral development. The cat, for instance, is capable of almost any type of motion, even to the extent of going around obstructions in his way, but, on the other hand, he still lacks much of the purposefulness of locomotion and frequently sits very still for hours at a time. The human being loses essentially all purposeful or voluntary motor functions on decortication.

FUNCTION OF THE CORD AND BRAIN STEM REFLEXES IN MAN

Though the foregoing discussions have concerned principally reflexes in animals rather than in man, the same principles of cord and brain stem function apply almost as well to man. Yet there are quantitative differences that must always be remembered.

First, man walks in an upright position and his limbs have become straightened to the point that almost no muscular strength is required to maintain the weight of the body against gravity. For instance, the direct line between the center of mass of the body and the direction of gravitational pull runs slightly behind the axes of the hip joints so that gravity tends to extend the hips and so that the ligaments of the hip joints, rather than the muscles, support the body against gravity. Likewise, the line of gravitational

pull runs slightly in front of the mid-position of the knee joints and well in front of the ankle joints. Here again, it is mainly tension in the ligaments and uncontracted muscles that maintains the weight of the body against gravity rather than postural tone.

Therefore, in man, contraction of postural muscles occurs principally to maintain equilibrium rather than to support the body against gravity. Yet, if man assumes an animal-like position, postural tone serves essentially the same functions as in lower animals.

In man with a spinal cord transection, most of the same reflexes as those that occur in lower animals can be elicited either wholly or partially. The only reflexes that often cannot be elicited in spinal man are the rhythmic reflexes; yet the reciprocal innervation that is required for rhythmic reflexes can be demonstrated. For instance, movement of an arm in one direction often causes simultaneous and directionally similar movement of the opposite leg, thus illustrating that appropriate reciprocal innervation is still present in the cord of man to cause at least crude types of diagonal movements necessary for the mark time reflex.

Also, stimulation in the subthalamic region in man causes rhythmic walking movements similar to those that occur in animals, illustrating that this same region of the brain subserves similar functions in man as in lower animals. However, a man who has lost large portions of the motor areas of his cortex cannot use these lower regions of the brain stem effectively enough actually to provide locomotion. This is a manifestation of the process called *encephalization* that has occurred in higher orders of animals, which suppresses many functions of the lower centers while the same functions are taken over, usually in a more complicated manner, by the higher centers. Thus, in man, the motor areas of the cortex are needed to provide progression in the act of locomotion and also to provide purposefulness of locomotion.

Nevertheless, in our subsequent discussions of the motor functions of the brain in man, we must always keep in mind the basic activities of the lower centers. The cord patterns of response are integrated into the overall control of muscular activity even when this control is initiated in the cerebral cortex. It is still the anterior motoneurons that have the final decisive power in the contraction of given muscles, and it is still the patterns of organization of the interneurons in the gray matter of the cord that provide many of the patterns of muscular contraction. Impulses from above seem to control the sequence in which these patterns of contraction occur, interspersed with other patterns generated in the brain itself.

REFERENCES

Barbeau, A., Chase, T. N., and Paulson, G. W. (eds.): Huntington's Chorea, 1872–1972. New York, Raven Press, 1973.

Brimblecombe, R. W.: Tremors and Tremorogenic Agents. Baltimore, The Williams & Wilkins Company, 1972.

Brodal, A. (ed.): Basic Aspects of Central Vestibular Mechanisms. New York, American Elsevier Publishing Co., Inc., 1971.

Calne, D. B. (ed.): Progress in the Treatment of Parkinsonism. New York, Raven Press, 1973.

Calne, D. B., Chase, T. N., and Barbeau, A. (eds.): Dopaminergic Mechanisms. (Advances in Neurology. Vol. 9.) New York, Raven Press, 1975.

Cooper, I. S.: Involuntary Movement Disorders. Hagerstown, Md., Harper & Row, Publishers, 1969.

Denny-Brown, D.: The Basal Ganglia: Their Relation to Disorders of Movement. New York, Oxford University Press, Inc., 1962.

Fischer, J. H.: The Labyrinth; Physiology and Functional Tests. New York, Grune & Stratton, Inc., 1956.

French, J. D.: The reticular formation. In Magoun, H. W. (ed.): Handbook of Physiology. Sec. 1, Vol. 2. Baltimore, The Williams & Wilkins Company, 1960, p. 1281.

Goldberg, J. M., and Fernandez, C.: Vestibular mechanisms. *Ann. Rev. Physiol.*, *37*:129, 1975.

Hornykiewicz, O.: Pharmacology and pathophysiology of dopaminergic neurons. *Adv. Cytopharmacol.*, *1*:369, 1971.

Kawamura, Y.: Neurogenesis of mastication. *Front. Oral Physiol.*, *1*:77, 1974.

Kidokoro, Y., Shuto, S., Kubota, K., and Sumino, R.: Reflex organization of cat masticatory muscles. *J. Neurophysiol.*, *31*:695, 1968.

Martin, J. P.: Basal Ganglia and Posture. Philadelphia, J. B. Lippincott Company, 1967.

Partridge, L. D., and Kim, J. H.: Dynamic characteristics of response in a vestibulomotor reflex. *J. Neurophysiol.*, *32*:485, 1969.

Precht, W.: Vestibular system. In Guyton, A. C. (ed.): MTP International Review of Science: Physiology. Vol. 3. Baltimore, University Park Press, 1974, p. 81.

Riklan, M.: L-Dopa and Parkinsonism. Springfield, Ill., Charles C Thomas, Publisher, 1973.

Sessle, B. J., and Kenny, D. J.: Control of tongue and facial motility: neural mechanisms that may contribute to movements such as swallowing and sucking. *Symp. Oral Sens. Percept.*, *4*:222, 1973.

Sherrington, C. S.: Decerebrate ridigity and reflex coordination of movements. *J. Physiol. (Lond.)*, *22*:319, 1898.

Suzuki, J. I.: Vestibular and spinal control of eye movements. *Bibl. Ophthalmol.*, *82*:109, 1972.

Thexton, A. J.: Some aspects of neurophysiology of dental interest. II. Oral reflexes and neural oscillators. *J. Dent.*, *2*:131, 1974.

Thoden, U., Magherini, P. C., and Pompeiano, O.: Cholinergic activaton of vestibular neurons leading to rapid eye movements in the mesencephalic cat. *Bibl. Ophthalmol.*, *82*:99, 1972.

Valdman, A. V. (ed.): Pharmacology and Physiology of the Reticular Formation. Progress in Brain Research. Vol. 20. New York, American Elsevier Publishing Co., Inc., 1967.

Wolfson, R. J.: The Vestibular System and Its Diseases. Philadelphia, University of Pennsylvania Press, 1966.

Young, L. R.: Cross coupling between effects of linear and angular acceleration on vestibular nystagmus. *Bibl. Ophthalmol.*, *82*:116, 1972.

11

Cortical and Cerebellar Control of Motor Functions

In preceding chapters we have been concerned with many of the subconscious motor activities integrated in the spinal cord and brain stem, especially those responsible for locomotion. In the present chapter we will discuss the control of motor function by the cerebral cortex and cerebellum, much of which is "voluntary" control in contradistinction to the subconscious control effected by the lower centers. Yet we will also see that at least some motor functions of the cerebral cortex and cerebellum are not entirely "voluntary."

PHYSIOLOGIC ANATOMY OF THE MOTOR AREAS OF THE CORTEX AND THEIR PATHWAYS TO THE CORD

Electrical stimulation anywhere within a large area of the cerebral cortex can at times cause muscle contraction. This area, illustrated by the shading in Figure 11–1, is called the *sensorimotor cortex*. This same area receives sensory signals from the somatic areas of the body.

However, the sensorimotor cortex can be divided into two separate areas: the *motor cortex*, which lies anterior to the central sulcus and the *somatic sensory cortex*, or *somesthetic cortex*, which lies posterior to the sulcus. The reason for this separation is a simple one: Electrical stimulation in the anterior region is far more likely to cause muscle contraction than stimulation in the posterior area. Conversely, stimulation in the posterior area is far more likely to cause a sensory experience. Yet, there is a very strong overlap between the two areas. This is exceedingly important, for as we shall see later in the chapter the motor

activities of the cortex are constantly controlled or modified by signals from the somatic sensory system. The area in Figure 11–1 immediately in front of the central sulcus, designated in the figure by the darkest shading, contains large numbers of *giant Betz cells,* or *pyramidal cells,* for which reason it is also called the *area pyramidalis.* This area causes motor movements following the least amount of electrical excitation and is therefore also called the *primary motor cortex.*

The Pyramidal Tract (Corticospinal Tract). One of the major pathways by which motor signals are transmitted from the motor areas of the cortex to the anterior motoneurons of the spinal cord is through the *pyramidal tract,* or *corticospinal tract,* which is illustrated in Figure 11–2. This tract origi-

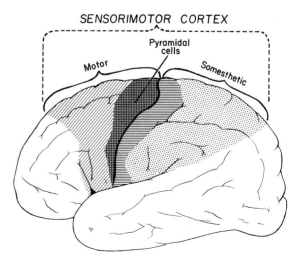

Figure 11–1. Relationship of the motor cortex to the somesthetic cortex.

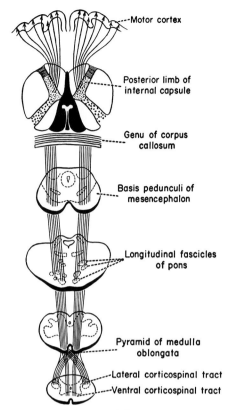

- - Motor cortex

Posterior limb of
internal capsule

Genu of corpus
callosum

Basis pedunculi of
mesencephalon

Longitudinal fascicles
of pons

Pyramid of medulla
oblongata

Lateral corticospinal tract

Ventral corticospinal tract

Figure 11–2. The pyramidal tract. (From Ranson and Clark: Anatomy of the Nervous System, 1959.)

nates in all the shaded areas in Figure 53–1, including both the motor and the somesthetic areas, about three-quarters from the motor area and about one-quarter from the somesthetic regions posterior to the central sulcus. The function of the fibers from the somesthetic cortex is probably not motor, but instead is to cause feedback control of sensory input to the nervous system, as was discussed in Chapter 7.

The most impressive fibers in the pyramidal tract are the large myelinated fibers that originate in the giant Betz cells of the motor area. These account for approximately 17,000 large fibers (mean diameter of about 16 microns) in the pyramidal tract from *each* side of the cortex. However, since each corticospinal tract contains more than a million fibers, only 2 per cent of the total number of corticospinal fibers are of this large type. The other 98 per cent are mainly fibers smaller than 4 microns diameter, 60 per cent of which are myelinated and 40 per cent unmyelinated.

The pyramidal tract passes downward through the *brain stem;* then it decussates mainly to the opposite side to form the *pyramids of the medulla.* By far the majority of the pyramidal fibers then descend in the *lateral corticospinal tracts* of the cord and terminate principally on interneurons at the bases of the dorsal horns of the cord gray matter. A few fibers, however,

do not cross to the opposite side but pass on down the cord ipsilaterally. Another small percentage passes ipsilaterally down the cord in the *ventral corticospinal tracts* but then mainly decussates to the opposite side farther down the cord.

Collaterals from the Pyramidal Tract in the Brain. Even before the pyramidal tract leaves the brain, many collaterals are given off as follows:

1. The axons from the giant Betz cells send short collaterals back to the cortex itself. It is believed that these collaterals mainly inhibit adjacent regions of the cortex when the Betz cells discharge, thereby "sharpening" the boundaries of the excitatory signal.

2. A large number of collateral fibers pass into the *striate body,* which is composed of the *caudate nucleus* and *putamen.* From here additional pathways extend down the brain stem and then into the spinal cord through the *extrapyramidal tracts,* which are discussed later in the chapter.

3. A moderate number of collaterals pass from the pyramidal tract into the *red nuclei.* From these, additional pathways pass down the cord through the *rubrospinal tract.*

4. A moderate number of collaterals also deviate from the pyramidal tract into the *reticular substance* of the brain stem; from here signals go to the cord via *reticulospinal tracts* and others go to the cerebellum via *reticulocerebellar tracts.*

5. A tremendous number of collaterals synapse in the pontile nuclei, which give rise to the *pontocerebellar fibers.* Thus, each time signals are transmitted from the motor cortex through the pyramidal tract, simultaneous signals are transmitted into the cerebellar hemispheres.

6. Many collaterals also terminate in the *inferior olivary nuclei,* and from here secondary *olivocerebellar fibers* transmit signals to most areas of the cerebellum.

Thus, the basal ganglia, the brain stem, and the cerebellum all receive strong signals from the pyramidal tract every time a signal is also transmitted down the spinal cord to cause a motor activity.

Importance of the Area Pyramidalis. The giant pyramidal cells of the *area pyramidalis* are very excitable. A much less degree of electrical stimulation is required in this area to cause motor movement than in any other area of the brain. Therefore, this area is called the *primary motor area* of the cortex. A single weak shock applied to a focal point in this area is sometimes strong enough to cause a definite motor movement somewhere in the body—for instance, a flick of a finger, deviation of the lip, or some other discrete movement; and a short train of stimuli almost always elicits a movement in some discrete part of the body. In almost no other region of the cortex can one be certain of achieving a motor response with such weak stimuli.

The Extrapyramidal Tracts. The extrapyramidal tracts are, collectively, all the tracts besides the pyramidal tract itself that transmit motor signals from the cortex to the spinal cord. In the above discussion of the collaterals from the pyramidal tract, we have noted some of these extrapyramidal pathways that pass through the striate nuclei, red nuclei, and reticular nuclei of the brain stem. In addition to these collateral fibers from the pyramidal tract, still many other fibers course directly from the cortex to these intermediate nuclei. For instance, large numbers of neurons project directly from the motor cortex into the *caudate nucleus* and then through the *putamen, globus pallidus, subthalamic nucleus, red nucleus, substantia nigra,* and *reticular nuclei of the brain stem* before passing into the spinal cord. The multiplicity of connections within these intermediate nuclei of the basal ganglia and reticular substance was presented in the preceding chapter.

The final pathways for transmission of extrapyramidal signals into the cord are the *reticulospinal tracts,* which lie in both the ventral and lateral columns of the cord; and, to a less extent, the *rubrospinal, tectospinal,* and *vestibulospinal tracts.*

THE FOUR MOTOR AREAS OF THE SENSORIMOTOR CORTEX

Four separate motor areas, which when stimulated are especially likely to cause contraction of specific muscles, have been found in the sensorimotor cortex. The precise locations of these in the human being have been mapped out only crudely because of the obvious impossibility of performing the necessary experiments to make accurate measurements. However, Figure 11–3 illustrates the somatotopical maps of the four separate motor areas in the monkey cortex, as described below:

1. The *primary motor area* (labeled Ms I in the figure), which is located immediately anterior to the central sulcus, with the feet areas extending down into the central sulcus, and the trunk extending toward the front of the brain. The tail and leg areas fold over the longitudinal fissure, and the head and tongue areas are located laterally in the posterior part of the frontal lobe.

2. The *supplementary motor area* (Ms II in the figure), which is located almost entirely on the medial wall of the hemisphere in the longitudinal fissure. This is illustrated in the upper portion of the figure, showing the medial hemisphere folded outward.

3. The *somatic sensorimotor area I* (Sm I), which is located immediately posterior to the central sulcus in the anterior gyrus of the parietal lobe. This area is coextensive with somatic sensory area I; the somatotopical map of the body representation is a mirror image of the map in the primary motor area immediately anterior to the central sulcus.

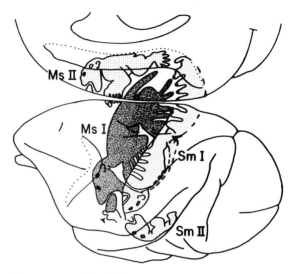

Figure 11–3. The different motor areas of the monkey cortex, illustrating especially the primary motor area (Ms I) located in the precentral gyrus. (The upper portion of the figure illustrates the medial surface of the cerebral hemisphere.) (From Woolsey, in Harlow and Woolsey (eds.): Biological and Biochemical Bases of Behavior. University of Wisconsin Press, 1958.)

4. The *somatic sensorimotor area II* (Sm II), which is located in the lateralmost portion of the parietal lobe immediately above the Sylvian fissure. This area is coextensive with somatic sensory area II.

Importance of the Different Motor Representations. Despite this multiplicity of motor representations in the cortex, very little is known about any of them except the primary motor area. Stimulation of the supplementary motor area (Ms II) seems to cause avoidance movements—that is, shrinking away from danger. Stimulation of somatic sensorimotor area II causes gross postural motor movements. Sensorimotor area I operates in association with the primary motor area, providing sensory signals that are the basis for many of the primary motor reactions.

The primary motor area is an extremely important one because even a weak stimulus usually elicits a muscle contraction somewhere in the body. Therefore, the remainder of this discussion will be concerned almost entirely with the primary motor area.

THE PRIMARY MOTOR CORTEX OF THE HUMAN BEING

Figure 11–4 gives an approximate map of the human brain showing the points in the primary motor cortex that cause muscle contractions in

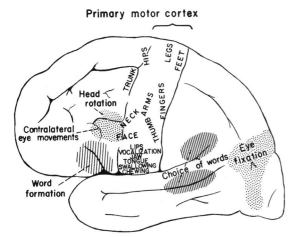

Figure 11–4. Representation of the different muscles of the body in the motor cortex and location of other cortical areas responsible for certain types of motor movements.

different parts of the body when electrically stimulated. These have been determined by electrical stimulation of the human brain in patients having brain operations under local anesthesia. Indeed, such stimulation is commonly used by the neurosurgeon to determine the location of the motor cortex, thus allowing him to avoid this area, if possible, during the operation.

Note in the figure that stimulation of the most lateral portions of the motor cortex causes muscular contractions related to swallowing, chewing, and facial movements, whereas stimulation of the midline portion of the motor cortex where it bends over into the longitudinal fissure, causes contraction of the legs, feet, or toes. The spatial organization is similar to that of the somatic sensory cortex I, which was shown in Figure 7–4 of Chapter 7.

Afferent Fibers that Excite the Primary Motor Cortex. The primary motor cortex is stimulated to action by signals from many different sources, including:

1. Subcortical fibers from adjacent regions of the cortex, especially from the somatic sensory areas and from the frontal areas—also subcortical fibers from the visual and auditory cortices.

2. Subcortical fibers that pass through the corpus callosum from the opposite cerebral hemisphere. These fibers connect corresponding areas of the motor cortices in the two sides of the brain.

3. Somatic sensory fibers derived directly from the ventrobasal complex of the thalamus. That is, every time that a sensory signal is transmitted into somatic sensory area I, collateral signals are also transmitted at less intensity into the primary motor area as well.

4. Tracts from the lateral nuclei of the thalamus,

which in turn receive tracts from both the basal ganglia and the cerebellum. These tracts provide signals that are necessary for coordination between the functions of the motor cortex, the basal ganglia, and the cerebellum.

5. Fibers from the nonspecific nuclei of the thalamus. These fibers control the general level of excitability of the motor cortex in the same manner that they also control the general level of excitability of most other regions of the cerebral cortex.

Vertical Columnar Arrangement of the Cells in the Motor Cortex. In Chapters 7 and 18 it is pointed out that the cells in the somatic sensory cortex and the visual cortex—and perhaps in all other parts of the brain as well—are organized in vertical columns of cells. In a like manner, the cells of the motor cortex are also organized in vertical columns—columns about 1 mm. in diameter and having several thousand cells in each column.

The columns of cells, in turn, are themselves arranged in six distinct layers, as is the arrangement throughout the cerebral cortex. The functions of these layers from outside inward are:

Layers I through IV are sensory; that is, they receive afferent fibers from other sources. The fibers from the nonspecific nuclei of the thalamus (from the "reticular activating system" that will be discussed in the following chapter) terminate in layers I and II. These fibers provide general enhancement of the degree of excitability of the motor cortex, as occurs also in other cortical regions of the brain when the reticular activating system is stimulated.

Layer IV is the main terminus and layer III the secondary terminus of the sensory afferents from the specific nuclei in the ventrobasal complex of the thalamus, the afferents from the sensory areas of the cortex, the afferents from the lateral nuclei of the thalamus that transmit signals from the cerebellum and the basal ganglia, and the corpus callosal afferents from the opposite cerebral hemisphere.

Layers V and VI are the origins of the efferent fibers or "output fibers," from the motor cortex. The large Betz cells that give rise to the long pyramidal tract fibers lie in layer V. Efferent fibers also pass from both layers V and VI to other areas of the brain.

Function of the Columns of Cells. Each column of cells seems to perform a specific motor function, such as stimulating a particular muscle or perhaps stimulating several synergistic muscles. The cells in each column seem to operate both as an integrative and an amplifying system. The integrative function of the column is its ability to combine signals from many different sources and to determine the appropriate output response. Specific cells within a column seem to be responsive to different types of input signals. For instance, some cells respond to somatic sensory signals related to joint movement, others to tactile stimuli, and still others to feedback signals from the cerebellum and basal ganglia. Also, the general level of activation of the motor cortex is provided by signals from the nonspecific nuclei of the thalamus.

The amplifying function of the column of cells allows weak input signals to cause stimulation of large numbers of output neurons. Direct electrical stimulation of a single output neuron in the motor cortex by means of a micropipette electrode will almost never excite a muscle contraction. Instead, at least several output neurons (preferably a large number) need to be excited simultaneously. Therefore, divergence of the signal within the column provides this needed motive power.

Degree of Representation of Different Muscle Groups in the Primary Motor Cortex. The different muscle groups of the body are not represented equally in the motor cortex. In general, the degree of representation is proportional to the discreteness of movement required of the respective part of the body. Thus, the thumb and fingers have large representations, as is true also of the lips, tongue, and vocal cords. The relative degrees of representation of the different parts of the body are illustrated in Figure 11–5, a figure constructed by Penfield and Rasmussen on the basis of stimulatory charts made of the human motor cortex during hundreds of brain operations.

When barely threshold stimuli are used, only small segments of the peripheral musculature ordinarily contract at a time. In the "finger" and "thumb" regions, which have tremendous representation in the cerebral cortex, threshold stimuli can sometimes cause single muscles or, at times, even single fasciculi of muscles to contract, thus illustrating that a high degree of control is exercised by this portion of the motor cortex over discrete muscular movement.

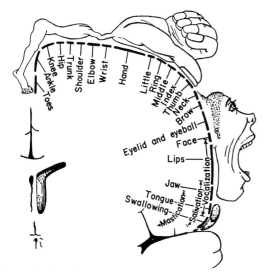

Figure 11–5. Degree of representation of the different muscles of the body in the motor cortex. (From Penfield and Rasmussen: The Cerebral Cortex of Man: A Clinical Study of Localization of Function. The Macmillan Co., 1968.)

On the other hand, threshold stimuli in the trunk region of the body might cause as many as 30 to 50 small trunk muscles to contract simultaneously, thus illustrating that the motor cortex does not control discrete trunk muscles but instead controls *groups* of muscles. Similarly, threshold stimuli in the lip, tongue, and vocal cord regions of the motor cortex cause contraction of minute muscular areas, whereas stimulation in the leg region ordinarily excites several synergistic muscles at a time, causing some gross movement of the leg. Also, it should be recognized that the finger muscles have far more representation in the motor cortex than do the muscles of the upper arm.

COMPLEX MOVEMENTS ELICITED BY STIMULATING THE CORTEX ANTERIOR TO THE MOTOR CORTEX—THE CONCEPT OF A "PREMOTOR CORTEX"

Electrical stimulation of the cerebral cortex for distances 1 to 3 centimeters in front of the primary motor cortex will often elicit complex contractions of groups of muscles. Occasionally, vocalization occurs, or rhythmic movements such as alternate thrusting of a leg forward and backward, coordinate moving of the eyes, chewing, swallowing, or contortion of parts of the body into different postural positions.

Some neurophysiologists have called this area the *premotor cortex* and have ascribed special capabilities to it to control coordinated movements involving many muscles simultaneously. One might also call the premotor cortex a *motor association area*. In fact, it is peculiarly organized to perform such a function for the following reasons: (1) It has long subcortical neuronal connections with the sensory association areas of the parietal lobe; (2) It has direct subcortical connections with the primary motor cortex; (3) It connects with areas in the thalamus contiguous with the thalamic areas that connect with the primary motor cortex; (4) The premotor area has direct connections with the basal ganglia.

Still another reason for the belief that there is a motor association area (a "premotor cortex") is that damage to this area causes loss of certain coordinate skills, as follows:

Broca's Area and Speech. Referring again to Figure 11–4, note that immediately anterior to the primary motor cortex and immediately above the Sylvian fissure is an area labeled "word formation." This region is called *Broca's area*. Damage to it does not prevent a person from vocalizing, but it does make it impossible for the person to speak whole words other than simple utterances such as "no" or "yes." A closely associated cortical area also causes appropriate respiratory function so that the vocal cords can be activated simultaneously with the movements of the mouth and tongue during speech. Thus, the activities that are related to Broca's area are highly complex.

The Voluntary Eye Movement Field. Immediately above Broca's area is a locus for controlling eye movements. Damage to this area prevents a person from voluntarily moving his eyes toward different objects. Instead, the eyes tend to lock on specific objects, an effect controlled by signals from the occipital region, as explained in Chapter 18. This frontal area also controls eyelid movements such as blinking.

Head Rotation Area. Still slightly higher in the "premotor region," electrical stimulation will elicit head rotation. This area is closely associated with the eye movement field and is presumably related to directing the head toward different objects.

Area for Hand Skills. In the frontal area immediately anterior to the primary motor cortex for the hands and fingers is a region neurosurgeons have observed to be an area for hand skills. That is, when tumors or other lesions cause destruction in this area, the hand movements become incoordinate and nonpurposeful, a condition called *motor apraxia.*

Summary of the Premotor Concept. It is clear that at least some areas anterior to the primary motor cortex can cause complex coordinate movements, such as for speech, for eye movements, for head movements, and perhaps even for hand skills. However, it should be remembered that all of these areas are closely connected with corresponding areas in the primary motor cortex, the thalamus, and the basal ganglia. Therefore, the complex coordinate movements almost certainly result from a cooperative effort of all these substructures.

EFFECTS OF LESIONS IN THE MOTOR AND PREMOTOR CORTEX

The motor cortex is frequently damaged—especially by the common abnormality called a "stroke," which is caused by loss of blood supply to the cortex. Also, experiments have been performed in animals to remove selectively different parts of the motor cortex.

Ablation of the Primary Motor Cortex. Removal of a very small portion of the primary motor cortex in a monkey causes paralysis of the represented muscles. If the sublying caudate nucleus is not damaged, gross postural and limb "fixation" movements can still be performed, but the animal loses voluntary control of discrete movements of the distal segments of the limbs—of the hands and fingers, for instance. This does not mean that the muscles themselves cannot contract, but that the animal's ability to control the fine movements is gone.

From these results one can conclude that the primary motor cortex is concerned mainly with voluntary initiation of finely controlled movements. On the other hand, the deeper motor areas, particularly the basal ganglia, seem to be responsible mainly for the involuntary and postural body movements.

Muscle Spasticity Caused by Ablation of Large Areas of the Motor Cortex—Extrapyramidal Lesions as the Basis of Spasticity. It should be recalled that the motor cortex gives rise to tracts that descend to the spinal cord through both the pyramidal tract and the extrapyramidal tract. These two tracts have opposing effects on the tone of the body muscles. The pyramidal tract causes continuous facilitation and, therefore, a tendency to increase muscle tone throughout the body. On the other hand, the extrapyramidal system transmits inhibitory signals through the basal ganglia and the bulboreticular system of the brain stem, with resultant inhibition of muscle action. When the motor cortex is destroyed, the balance between these two opposing effects may be altered. If the lesion is located discretely in the primary motor cortex where the large Betz cells lie, very little change in muscle tone results because both pyramidal and extrapyramidal elements are affected about equally. On the other hand, the usual lesion is very large and involves large portions of the sensorimotor cortex, both anterior and posterior to the primary motor area, and both of these regions normally transmit inhibitory signals through the extrapyramidal tracts. Therefore, loss of extrapyramidal inhibition is the dominant feature, thus leading to muscle spasm.

If the lesion involves the basal ganglia as well as the motor cortex itself, the spasm is even more intense because the basal ganglia normally provide additional very strong inhibition of the bulboreticular system, and loss of this inhibition further exacerbates the reticular excitation of the muscles. In patients with strokes, the lesion almost invariably affects both the motor cortex itself and the sub-lying basal ganglia, so that very intense spasm normally occurs in the muscles of the opposite side of the body.

The muscle spasm that results from damage to the extrapyramidal system is different from the spasticity that occurs in decerebrate rigidity. In decerebrate rigidity the spasm is of the antigravity muscles and is called *extensor spasm*. On the other hand, the spasm resulting from lesions of the extrapyramidal system usually involves the flexors as well, causing intense stiffening of the limbs and other parts of the body.

The Babinski Sign. Destruction of the foot region of the area pyramidalis or transection of the foot portion of the pyramidal tract causes a peculiar response of the foot called the *Babinski sign*. This response is demonstrated when a firm tactile stimulus is applied to the sole of the foot: The great toe extends upward and the other toes fan outward. This is in contradistinction to the normal effect in which all the toes bend downward. Also, the Babinski sign does not occur when the damage is only in the extrapyramidal system. Therefore, the sign is often used clinically to detect damage specifically in the pyramidal portion of the motor control system. Despite the clinical significance of the Babinski sign, however, its physiological mechanism is not known.

STIMULATION OF THE SPINAL MOTONEURONS BY MOTOR SIGNALS FROM THE BRAIN

Figure 11-6 shows several different motor tracts entering a segment of the spinal cord from the brain. The corticospinal tract (pyramidal tract) terminates mainly on small interneurons in the base of the dorsal horns, although as

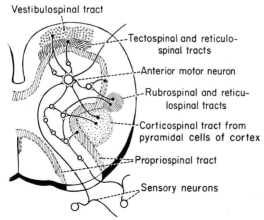

Figure 11-6. Convergence of all the different motor pathways on the anterior motoneurons.

many as 15 per cent may also terminate directly on the anterior motoneurons themselves. From the primary interneurons, most of the motor signals are transmitted through still other interneurons before finally exciting the anterior motoneurons.

Figure 11-6 shows several other descending tracts from the brain, collectively called the extrapyramidal tracts, which also carry signals to the anterior motoneurons: (1) the rubrospinal tract, (2) the reticulospinal tract, (3) the tectospinal tract, and (4) the vestibulospinal tract. In addition, sensory signals arriving through the dorsal sensory roots, as well as signals transmitted from segment to segment of the spinal cord via the propriospinal tracts, also stimulate the anterior motoneurons. In general, the extrapyramidal tracts terminate farther anteriorly in the gray matter of the spinal cord than does the corticospinal tract; a larger share of these fibers terminate directly on the anterior motoneurons. Also, some terminate on *inhibitory neurons,* which in turn inhibit the anterior motoneurons, an effect opposite to the excitatory effect of the corticospinal tract.

The corticospinal tract seems to cause very specific muscle contractions; neurophysiological recordings have demonstrated that the intensity of muscle contraction—everything else being equal—is directly proportional to the nervous energy transmitted through the corticospinal tract. On the other hand, the extrapyramidal tracts terminate in the cord gray matter near the anterior motoneurons and provide less specific muscle contractions. Instead, they provide such effects as general facilitation, general inhibition, or gross postural signals, all of which provide the background against which the corticospinal system operates. Finally, the sensory and propriospinal signals also add their input to the total melee of spinal integration.

Patterns of Movement Elicited by Spinal Cord Centers. From Chapter 9, recall that the spinal cord can provide specific reflex patterns of movement in response to sensory nerve stimulation. Many of these patterns are also important when the anterior motoneurons are excited by signals from the brain. For instance, the stretch reflex is functional at all times, helping to damp the motor movements initiated from the brain and probably providing at least part of the motive power required to cause the muscle contractions employing the servo-assist mechanism that was described in Chapter 9.

Also, when a brain signal excites an agonist muscle, it is not necessary to transmit an inverse signal to the antagonist at the same time;

this transmission will be achieved by the reciprocal innervation circuit that is always present in the cord for coordinating the functions of antagonistic pairs of muscles.

Finally, parts of the other reflex mechanisms such as withdrawal, stepping and walking, scratching, postural mechanisms, and so forth, are at times activated by signals from the brain. Thus, very simple signals from the brain can lead, at least theoretically, to many of our normal motor activities, particularly for such functions as walking and the attainment of different postural attitudes of the body.

On the other hand, at times it is important to suppress the cord mechanisms to prevent their interference with the performance of patterns of motor activity generated within the brain itself. It has been suggested that this is the specific function of some of the inhibitory signals transmitted through some reticulospinal fibers.

THE CEREBELLUM AND ITS MOTOR FUNCTIONS

The cerebellum has long been called a *silent area* of the brain principally because electrical excitation of this structure does not cause any sensation and rarely any motor movement. However, as we shall see, removal of the cerebellum does cause the motor movements to become highly abnormal—so much so that some very prominent neurophysiologists consider the cerebellum to be as important as all other motor control elements of the nervous system. The cerebellum is especially vital to the control of very rapid muscular activities such as running, typing, playing the piano, and even talking. Loss of this area of the brain can play havoc with each of these activities even though its loss causes paralysis of no muscles.

But how is it that the cerebellum can be so important when it has no direct control over muscle contraction? The answer to this is that it *monitors and makes corrective adjustments in the motor activities elicited by other parts of the brain.* It receives continuously updated information from the peripheral parts of the body to determine the instantaneous status of each part of the body—its position, its rate of movement, forces acting on it, and so forth. The cerebellum *compares* the actual physical status of each part of the body as depicted by the sensory information with the status that is intended by the motor system. If the two do not compare favorably, then appropriate corrective signals are transmitted instantaneously back into the motor

system to increase or decrease the levels of activation of the specific muscles.

Since the cerebellum must make major motor corrections extremely rapidly *during the course of motor movements*, a very extensive and rapidly acting cerebellar input system is required both from the peripheral parts of the body and from the cerebral motor areas. Also, an extensive output system feeding equally as rapidly into the motor system is necessary to provide the necessary corrections of the motor signals.

THE INPUT SYSTEM TO THE CEREBELLUM

The human cerebellum is generally divided into two major lobes, as illustrated in Figure 11–7, the *anterior lobe*, which is small, and the *posterior lobe*, which is much larger. The posterior cerebellum is greatly enlarged bilaterally to form the *cerebellar hemispheres*, which are also known as the *neocerebellum* (new cerebellum) because they represent a phylogenetically new portion of the cerebellum. The older portions of the cerebellum, including the small midline section of the posterior cerebellum and the entire anterior cerebellum, are called the *paleocerebellum* (old cerebellum).

The Afferent Pathways. The basic afferent pathways to the cerebellum are also illustrated in Figure 11–7. An extensive and important afferent pathway is the *corticocerebellar pathway*, which originates mainly in the *motor cortex* (but to a lesser extent, in the sensory cortex as well) and then passes by way of the *pontile nuclei* and *pontocerebellar tracts* directly to the cortex of the cerebellum. In addition, important afferent tracts originate in the

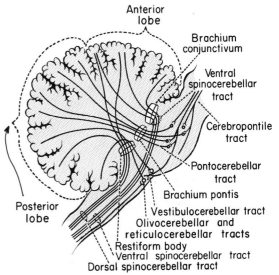

Figure 11–7. The principal afferent tracts to the cerebellum.

brain stem; they include: (a) an extensive *olivo-cerebellar* tract, which passes from the *inferior olive* to all parts of the cerebellum; this tract is excited by fibers from the *motor cortex,* the *basal ganglia,* widespread areas of the *reticular formation,* and the spinal cord through the *spino-olivary tract;* (b) *ves-tibulocerebellar fibers,* some of which originate in the vestibular apparatus itself; most of these terminate in the *flocculonodular lobe* and *fastigial nucleus* of the cerebellum; (c) *reticulocerebellar fibers,* which origi-nate in different portions of the reticular formation and terminate mainly in the midline structures of the paleocerebellum.

The cerebellum also receives important sensory signals directly from the peripheral parts of the body, which reach the cerebellum by way of the *ventral* and *dorsal spinocerebellar* tracts illustrated in Figures 11–7 and 11–8. The signals transmitted in these tracts originate in the muscle spindles, the Golgi tendon organs, and the large tactile receptors of the skin and joints, and they apprise the cerebellum of the momentary status of muscle contraction, degree of tension on the muscle tendons, positions of the parts of the body, and forces acting on the surfaces of the body. All of this information keeps the cerebellum constantly apprised of the instantaneous physical status of the body.

Note in Figure 11–8 that the nerve fibers from the sensory receptors terminate on Clarke's cells at the bases of the dorsal horns and that most of these fibers pass ipsilaterally up to the cerebellum. These path-ways can transmit impulses at velocities over 100 meters per second, which is the most rapid conduc-tion of any pathway in the entire central nervous sys-tem. This extremely rapid conduction is also impor-

Figure 11–9. The sensory projection areas, called "homunculi," on the cortex of the cerebellum. (From Snider: *Sci. Amer., 199*:4, 1958. Copyright © 1958 by Scientific American, Inc. All rights reserved.)

tant for the instantaneous apprisal of the cerebellum of changes that take place in the status of the body.

In addition to the signals in the spinocerebellar tracts, other signals are transmitted through the dor-sal columns to the medulla and then relayed from there to the cerebellum. Likewise, signals are trans-mitted through the *spinoreticular pathway* to the re-ticular substance of the brain stem and through the *spino-olivary pathway* to the inferior olivary nucleus and then relayed to the cerebellum. Thus, the cere-bellum collects continual information about all parts of the body even though it is operating at a subcon-scious level.

Spatial Localization of Sensory Input to the Cerebellum. Afferent fibers entering the cerebel-lum terminate in distinct spatially oriented areas of the cerebellar cortex. Figure 11–9 illustrates the loci of two different "homunculi," as recorded in the monkey, which show the terminations of sensory fibers from all parts of the body. Figure 11–10 illus-trates the human cerebellum, showing the approxi-mate sensory terminations based on anatomical data and extrapolation from animals. Note especially that there are two separate representations of the body in the cerebellum. One of these lies mainly in the an-terior cerebellum but extends also into the upper part of the posterior cerebellum, and the other is split in half and lies entirely in the posterior cerebellum.

It is also important to note that the signals from the motor cortex project to corresponding points in (a) the peripheral muscles and joints of the body, and (b) the sensory representations for the same muscles and joints in the cerebellum. Therefore, each respective point in the cerebellum in reality represents a specific muscle or a specific joint; simultaneously it receives information directly from the motor cortex concern-

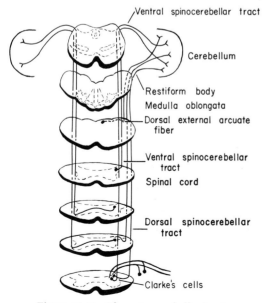

Ventral spinocerebellar tract

Cerebellum

Restiform body

Medulla oblongata

Dorsal external arcuate fiber

Ventral spinocerebellar tract

Spinal cord

Dorsal spinocerebellar tract

Clarke's cells

Figure 11–8.   The spinocerebellar tracts.

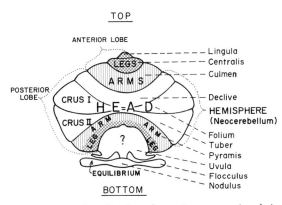

Figure 11–10. Localization of somatic sensory signals in the cerebellum of the human being.

ing the motor signals to activate the muscle or joint and from the muscle or joint concerning the effect actually produced. Then it projects signals back into the motor pathway to the same respective topographical part of the system.

The Equilibrium Area of the Cerebellum. Note in Figure 11–10 at the lowest part of the cerebellum (or most posterior part) an area labeled "equilibrium." This is the flocculonodular lobe of the cerebellum, a very old part that connects through bidirectional pathways with the vestibular nuclei. As was discussed in the previous chapter, this area is concerned almost entirely with equilibrium, and its destruction causes serious loss of equilibrium particularly when rapid movements are being performed.

OUTPUT SIGNALS FROM THE CEREBELLUM

The Deep Cerebellar Nuclei and the Efferent Pathways. Located deep in the cerebellar mass are four *deep cerebellar nuclei*–the *dentate, globose, emboliform,* and *fastigial nuclei.* These nuclei receive signals from two different sources: (1) the cerebellar cortex, and (2) all the sensory afferent tracts to the cerebellum. Each time an input signal arrives in the cerebellum, it goes both to the cerebellar cortex and also directly to the deep nuclei through collateral fibers; then, a short time later, the cerebellar cortex relays its output signals also to the the deep nuclei. Thus, all the input signals that enter the cerebellum eventually end in the deep nuclei. We shall discuss this circuit in greater detail below.

All of the efferent tracts from the cerebellum arise in the deep nuclei—none from the cerebellar cortex, which transmits its output signals only through the deep nuclei. Efferent signals are transmitted to many portions of the motor system including (1) the motor cortex, (2) the basal ganglia, (3) the red nucleus, (4) the reticular formation of the brain stem, and (5) the

vestibular nuclei. The important tracts, illustrated in Figure 11–11, are the following:

1. To the Motor Cortex. Fibers originate in the dentate nuclei and pass to the ventrolateral nucleus of the thalamus where they synapse with second order neurons that pass directly to the motor cortex.

2. To the Basal Ganglia. Signals pass from the dentate nucleus to the centromedian nucleus of the thalamus from which they are relayed to the striate body of the basal ganglia.

3. To the Red Nucleus. Fibers originating also in the dentate nucleus terminate in the *red nucleus*. This in turn transmits signals to the spinal cord through the rubrospinal tract, and it also sends short axons into the reticular formation.

4. To the Reticular Formation. Fibers enter the reticular formation, probably from all four of the deep cerebellar nuclei—the dentate, globose, and emboliform nuclei through the brachium conjunctivum into the upper part of the reticular formation, and from the fastigial nuclei into the lower reticular formation via the restiform body.

5. To the Vestibular Nuclei. As has already been pointed out in the previous chapter, the *fastigial nuclei* have bidirectional connections with the vestibular nuclei. The fastigial nuclei subserve primarily the flocculonodular lobe of the cerebellum and other closely allied regions of the older cerebellum.

THE NEURONAL CIRCUIT OF THE CEREBELLUM

The structure of the cerebellar cortex is entirely different from the cerebral cortex. Furthermore, each part of the cerebellar cortex has a neuronal organization almost precisely the same as that in all other parts.

The human cerebellum is actually a large folded sheet, approximately 17 cm. wide by 120

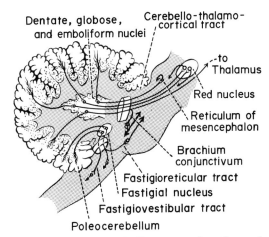

Figure 11–11. Principal efferent tracts from the cerebellum.

cm. long, the folds lying crosswise, as illustrated in Figures 11–9 and 11–10. Each fold is called a *folium.*

The Functional Unit of the Cerebellar Cortex—the Purkinje Cells. The cerebellum has approximately 30 million nearly identical functional units, one of which is illustrated in Figure 11–12. This functional unit centers around the Purkinje cell, of which there are also 30 million in the cerebellar cortex.

Note to the far right in Figure 11–12 the three major layers of the cerebellum: the *molecular layer,* the *Purkinje cell layer,* and the *granular cell layer.* In addition to these layers, the deep nuclei are located far within the center of the cerebellar mass.

The Neuronal Circuit of the Functional Unit. As illustrated in Figure 11–12, the output from the functional unit is from a deep nuclear cell. However, this cell is continually under the influence of both excitatory and inhibitory influences. The excitatory influences arise from direct connections with the afferent fibers that enter the cerebellum. The inhibitory influences arise entirely from the Purkinje cells in the cortex of the cerebellum.

The afferent inputs to the cerebellum are of two types, one called the *climbing fiber type* and the other called the *mossy fiber type.* There is one climbing fiber for about 10 Purkinje cells. After sending collaterals to several deep nuclear cells, the climbing fiber projects all the way to the molecular layer of the cerebellar cortex where it makes about 300 synapses with the dendrites of each Purkinje cell. This climbing fiber is distinguished by the fact that a single impulse in it will always cause a single action potential in each Purkinje cell with which it connects. Another distinguishing feature of the climbing fibers is that they all originate in the inferior olive of the medulla.

The mossy fibers also send collaterals to excite the deep nuclear cells. Then these fibers proceed to the granular layer of the cortex where they synapse with hundreds of *granule cells.* These in turn send their very small axons, less than 1 micron in diameter, up to the outer surface of the cerebellar cortex to enter the surface-lining molecular layer. Here the axons divide into two branches that extend 1 to 2 millimeters in each direction parallel to the folia. There are literally millions of these *parallel nerve fibers* in each small segment of the cerebellar cortex (there are about 1000 granule cells for every Purkinje cell). It is into this molecular layer that the dendrites of the Purkinje cells project, and each Purkinje cell synapses with 80,000 to 200,000 of these parallel fibers. Yet, the mossy fiber input to the Purkinje cell is quite different from the climbing fiber input because stimulation of a single mossy fiber will never elicit an action potential in the Purkinje cell; instead, large numbers of mossy fibers must be stimulated simultaneously to activate the Purkinje cell. Furthermore, this activation usually takes the form of prolonged facilitation or excitation that, when it reaches threshold for stimulation, causes repetitive Purkinje cell firing rather than the single action potential occurring in response to the climbing fiber input.

Thus, the Purkinje cells are stimulated by two types of input circuits—one that causes a highly specific output in response to the incoming signal and the other that causes a less specific but tonic type of response. It should be noted that the greater proportion of the afferent input to the cerebellum is of the mossy fiber type because this represents the afferent input from all of the cerebellar afferent tracts besides those from the inferior olive.

Balance Between Excitation and Inhibition in the Deep Cerebellar Nuclei. Referring again to the circuit of Figure 11–12, one should note that direct stimulation of the deep nuclear cells by both the climbing and the mossy fibers excites them, whereas the signals arriving from the Purkinje cells inhibit them. Normally, there is a continual balance between these two effects so that the degree of output from the deep nuclear cell remains relatively constant. On the other hand, in the execution of rapid motor movements, the *timing* of the two effects on the

Figure 11–12. Basic neuronal circuit of the cerebellum. Also shown in the upper right hand corner are the three major layers of the cerebellar cortex.

deep nuclei is such that the excitation appears before the inhibition. Also, the relative balance between excitation and inhibition probably changes. In this way, very rapid excitatory and inhibitory transient signals can be fed back into the motor pathways to correct motor movements that are going awry. The inhibitory portions of these signals resemble delay-line negative feedback signals of the type that are very effective in providing damping. That is, when the motor system is excited, a negative feedback signal occurs after a short delay to stop the muscle movement from overshooting its mark, the usual cause of oscillation.

Other Inhibitory Cells in the Cerebellar Cortex. In addition to the granule cells and Purkinje cells, three other types of neurons are also located in the cerebellar cortex: *basket cells, stellate cells,* and *Golgi cells.* All of these are inhibitory cells with very short axons. After being excited, they inhibit either the Purkinje cells in the case of the stellate and basket cells, or the granule cells in the case of the Golgi cells. There is a strong possibility that this inhibition provides a sharpening of the signal. That is, these cells possibly or probably prevent crosstalk between individual functional units of the cerebellum.

Special Features of the Cerebellar Neuronal Circuit. A special feature of the cerebellum is that there are no reverberatory pathways in the cerebellar neuronal circuits, so that the input-output signals of the cerebellum are very rapid transients that never persist for long periods of time.

Another special feature is that most of the cells of the cerebellum are constantly active. This is especially true of the deep nuclear cells; they continually send output signals to the other areas of the motor system. The importance of this is that decrease of the nuclear cell firing rate can provide an inhibitory output signal from the cerebellum, while an increase in firing rate can provide an excitatory output signal.

FUNCTION OF THE CEREBELLUM IN VOLUNTARY MOVEMENTS

The cerebellum functions only in association with motor activities initiated elsewhere in the central nervous system. These activities may be initiated originally in the spinal cord, in the reticular formation, in the basal ganglia, or in the major areas of the cerebral cortex. We will discuss, first, the operation of the cerebellum in association with the motor cortex for the control of voluntary movements.

Figure 11–13 illustrates the basic cerebellar pathways involved in cerebellar control of voluntary movements. When motor impulses are transmitted from the cerebral cortex downward through the pyramidal and extrapyramidal tracts to excite the muscles, collateral impulses are transmitted simultaneously into the cerebellum through the pontocerebellar and olivocerebellar tracts. Therefore, for every motor movement that is performed, not only do the muscles receive activating signals, but the cerebellum receives similar signals at the same time.

When the muscles respond to the motor signals, the muscle spindles, Golgi tendon apparatuses, joint receptors, and other peripheral receptors transmit signals upward mainly through the spinocerebellar and spino-olivary pathways to terminate in the cerebellum.

After the signals from the periphery and those from the motor cortex are integrated, efferent impulses are transmitted from the cerebellar cortex to the dentate nuclei and thence upward through the ventrolateral nuclei of the thalamus back to the motor cortex where the stimulus first originated.

"Error Control" by the Cerebellum. One will readily recognize that the circuit described above represents a complicated feedback circuit beginning in the motor cortex and also returning to the motor cortex. Furthermore,

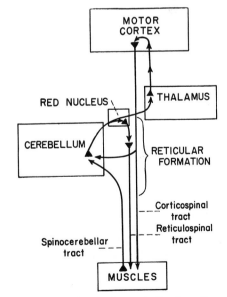

Figure 11–13. Pathways for cerebellar "error" control of voluntary movements.

experiments have shown that the cerebellum operates in much the same manner as a servo-mechanism such as that used in (a) industrial control systems, (b) the control system of an anti-aircraft gun, or (c) the control system of the automatic pilot. That is, the cerebellum seems to compare the "intentions" of the cortex with the "performance" by the parts of the body, and, if the parts are not moving according to the intentions of the cortex, the "error" between these two is calculated by the cerebellum so that appropriate and immediate corrections can be made. Thus, if the cortex has transmitted a signal intending the limb to move to a particular point, but the limb begins to move too fast and obviously is going to overshoot the point of intention, the cerebellum can initiate "braking impulses" to slow down the movement of the limb and stop it at the point of intention.

Ordinarily, the motor cortex transmits far more impulses than are needed to perform each intended movement, and the cerebellum therefore must act to inhibit the motor cortex at the appropriate time after the muscle has begun to move. The cerebellum automatically assesses the rate of movement and calculates the length of time that will be required to reach the point of intention. Then appropriate inhibitory impulses are transmitted to the motor cortex to inhibit the agonist muscle and to excite the antagonist muscle. In this way, appropriate "brakes" are applied to stop the movement at the precise point of intention.

Experiments have demonstrated two important characteristics of the cerebellar feedback system:

1. When a person performs a particular act, such as moving a heavy weight rapidly to a new position, at first he is unable to judge the degree of inertia that will be involved in the movement. Therefore, he almost always overshoots the point of intention on his first trial. However, after several trials, he can stop the movement at the precise point. This illustrates that learned knowledge of the inertia of the system is an important feature of the cerebellar feedback mechanism, though it is likely that this learning occurs in the cerebral cortex rather than in the cerebellum.

2. When a rapid movement is made toward a point of intention, the agonist muscle contracts strongly throughout the early course of movement. Then, suddenly, shortly before the point of intention is reached, the agonist muscle becomes completely inhibited while the antagonist muscle becomes strongly excited. Furthermore, the point at which this reversal of excitation occurs depends on the rate of movement and on the previously learned knowledge of the inertia of the system. The faster the movement and the greater the inertia, the earlier the reversal point appears in the course of movement.

Since all these events transpire much too rapidly for the motor cortex to reverse the excitation "voluntarily," it is evident that the excitation of the antagonist muscle toward the end of a movement is an entirely automatic and subconscious function and is not a "willed" contraction of the same nature as the original contraction of the agonist muscle. We shall see below that in patients with serious cerebellar damage, excitation of the antagonist muscles does not occur at the appropriate time but instead always too late. Therefore, it is almost certain that one of the major functions of the cerebellum is automatic excitation of antagonist muscles at the end of a movement while at the same time inhibiting agonist muscles that have started the movement.

The "Damping" Function of the Cerebellum. One of the by-products of the cerebellar feedback mechanism is its ability to "damp" muscular movements. To explain the meaning of "damping" we must first point out that essentially all movements of the body are "pendular." For instance, when an arm is moved, momentum develops, and the momentum must be overcome before the movement can be stopped. And, because of the momentum, all pendular movements have a tendency to overshoot. If overshooting does occur in a person whose cerebellum has been destroyed, the conscious centers of the cerebrum eventually recognize this and initiate a movement in the opposite direction to bring the arm to its intended position. But again the arm, by virtue of its momentum, overshoots, and appropriate corrective signals must again be instituted. Thus, the arm oscillates back and forth past its intended point for several cycles before it finally fixes on its mark. This effect is called an *action tremor,* or *intention tremor.*

However, if the cerebellum is intact, appropriate subconscious signals stop the movement precisely at the intended point, thereby preventing the overshoot and also the tremor. This is the basic characteristic of a damping system. All servocontrol systems regulating pendular elements that have inertia must have damping circuits built into the servomechanisms. In the motor control system of our central nervous system, the cerebellum seems to provide much of this damping function.

Relationship of Cerebellar Damping to Damping Caused by the Stretch Reflex. The stretch reflex, which is strictly a cord reflex, also provides much of the damping of body movements, as pointed out in Chapter 9. The cerebellar damping mechanism seems to be superimposed onto the basic cord damping mechanism. The muscle spindles excite both these functions. Rapid stretch of a muscle transmits spindle signals both directly to the anterior motoneuron to cause the damping action of the stretch reflex and simultaneously to the cerebellum to cause additional damping. The cerebellum probably provides its damping action by transmitting reflex signals into the reticular formation and vestibular nuclei and thence back down the cord to stimulate or inhibit both the alpha and the gamma motoneurons.

The cerebellar damping mechanism at times supports the stretch reflex damping system and at other times inhibits it, thus illustrating that the cerebellar system has considerable latitude of control that makes it adaptable to more complex motor activities than is true of the stretch reflex.

Function of the Cerebellum in Prediction. Another important by-product of the cerebellar feedback mechanism is its ability to help the central nervous system predict the future positions of moving parts of the body. Without the cerebellum a person "loses" his limbs *when they move rapidly,* indicating that feedback information from the periphery probably must be analyzed by the cerebellum if the brain is to keep up with the motor movements. Thus, the cerebellum detects from the incoming proprioceptive signals the rapidity with which the limb is moving and then seems to predict from this the projected time course of movement. This allows the cerebellum, operating through the cerebellar output circuits to inhibit the agonist muscles and to excite the antagonist muscles when the movement approaches the point of intention.

Without the cerebellum this predictive function is so deficient that moving parts of the body move much farther than the point of intention. This failure to control the distance that the parts of the body move is called *dysmetria,* which means simply poor control of the distance of movement. As would be expected, dysmetria is much more pronounced in rapid movements than in slow movements.

Failure of Smooth "Progression of Movements." One of the most important features of normal motor function is one's ability to progress from one movement to the next in an orderly succession. When the cerebellum be-

comes dysfunctional and the person loses his subconscious ability to predict ahead of time how far the different parts of his body will move in a given time, he becomes unable also to control the beginning of the next movement. As a result, the succeeding movement may begin much too early or much too late. Therefore, movements such as those required for writing, running, or even talking all become completely incoordinate, lacking completely in the ability to progress in an orderly sequence from one movement to the next.

Extramotor Predictive Functions of the Cerebellum. The cerebellum also plays a role in predicting other events besides simply movements of the body. For instance, the rates of progression of both auditory and visual phenomena can be predicted. As an example, a person can predict from the changing visual scene how rapidly he is approaching an object. A striking experiment that demonstrates the importance of the cerebellum in this ability is the effect of removing the "head" portion of the cerebellum in monkeys. Such a monkey occasionally charges the wall of a corridor and literally bashes its brains out because it is unable to predict when it will reach the wall.

Unfortunately, we are only now beginning to learn about these extramotor predictive functions of the cerebellum. It is quite possible that the cerebellum provides a "time base" against which signals from other parts of the central nervous system can be compared. It is often stated that the cerebellum is especially important in interpreting spatiotemporal relationships in sensory information.

FUNCTION OF THE CEREBELLUM IN INVOLUNTARY MOVEMENTS

The cerebellum functions in involuntary, subconscious, or postural movements in almost exactly the same manner as it does in voluntary movements except that slightly different pathways are involved, as shown in Figure 11–14. The extrapyramidal signals that originate in the motor cortex, basal ganglia, or reticular formation to cause involuntary movements pass mainly into the inferior olive and thence into the cerebellum, primarily to the paleocerebellum. Then as the muscle movements occur, proprioceptive information from the muscles, joints, and other peripheral parts of the body passes to the cerebellum, thus providing the same type of "error" control for involuntary movements as is provided for voluntary movements, as discussed above. Signals then feed from the cerebellum back to the *motor cortex, basal ganglia,* and *reticular formation.* They feed back into the basal ganglia mainly by way of the *emboliform*

Figure 11–14. Pathways for cerebellar "error" control of involuntary movements.

nuclei, then upward through the *centromedian nuclei* of the thalamus, and thence into the *putamen.*

One of the principal pathways through which corrective signals are transmitted to the muscles is *reticulospinal fibers* that control the *gamma efferent system* to the muscle spindles. Indeed, the cerebellum is one of the most powerful of all the activators of this system, which indicates a special importance of the gamma efferents in cerebellar functions.

Function of the Cerebellum for Control of Spinal Reflex Movements. Even movements elicited by spinal reflexes are modified to some extent by the cerebellum. For instance, in the absence of the cerebellum, sudden movement of a limb by some extraneous force is met with almost no resistance, but in the presence of the cerebellum the stretch reflexes oppose the movement almost instantaneously. Thus, the cerebellum, operating through a cerebellar-reticular feedback system, greatly enhances the power of the spinal stretch reflex.

On the other hand, many movements integrated in the spinal cord, such as scratching and cleaning of the face with the paws, can be performed completely coordinately in the absence of a cerebellum.

FUNCTION OF THE CEREBELLUM IN EQUILIBRIUM

In the discussion of the vestibular apparatus and of the mechanism of equilibrium in Chapter 10, it was

pointed out that the flocculonodular lobes of the cerebellum are required for proper integration of the equilibratory impulses. Removal of the *nodulus* in particular causes almost complete loss of equilibrium, and removal of the *flocculus* causes temporary loss. The symptoms of mal-equilibrium are essentially the same as those that result from destruction of the semicircular canals. This indicates that these areas of the cerebellum are particularly important for integration of *changes in direction of motion* as detected by the semicircular canals, but not so important for integrating static signals of equilibrium from the maculae in the utricles and saccules. This is in keeping with the other functions of the cerebellum; that is, the semicircular canals allow the central nervous system to *predict* ahead of time that rotational movements of the body are going to cause mal-equilibrium, and this predictive function causes appropriate muscles to contract to prevent the person from losing equilibrium even before this state develops. This is very much the same as the predictive function of the cerebellum for coordination of rapid voluntary movements.

CLINICAL ABNORMALITIES OF THE CEREBELLUM

Destruction of small portions of the cerebellar cortex causes no detectable abnormality in motor function. In fact, several months after as much as half the cerebellar cortex has been removed, the motor functions appear to be almost entirely normal—but only as long as the person performs all movements very slowly. Thus, the remaining areas of the cerebellum compensate tremendously for loss of part of the cerebellum.

To cause serious and continuous dysfunction of the cerebellum, the cerebellar lesion must usually involve the deep cerebellar nuclei—the *dentate, emboliform, globose,* and *fastigial nuclei*—as well as the cerebellar cortex.

Dysmetria and Ataxia. Two of the most important symptoms of cerebellar disease are dysmetria and ataxia. It was pointed out above that in the absence of the cerebellum a person cannot predict ahead of time how far his movements will go. Therefore, the movements ordinarily overshoot their intended mark. This effect is called *dysmetria,* and it results in incoordinate movements which are called *ataxia.*

Dysmetria and ataxia can also result from lesions in the spinocerebellar tracts, for the feedback information from the moving parts of the body is essential for accurate control of the muscular movements.

Past Pointing. Past pointing means that in the absence of the cerebellum a person ordinarily moves his hand or some other moving part of his body considerably beyond the point of intention. This probably results from the following effect: The motor cortex normally transmits more impulses to the muscles to perform a given motor function than are actually needed. The cerebellum automatically corrects this by inhibiting the movement after it has begun. However, if the cerebellum is not available to cause this inhibition, the movement ordinarily goes far beyond the intended point. Therefore, past pointing is actually a manifestation of dysmetria.

Failure of Progression. *Dysdiadochokinesia.* When the motor control system fails to predict ahead of time where the different parts of the body will be at a given time, it temporarily "loses" the parts during rapid motor movements. As a result, the succeeding movement may begin much too early or much too late so that no orderly "progression of movement" can occur. One can demonstrate this readily in a patient with cerebellar damage by having him turn one of this hands upward and downward at a rapid rate. He rapidly "loses" his hand and does not know its position during any portion of the movement. As a result, a series of jumbled movements occurs instead of the normal coordinate upward and downward motions. This is called dysdiadochokinesia.

Dysarthria. Another instance in which failure of progression occurs is in talking, for the formation of words depends on rapid and orderly succession of individual muscular movements in the larynx, mouth, and respiratory system. Lack of coordination between these and inability to predict either the intensity of the sound or the duration of each successive sound cause jumbled vocalization, with some syllables loud, some weak, some held long, some held for a short interval, and resultant speech that is almost completely unintelligible. This is called dysarthria.

Intention Tremor. When a person who has lost his cerebellum performs a voluntary act, his muscular movements are jerky; this reaction is called an *intention tremor* or an *action tremor,* and it results from failure of the cerebellar system to damp the motor movements. Tremor is particularly evident when the dentate nuclei or the brachium conjunctivum is destroyed, but it is not present when the spinocerebellar tracts from the periphery to the cerebellum are destroyed. This indicates that the feedback pathway from the cerebellum to the motor cortex is a principal pathway for damping of muscular movements.

Cerebellar Nystagmus. Cerebellar nystagmus is a tremor of the eyeballs that occurs usually when a person attempts to fixate his eyes on a scene to the side of this head. This off-center type of fixation results in rapid tremorous movements of the eyes rather than a steady fixation, and it is probably another manifestation of the failure of damping by the cerebellum. It also occurs especially when the flocculonodular lobes are damaged; and in this instance it is associated with loss of equilibrium, presumably because of dysfunction of the pathways through the cerebellum from the semicircular canals. Nystagmus resulting from damage to the semicircular canals was discussed in Chapter 10.

Rebound. If a person with cerebellar disease is asked to contract his arm tightly while the physician holds it back at first and then lets go, the arm will fly back until it strikes the face instead of being automatically stopped. This is called rebound, and it results from loss of the cerebellar component of the stretch reflex. That is, the normal cerebellum ordinarily instantaneously and powerfully sensitizes the spinal cord reflex mechanism whenever a portion of the body begins to move unexpectedly in an unwilled direction. But, without the cerebellum, activation of the antagonist muscles fails to occur, thus allowing over-movement of the limb.

Hypotonia. Loss of the deep cerebellar nuclei, particularly the dentate nuclei, causes moderate decrease in tone of the peripheral musculature on the side of the lesion, though after several months the motor cortex usually compensates for this by an increase in its intrinsic activity. The hypotonia results from loss of facilitation of the motor cortex by the tonic discharge of the dentate nuclei.

SENSORY FEEDBACK CONTROL OF MOTOR FUNCTIONS

Everyone who has ever studied the relationship of the somatic sensory areas to the motor areas of the cortex has been impressed by the close functional interdependence of the two areas. Anatomically, the characteristic pyramidal cells of the motor cortex extend backward into the anterior lip of the postcentral gyrus where they intermingle with the large numbers of granule cells of the somatic sensory cortex. Likewise, the granule cells of the sensory cortex extend anteriorly into the precentral gyrus, the *area pyramidalis.* Thus the two areas fade into each other with many somatic sensory fibers actually terminating directly in the motor cortex and some motor signals originating in the sensory cortex.

Furthermore, when a portion of the somatic sensory cortex in the postcentral gyrus is removed, the muscles controlled by the motor cortex immediately anterior to the removed area often lose much of their coordination. This observation illustrates that the somatic sensory area plays a major role in the control of motor functions. The overall mechanism by which sensory feedback plays this role has been postulated to be the following:

THE SENSORY "ENGRAM" FOR MOTOR MOVEMENTS

A person performs a motor movement mainly to achieve a purpose. It is primarily in the sensory and sensory association areas that he experiences effects of motor movements and records "memories" of the different patterns of motor movements. These are called sensory engrams of the motor movements. When he wishes to achieve some purposeful act, he presumably calls forth one of these engrams and then sets the motor system of the brain into action to reproduce the sensory pattern that is laid down in the engram.

The Proprioceptor Feedback Servomechanism for Reproducing the Sensory Engram. From the earlier discussion of cerebellar function, it is clear how proprioceptor signals from the periphery can affect motor activity. However, in addition to the feedback pathways through the cerebellum, more slowly acting feedback pathways also pass from proprioceptors to the sensory areas of the cerebral cortex and thence back to the motor cortex. Each of these feedback pathways is capable of modifying the motor response. For instance, if a person learns to cut with scissors, the movements involved in this process cause a particular sequential pattern of proprioceptive impulses to pass to the somatic sensory area. Once this pattern has been "learned" by the sensory cortex, the memory engram of the pattern can be used to activate the motor system to perform the same sequential pattern whenever it is required.

To do this, the proprioceptor signals from the fingers, hands, and arms are compared with the engram, and if the two do not match each other, the difference, called the "error," supposedly initiates additional motor signals that automatically activate appropriate muscles to bring the fingers, hands, and arms into the necessary sequential attitudes for performance of the task. Each successive portion of the engram presumably is projected according to a time sequence, and the motor control system automatically follows from one point to the next so that the fingers go through the precise motions necessary to duplicate exactly the sensory engram of the motor activity.

Thus, one can see that the motor system in this case actually acts as a servomechanism, for it is not the motor cortex itself that controls the pattern of activity to be accomplished. Instead, the pattern is located in the sensory part of the brain, and the motor system merely "follows" the pattern, which is the definition of a servomechanism. If ever the motor system fails to follow the pattern, sensory signals are fed back to the cerebral cortex to apprise the sensorium of this failure, and appropriate corrective signals are transmitted to the muscles.

Other sensory signals besides somesthetic signals are also involved in motor control, particularly visual signals. However, these other sensory systems are often slower to recognize error than is the somatic proprioceptor system. Therefore, when the sensory engram depends on visual feedback for control purposes, the motor movements are usually considerably slowed in comparison with those that depend on somatic feedback.

An extremely interesting experiment that demonstrates the importance of the sensory engram for control of motor movements is one in which a monkey has been trained to perform some complex activity and then various portions of his cortex are removed. Removal of small portions of the motor cortex that control the muscles normally used for the activity does not prevent the monkey from performing the activity. Instead he automatically uses other muscles in place of the paralyzed ones to perform the same activity. On the other hand, if the corresponding somatic sensory cortex is removed but the motor cortex is left intact, the monkey loses all ability to perform the activity. Thus, this experiment demonstrates that the motor system acts automatically as a servomechanism to use whatever muscles are available to follow the pattern of the sensory engram, and if some muscles are missing, other muscles are substituted automatically. The experiment also demonstrates forcefully that the somatic sensory cortex is essential to at least some types of "learned" motor performance.

ESTABLISHMENT OF "SKILLED" MOTOR PATTERNS

Many motor activities are performed so rapidly that there is insufficient time for sensory feedback signals to control these activities. For instance, the movements of the fingers during typing occur much too rapidly for somatic sensory signals to be transmitted either to the somatic sensory cortex or even directly to the motor cortex and for these then to control each discrete movement. It is believed that the patterns for control of these rapid coordinate muscular movements are established in the motor system itself, probably involving complex circuitry in the primary motor cortex, the so-called premotor area of the cortex, the basal ganglia, and even the cerebellum. Indeed, lesions in any of these areas can destroy one's ability to perform rapid coordinated muscular contractions, such as those required during the act of typing, talking, or writing by hand.

Role of Sensory Feedback During Establishment of the Rapid Motor Patterns. Even a highly skilled motor activity can be performed the very first time if it is performed extremely slowly—slowly enough for sensory feedback to guide the movements through each step. However, to be really useful, many skilled motor activities must be performed rapidly. This probably is achieved by successive performance of the same skilled activity until finally an engram of the skilled activity is laid down in the motor system as well as in the sensory system. This motor engram causes a precise set of muscles to go through a specific sequence of movements required to perform the skilled activity. Therefore, such an engram is called a *pattern of skilled motor function,* and the motor areas are primarily concerned with this.

After a person has performed a skilled activity many times, the motor pattern of this activity can thereafter cause the hand or arm or other part of the body to go through the same pattern of activity again and again, now entirely *without* sensory feedback control. However, even though sensory feedback control is no longer present, the sensory system still determines whether or not the act has been performed correctly. This determination is made in retrospect rather than while the act is being performed. If the pattern has not been performed correctly, information from the sensory system supposedly can help to correct the pattern the next time it is performed.

Thus, eventually, hundreds of patterns of different coordinate movements are laid down in the motor system, and these can be called upon one at a time in different sequential orders to perform literally thousands of complex motor activities.

An interesting experiment that demonstrates the applicability of these theoretical methods of muscular control is one in which the eyes are made to "follow" an object that moves around and around in a circle. At first, the eyes can follow the object only when it moves around the circle slowly, and even then the movements of the eyes are extremely jerky. Thus, sensory feedback is being utilized to control the eye movements for following the object. However, after a few seconds, the eyes begin to follow the moving object rather faithfully, and the rapidity of movement around the circle can be increased to many times per second, and still, the eyes continue to follow the object. Sensory feedback control of each stage of the eye movements at these rapid rates would be completely impossible. Therefore, by this time, the eyes have developed a pattern of movement that is not dependent upon step-by-step sensory feedback. Nevertheless, if the eyes should fail to follow the object around the circle, the sensory system would immediately become aware of this and presumably could make corrections in the pattern of movement.

EFFECT OF DIFFERENT MUSCULAR LOADS ON THE PERFORMANCE OF SKILLED MOTOR ACTIVITIES

All of us know that a person can move his hand around and around in a circle whether the hand be empty or loaded with a 10-pound weight. That is, the load makes little difference in the faithfulness of performance of the required activity. The reason for this is that the motor activity is probably controlled by a servo feedback mechanism that monitors the performance of the motor act constantly, and, if the performance is not according to the sensory engram of the required movement, appropriate "error" signals are automatically transmitted into the motor system to achieve the desired result. One can see, therefore, the practical significance of the servomechanism type of control of muscular activity.

Unfortunately, we still do not know all the neuronal circuitry that allows the pattern of movement to be dissociated from the muscle load. If the motor activity is performed very slowly, obviously feedback through the sensory cortex can provide adjustment of muscle forces so that the effects of load can be compensated. After a pattern of motor function has been established, however, precise patterns can be executed entirely subconsciously, despite widely varying loads. Even after loss of the cerebellum this can still be achieved, though not very well for rapid movements. Therefore, by the process of elimination, we can perhaps point to the basal ganglia as likely major components of the servomechanism for dissociating load from muscle performance. Another reason for implicating the basal ganglia is that their circuitry is ideally organized for this purpose, having tremendous numbers of interlacing feedback pathways and also receiving strong feedback sensory signals from all parts of the body. This, however, is entirely hypothetical, though it is an approach to one of the most important questions in the field of motor neurophysiology.

INITIATION OF VOLUNTARY MOTOR ACTIVITY

Because of the spectacular properties of the primary motor cortex and of the instantaneous muscle contractions that can be achieved by stimulating this area, it has become customary to think that the initial brain signals that elicit voluntary muscle contractions begin in the primary motor cortex. However, this almost certainly is far from the truth. Indeed, experiments have shown that the cerebellum and the basal ganglia are activated at almost exactly the same time that the motor cortex is activated, and all of these are activated even *before* the voluntary movement occurs. Furthermore, there is no known mechanism by which the motor cortex can conceive the entire sequential pattern that is to be achieved by the motor movements.

Therefore, we are left with an unanswered question: What is the locus of the initiation of voluntary motor activity? In the following chapter we will learn that the reticular formation of the brain stem and much of the thalamus play essential roles in activating all other parts of the brain. Therefore, it is very likely that these areas provide the initial signals that lead to subsequent activity in the motor cortex, the basal ganglia, and the cerebellum at the onset of voluntary movement. Here again, we come to a circular question: What is it that initiates the activity in the brain stem and the thalamus? We do know part of the answer to this: The activity is initiated by continual sensory input into these areas, including sensory input from the peripheral receptors of the body and from the cortical sensory storage, or memory, areas. Much of motor activity is almost reflex in nature, occurring instantly after an incoming sensory signal from the periphery. But so-called voluntary activity occurs minutes, hours, or even days after the initiating sensory input—after analysis, storage of memories, recall of the memories, and finally initiation of a motor response. We shall see in Chapter 13 that the control of motor activity is strongly influenced by these prolonged procedures of cerebration. Furthermore, damage to the essential areas of the cerebral cortex for analysis of sensory information leads to serious deficits and abnormalities of voluntary muscle control.

Therefore, for the present, let us conclude that the immediate energy for eliciting voluntary motor activity probably comes from the basal regions of the brain. These, in turn, are under the control of the different sensory inputs, the memory storage areas, and the associated areas of the brain that are devoted to the processes of analysis, a mechanism frequently called *cerebration*.

REFERENCES

Allen, G. I., and Tsukahara, N.: Cerebrocerebellar communication systems. Physiol. Rev., 54:957, 1974.

Asanuma, H.: Cerebral cortical control of movement. Physiologist, 16:143, 1973.
Asanuma, H.: Recent developments in the study of the columnar arrangement of neurons within the motor cortex. Physiol. Rev., 55:143, 1975.
Barr, M. L: The Human Nervous System, 2nd Ed. Hagerstown, Md., Harper & Row, Publishers, 1974.
Brooks, V. B., and Stoney, S. D., Jr.: Motor mechanisms: the role of the pyramidal system in motor control. Ann. Rev. Physiol., 33:337, 1971.
Cohen, B., and Highstein, S. M.: Cerebellar control of the vestibular pathways to oculomotor neurons. Prog. Brain Res., 37:411, 1972.
Cooper, I. S., Riklan, M., and Snider, R. S. (eds.): The Cerebellum, Epilepsy, and Behavior. New York, Plenum Publishing Corporation, 1974.
Eccles, J. C.: The Understanding of the Brain. New York, McGraw-Hill Book Company, 1973.
Eccles, R. M., Shealy, C. N., and Willis, W. D.: Patterns of innervation of kitten motoneurones. J. Physiol. (Lond.), 165:392, 1963.
Eliasson, S. G., Prensky, A. L., and Hardin, W. B., Jr. (eds.): Neurological Pathophysiology. New York, Oxford University Press, 1974.
Evarts, E. V.: Activity of pyramidal tract neurons during postural fixation. J. Neurophysiol., 32:375, 1969.
Evarts, E. V.: Brain mechanisms in movement. Sci. Amer., 229:96, 1973.
Evarts, E. V., and Thach, W. T.: Motor mechanisms of the CNS: cerebrocerebellar interrelations. Ann. Rev. Physiol., 31:451, 1969.
Fox, C. A., and Snider, R. S.: The Cerebellum. Progress in Brain Research. Vol. 25. New York, American Elsevier Publishing Co., Inc., 1967.
Granit, R.: The Basis of Motor Control. New York, Academic Press, Inc., 1970.
Grillner, S.: Locomotion in vertebrates: central mechanisms and reflex interaction. Physiol. Rev., 55:247, 1975.
Hunt, C. C., and Kuno, M.: Properties of spinal interneurones. J. Physiol. (Lond.), 147:346, 1959.
Langworthy, O. R.: The Sensory Control of Posture and Movement. Baltimore, The Williams & Wilkins Company, 1970.
Lenman, J. A. R.: Clinical Neurophysiology. Philadelphia, J. B. Lippincott Company, 1975.
Llinas, R., Bloedel, J. E., and Hillman, D. E.: Functional characterization of neuronal circuitry of frog cerebellar cortex. J. Neurophysiol., 32:847, 1969.
Llinas, R.: Eighteenth Bowditch lecture. Motor aspects of cerebellar control. Physiologist, 17:19, 1974.
Massion, J.: The mammalian red nucleus. Physiol. Rev., 47:383, 1967.
Merritt, H. H.: A Textbook of Neurology. Philadelphia, Lea & Febiger, 1973.
Mettler, F. A.: Muscular tone and movement: their cerebral control in primates. Neurosci. Res., 1:175, 1968.
O'Connell, A. L., and Gardner, E. B.: Understanding the Scientific Bases of Human Movement. Baltimore, The Williams & Wilkins Company, 1972.
Oscarsson, O.: Functional organization of the spino- and cuneocerebellar tracts. Physiol. Rev., 45:495, 1965.
Paillard, J.: The patterning of skilled movements. In Magoun, H. W. (ed.): Handbook of Physiology. Sec. 1, Vol. 3. Baltimore, The Williams & Wilkins Company, 1960, p. 1489.
Penfield, W., and Rasmussen, T.: The Cerebral Cortex of Man. New York, The Macmillan Company, 1950.
Porter, R.: Functions of the mammalian cerebral cortex in movement. Prog. Neurobiol., 1:3, 1973.
Porter, R.: The neurophysiology of movement performance. In Guyton, A. C. (ed.): MTP International Review of Science: Physiology. Vol. 3. Baltimore, University Park Press, 1974, p. 151.
Stark, L., Ida, M., and Willis, P. A.: Dynamic characteristics of the motor coordination system in man. Biophys. J., 1:279, 1961.
Woody, C. D.: Aspects of the electrophysiology of cortical processes related to the development and performance of learned motor responses. Physiologist, 17:49, 1974.

12

Activation of the Brain—the Reticular Activating System; the Diffuse Thalamocortical System; Brain Waves; Epilepsy; Wakefulness and Sleep

In the previous chapters of this section on neurophysiology we have discussed, first, the somatic sensory mechanisms of the nervous system and, second, the motor mechanisms. In the present chapter we will consider the functions of the *reticular activating system,* a system that controls the overall degree of central nervous system activity, including control of wakefulness and sleep, and control of at least part of our ability to direct attention toward specific areas of our conscious minds.

Figure 12–1A illustrates the extent of this system, showing that it begins in the lower brain stem and extends upward through the mesencephalon and thalamus to be distributed throughout the cerebral cortex. Impulses are transmitted from the ascending reticular activating system to the cortex by two different pathways. One pathway passes upward from the brain stem portion of the reticular formation to the intralaminar, midline, and reticular nuclei of the thalamus and thence through diverse pathways to essentially all parts of the cerebral cortex as well as the basal ganglia. A second and probably much less important pathway is through the subthalamic, hypothalamic, and adjacent areas.

FUNCTION OF THE RETICULAR ACTIVATING SYSTEM IN WAKEFULNESS

Diffuse electrical stimulation in the *mesencephalic, pontile and upper medullary portions of the reticular formation*—an area also called the *bulboreticular facilitatory area* and discussed in Chapter 10 in relation to the motor functions of the nervous system—causes immediate and marked activation of the cerebral cortex and even causes a sleeping animal to awaken instantaneously. Furthermore, when this brain stem portion of the reticular formation is damaged severely, as occurs (a) when a *brain tumor* develops in this region, (b) when serious *hemorrhage* occurs, or (c) in diseases such as *encephalitis lethargica* (sleeping sickness), the person passes into coma and is completely nonsusceptible to normal awakening stimuli.

Function of the Brain Stem Portion of the Reticular Activating System. Electrical stimuli applied to different portions of the reticular activating system have shown that the brain stem portion functions quite differently from the thalamic portion. Electrical stimulation of the

Figure 12–1. (A) The ascending reticular activating system schematically projected on a monkey brain. (From Lindsley: Reticular Formation of the Brain. Little, Brown and Co.) (B) Convergence of pathways from the cerebral cortex and from the spinal afferent systems on the reticular activating system. (From French, Hernandez-Peon, and Livingston: *J. Neurophysiol., 18*:74, 1955.)

brain stem portion causes generalized activation of the entire brain, including activation of the cerebral cortex, thalamic nuclei, basal ganglia, hypothalamus, other portions of the brain stem, and even the spinal cord. Furthermore, once the brain stem portion is stimulated, the degree of activation throughout the nervous system remains high for as long as a half minute or more after the stimulation is over. Therefore, *it is believed that the brain stem portion of the reticular activating system is basically responsible for normal wakefulness of the brain.*

Function of the Thalamic Portion of the Activating System. Electrical stimulation in different areas of the thalamic portion of the activating system (if the stimulation is not too strong) activates specific regions of the cerebral cortex more than others. This is distinctly different from stimulation in the brain stem portion, which activates all the brain at the same time. Therefore, it is believed that the thalamic portion of the activating system has two specific functions: first, it relays most of the diffuse facilitatory signals from the brain stem to all parts of the cerebral cortex to cause generalized activation of the cerebrum; second, stimulation of selected points in the thalamic activating system causes specific activation of certain areas of the cerebral cortex in distinction to the other areas. This selective activation of specific cortical areas possibly or probably plays an important role in our ability to direct our attention to certain parts of our mental activity, which is discussed later in the chapter.

THE AROUSAL REACTION—SENSORY ACTIVATION OF THE RETICULAR ACTIVATING SYSTEM

When an animal is asleep, the level of activity of the reticular activating system is greatly decreased; yet almost any type of sensory signal can immediately activate the system. For instance, proprioceptive signals from the joints and muscles, pain impulses from the skin, visual signals from the eyes, auditory signals from the ears, or even visceral sensations from the gut can all cause sudden activation of the reticular activating system and therefore arouse the animal. This is called the *arousal reaction.*

Some types of sensory stimuli are more potent than others in eliciting the arousal reaction, the most potent being pain and proprioceptive somatic impulses.

Anatomically, the reticular formation of the brain stem is admirably constructed to perform the arousal functions. It receives tremendous numbers of signals either directly or indirectly from the *spinoreticular tracts,* the *spinothalamic tracts,* the *spinotectal tracts,* the *auditory tracts,* the *visual tracts,* and others, so that almost any sensory stimulus in the body can activate it. The reticular formation in turn can transmit signals both upward into the brain and downward into the spinal cord. Indeed, many of the fibers originating from cells in the reticular formation divide, with one branch of the fiber passing upward and the other branch passing downward, as was explained in Chapter 10.

STIMULATION OF THE RETICULAR ACTIVATING SYSTEM BY THE CEREBRAL CORTEX

In addition to activation of the reticular activating system by sensory impulses, the cerebral cortex can also stimulate this system. Direct fiber pathways pass into the reticular activating areas, as shown in Figure 12–1B, from almost all parts of the cerebrum but particularly from (1) the *sensorimotor cortex* of the pre- and postcentral gyri, (2) the *frontal cortex,* (3) the *cingulate gyrus,* (4) the *hippocampus* and *other structures of the rhinencephalon,* (5) the *hypothalamus,* and (6) the *basal ganglia.* Because of

an exceedingly large number of nerve fibers that pass from the motor regions of the cerebral cortex to the reticular formation, motor activity in particular is associated with a high degree of wakefulness, which partially explains the importance of movement to keep a person awake. However, intense activity of any other part of the cerebrum can also activate the reticular activating system and consequently can cause a high degree of wakefulness.

THE DIFFUSE THALAMOCORTICAL SYSTEM

At this point it is important that we explain some of the interrelationships between the thalamus and the cerebral cortex. The thalamus is the main entryway for essentially all sensory nervous signals to the cortex, with the exception of signals from the olfactory system. In Chapters 7 and 8 we have already discussed the transmission of the somatic signals through the thalamus to the cerebral cortex, and we shall see in Chapters 18, 19, and 20 that all the signals from the visual, auditory, and taste systems are also relayed through the thalamus before reaching the cortex. In the following chapter we shall discuss the two-way communication between essentially all parts of the cerebral cortex and the thalamus. For all of these functions of the thalamus, there are very definite nuclei that are called the *specific nuclei of the thalamus;* the combination of these nuclei and their connecting areas in the cortex is called the *specific thalamocortical system.* It is this system of which we usually speak when we discuss the transmission of sensory information into the cerebral cortex.

In addition to the specific thalamocortical system, there is a separate system, partially separated from the specific system, called the *diffuse thalamocortical system,* or the *generalized thalamocortical system,* or the *nonspecific thalamocortical system.* This system is subserved by *diffuse thalamic nuclei* and also by *diffuse fiber projections* from the thalamus to the cortex. In general, the thalamic neurons of this system are not collected into discrete nuclei as are the neurons of the specific system. Instead, they lie mainly between the specific nuclei or on the outer surface of the thalamus; they are divided into three separate groups: (1) the *intralaminar nuclei,* which are diffuse collections of neurons that lie in the middle of the thalamic mass between the specific nuclei; (2)

the *midline nuclei,* which are small collections of neurons in the midline of the thalamus where the two halves of the thalamus come together and which seem to have little organization; and (3) the *reticular nuclei* of the thalamus, which form a thin shell of diffuse neurons that lies over the surface of the thalamus and through which all the pathways from the thalamus to the cerebral cortex must pass. All of these nuclei make multiple connections with the specific thalamic nuclei. They also project very small fibers to all parts of the cerebral cortex, with the exception of small portions of the temporal lobes that are mainly associated with the limbic system, a very old part of the brain which plays major roles in behavior, emotions, and so forth as will be discussed in Chapter 14.

The diffuse system of the thalamus is continuous with the upper end of the reticular formation in the brain stem and receives much of its input from this source. However, it is also an important terminus of one of the very important somatic sensory pathways, the *paleo-spinothalamic pathway for pain*—the pathway that transmits the intolerable type of burning, aching pain. This is the same pathway that transmits the major sensory signals into much of the reticular formation of the brain stem as well.

Control Functions of the Diffuse Thalamocortical System. One can well understand from the above description of the diffuse thalamic nuclei that they lie in propitious locations for affecting the levels of activity of all of the specific nuclei of the thalamus. It is also clear that they are properly located to relay control functions from the brain stem reticular formation to the cerebrum, and that they in turn can receive much helpful input information from the specific nuclei of the thalamus. Perhaps most important of all, however, is that these nuclei have a specific capability to control the level of activity of the entire cerebral cortex itself; this is mediated by signals that play on the cerebral cortex through the diffuse thalamocortical projections.

Effect of the Diffuse Thalamic System on Cortical Activity. Activation of the cortex by the diffuse thalamic system is entirely different from activation by the specific system. Some of the differences are the following:

1. Stimulation of a specific thalamic nucleus activates the cortex within 1 to 2 milliseconds, whereas stimulation of the diffuse system causes no activation for approximately the first 25 milliseconds. The activation level builds up over a period of several hundred milliseconds if the stimulation is continued.

2. At the end of stimulation of the thalamus, the activation of the cortex by the specific nuclei dies away within another few milliseconds, whereas the activation by the diffuse system sometimes continues as an "after-discharge" for as long as 30 seconds.

3. Signals from the specific nuclei to the cortex activate mainly layer IV of the cortex, as was explained in Chapter 7, whereas activation of the diffuse thalamic system activates mainly layers I and II of the cortex. Since this latter activation is prolonged and because layers I and II are the loci of many of the dendrites of the deeper cortical neurons, it is supposed that the stimulation by the diffuse thalamic system mainly causes partial depolarization of large numbers of dendrites near the surface of the cortex; this in turn causes a generalized increase in the degree of facilitation of the cortex. When the cortex is thus facilitated by the diffuse thalamic system, specific signals that enter the cortex from other sources are exuberantly received.

Figure 12–2 illustrates the major differences between the specific and the diffuse thalamocortical systems. It shows the response of the visual cortex to (a) stimulation of a specific thalamic nucleus, and (b) stimulation of the diffuse thalamocortical system. In the upper record, elicited by stimulation of the lateral geniculate body, the specific nucleus for vision, the response occurred within a few milliseconds after the stimulus. Also, it began with a record below the line, indicating positivity on the surface of the cortex; this is the type of record that occurs when the deeper layers of the cortex are stimulated first—in this case, layer IV of the cortex. In the lower record, the stimulus was

Figure 12–2. Comparison of the response of the visual cortex following stimulation of the lateral geniculate body (record A), which is part of the specific thalamocortical system, with the response of the visual cortex following stimulation of the visual portion of the diffuse thalamocortical system (record B). Note in record B the long latent period before appearance of the diffuse response and also the prolonged duration of the response.

applied to the visual region of the diffuse thalamic nuclei. Note the very long latent period, the long response, and the fact that the response is entirely above the line (indicating negativity) which means that the superficial layers of the cortex were stimulated by this signal.

Another feature of stimulation of the diffuse system is the phenomenon called the *recruiting response*. When this system is stimulated repetitively at a frequency of about 10 to 12 cycles per second, the first response is relatively weak, the second a little stronger, the third still stronger, and so forth, the response becoming considerably stronger for the first 4 to 10 stimuli. That is, the system "recruits" more and more cortical synapses into the pattern of response with the repetitive stimulation.

In summary, the diffuse thalamocortical system controls the overall degree of activity of the cortex. It probably can at times facilitate activity in regional areas of the cortex distinct from the remainder of the cortex. Collateral signals control the level of activity in the specific nuclei of the thalamus, the basal ganglia, the hypothalamus, and other structures of the cerebrum as well.

ATTENTION

So long as a person is awake, he has the ability to direct his attention to specific aspects of his mental environment. Furthermore, his degree of attention can change remarkably from (a) almost no attention at all to (b) broad attention to almost everything that is going on, or to (c) intense attention to a minute facet of his momentary mental experience.

Unfortunately, the basic mechanisms by which the brain accomplishes its diverse acts of attention are not known. However, a few clues are beginning to fall into place, as follows:

Brain Stem Control of Overall Attentiveness. In exactly the same way that a person can change from a state of sleep to a state of wakefulness, there can be all degrees of wakefulness, from wakefulness in which a person is nonattentive to almost all his surroundings to an extremely high degree of wakefulness in which the person reacts instantaneously to almost any sensory experience. These changes in degree of *overall attentiveness* seem to be caused primarily by changes in activity of the brain stem portion of the reticular activating system. Thus, control of the general level of attentiveness is

probably exerted by the same mechanism that controls wakefulness and sleep, the control center for which is located in the mesencephalon and upper pons.

Function of the Thalamus in Attention. Earlier in the chapter it was pointed out that stimulation of a single specific area in the thalamic portion of the reticular activating system, when the stimulus intensity is not too strong, activates only a specific area of the cerebral cortex. Since the cerebral cortex is one of the most important areas of the brain for conscious awareness of our surroundings, one can surmise that the ability of specific thalamic areas to excite specific cortical regions might be one of the mechanisms by which a person can direct his attention to specific aspects of his mental environment, whether these be immediate sensory experiences or stored memories.

Relation of Centrifugal Control of Sensory Information to Attention. Nervous pathways extend centrifugally from almost all sensory areas of the brain toward the lower centers to control the intensity of sensory input to the brain. For instance, the auditory cortex can either inhibit or facilitate signals from the cochlea, the visual cortex can control the signals from the retina in the same way, and the somesthetic cortex can control the intensities of signals from the somatic areas of the body.

Thus, it is likely that activated regions of the cortex control their own sensory input under some conditions. This is another means by which the brain might direct its attention to specific phases of its mental activity.

POSSIBLE "SCANNING" AND "PROGRAMMING" FUNCTIONS OF THE BRAIN'S ACTIVATING SYSTEM

At this point it is important to refer back to the analogy drawn in Chapter 4 between the functions of the central nervous system and of a general purpose computer. Almost all complex computers, particularly those that are capable of storing information and then recalling this information at later times, have a control center called a "programming unit" that directs the attention of different parts of the computer to specific information stored in other parts of the computer. It is quite likely that the activating system of the brain, particularly the thalamic part, operates in much the same way as the programming unit of a computer for the following reasons:

1. The ability of the activating system to direct one's attention to specific mental activities is analogous to the ability of the programming unit to call

forth information that has been stored in the memory of the computer or to call forth information that is given to the computer at its input, information that is comparable to sensory information in the human being.

2. The programming unit can "find information" when its exact locus is not known. In the computer, this is achieved by dictating certain qualities required of the information and then searching through hundreds or thousands of stored bits of information until the appropriate information is found, a function called *scanning*. We know from psychological tests that our own brain can perform this same function, though we do not know how it does so. Yet, since the thalamus perhaps plays a role in directing our attention to stored information in specific areas of the cortex, it is reasonable to postulate that the thalamus, probably operating in conjunction with other basal areas of the brain, plays a major role in this scanning operation.

3. The programming unit of a computer determines the sequence of processing of information. Our brain can also control its thoughts in orderly sequence. Here again, mainly on the basis of anatomical considerations and on the basis of the fact that the reticular activating system is the primary controller of cerebral activity, it can be surmised, until we know more about the subject, that the reticular activating system is the primary controller of our orderly sequence of thoughts.

It is obviously premature to suggest an anatomical locus for the scanning function of the brain; indeed, this function probably requires complex circuitry that involves several loci. However, good candidates for this function are the centrum medianum and the medial dorsal nucleus of the thalamus, both of which are located in the middle of each half of the thalamus. They are large nuclei surrounded on all sides by the diffuse thalamic system, and they make multiple bidirectional connections with essentially all parts of the thalamus. Obviously, they are propitiously located for playing major roles in determining attention, drive, and so forth.

EFFECT OF BARBITURATE ANESTHESIA ON THE RETICULAR ACTIVATING SYSTEM

The barbiturates have a specific depressant effect on the brain stem portion of the reticular activating system. Therefore, barbiturates obviously can either depress brain activity or even cause sleep. Yet it is especially interesting that barbiturate anesthesia does not block transmission in most of the specific sensory systems and also does not entirely block function of the thalamic portion of the reticular activating system. It is probable that many other clinically used anesthetics also have specific depressant effects on the brain stem portion of the reticular activating system and in this way cause general anesthesia.

BRAIN WAVES

Electrical recordings from the surface of the brain or from the outer surface of the head demonstrate continuous electrical activity in the brain. Both the intensity and patterns of this electrical activity are determined to a great extent by the overall level of excitation of the brain resulting from functions in the reticular activating system. The undulations in the recorded electrical potentials, shown in Figure 12–3, are called *brain waves,* and the entire record is called an *electroencephalogram* (EEG).

The intensities of the brain waves on the surface of the scalp range from zero to 300 microvolts, and their frequencies range from once every few seconds to 50 or more per second. The character of the waves is highly dependent on the degree of activity of the cerebral cortex, and the waves change markedly between the states of wakefulness and sleep.

Much of the time, the brain waves are irregular, and no general pattern can be discerned in the EEG. However, at other times, distinct patterns do appear. Some of these are characteristic of specific abnormalities of the brain, such as epilepsy, which is discussed later. Others occur even in normal persons and can be classified into *alpha, beta, theta,* and *delta waves,* which are all illustrated in Figure 12–3.

Alpha waves are rhythmic waves occurring at a frequency between 8 and 13 per second and are found in the EEG's of almost all normal persons when they are awake in a quiet, resting state of cerebration. These waves occur most intensely in the occipital region but can also be recorded at times from the parietal and frontal regions of the scalp. Their voltage usually is about 50 microvolts. During sleep the alpha waves disappear entirely, and when the awake person's attention is directed to some specific type of mental activity, the alpha waves are replaced by asynchronous, higher frequency but lower voltage waves. Figure 12–4 illustrates the effect on the alpha waves of simply opening the eyes in bright light and

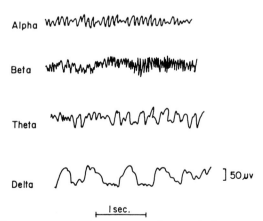

Figure 12–3. Different types of normal electroencephalographic waves.

Eyes open   Eyes closed

Figure 12–4. Replacement of the alpha rhythm by an asynchronous discharge on opening the eyes.

then closing the eyes again. Note that the visual sensations cause immediate cessation of the alpha waves and that these are replaced by low voltage, asynchronous waves.

Beta waves occur at frequencies of more than 14 cycles per second and as high as 25 and rarely 50 cycles per second. These are most frequently recorded from the parietal and frontal regions of the scalp, and they can be divided into two major types, *beta I* and *beta II*. The beta I waves, which are illustrated in Figure 12–3, have a frequency about twice that of the alpha waves, and these are affected by mental activity in very much the same way as the alpha waves—that is, they disappear and in their place appears an asynchronous but low voltage recording. The beta II waves, on the contrary, appear during *intense* activation of the central nervous system or during tension. Thus, one type of beta wave is inhibited by cerebral activity while the other is elicited.

Theta waves have frequencies between 4 and 7 cycles per second. These occur mainly in the parietal and temporal regions in children, but they also occur during emotional stress in some adults, particularly during disappointment and frustration. They can often be brought out in the EEG of a frustrated person by allowing him to enjoy some pleasant experience and then suddenly removing this element of pleasure; this causes approximately 20 seconds of theta waves. These same waves also occur in many brain disorders.

Delta waves include all the waves of the EEG below 3½ cycles per second and sometimes as low as 1 cycle every 2 to 3 seconds. These occur in deep sleep, in infancy, and in very serious organic brain disease. And they occur in the cortex of animals that have had subcortical transections separating the cerebral cortex from the thalamus. Therefore, delta waves can occur strictly in the cortex independently of activities in lower regions of the brain.

ORIGIN OF THE DIFFERENT TYPES OF BRAIN WAVES

The discharge of a single neuron or single nerve fiber in the brain cannot be recorded from the surface of the head. Instead, for an electrical potential to be recorded all the way through the skull, large portions of nervous tissue must emit electrical current simultaneously. There are two ways in which this can occur. First, tremendous numbers of nerve fibers can discharge in synchrony with each other, thereby generating very strong electrical currents. Second, large numbers of neurons can partially discharge,

though not emit action potentials; furthermore, these partially discharged neurons can give prolonged periods of current flow that can undulate slowly with changing degrees of excitability of the neurons. Simultaneous electrical measurements within the brain while recording brain waves from the scalp indicate that it is the second of these that causes the usual brain waves.

To be more specific, the surface of the cerebral cortex is composed almost entirely of a mat of dendrites from neuronal cells in the lower layers of the cortex. When signals impinge on these dendrites, they become partially discharged, emitting negative potentials characteristic of excitatory postsynaptic potentials, as discussed in Chapter 4. This partially discharged state makes the neurons of the cortex highly excitable, and the negative potential is simultaneously recorded from the surface of the scalp, indicating this high degree of excitability.

One of the important sources of signals to excite the outer dendritic layer of the cerebral cortex is the ascending reticular activating system. Therefore, brain wave intensity is closely related to the degree of activity in either the brain stem or the thalamic portions of the reticular activating system.

Origin of Delta Waves. Transection of the fiber tracts from the thalamus to the cortex, which blocks the reticular activating system fibers, causes delta waves in the cortex. This indicates that some synchronizing mechanism can occur in the cortical neurons themselves—entirely independently of lower structures in the brain—to cause the delta waves.

Delta waves also occur in very deep "slow wave" sleep; and this suggests that the cortex is then released from the activating influences of the reticular activating system, as was explained earlier in the chapter.

Origin of the Alpha Waves. Alpha waves will *not* occur in the cortex without connections with the thalamus. Also, stimulation in the diffuse thalamic nuclei often sets up waves in the diffuse thalamocortical system at a frequency of between 8 and 13 per second, the natural frequency of the alpha waves. Therefore, it is assumed that the alpha waves result from spontaneous activity in the diffuse thalamocortical system, which causes both the periodicity of the alpha waves and the synchronous activation of literally millions of cortical neurons during each wave.

EFFECT OF VARYING DEGREES OF CEREBRAL ACTIVITY ON THE BASIC RHYTHM OF THE ELECTROENCEPHALOGRAM

There is a general relationship between the degree of cerebral activity and the average frequency of the electroencephalographic rhythm, the frequency increasing progressively with higher and higher degrees of activity. This is illustrated in Figure 12–5, which shows the existence of delta waves in stupor,

Figure 12–5. Effect of varying degrees of cerebral activity on the basic rhythm of the EEG. (From Gibbs and Gibbs: Atlas of Electroencephalography. Addison-Wesley, 1974.)

surgical anesthesia, and sleep; theta waves in psychomotor states and in infants; alpha waves during relaxed states; and beta waves during periods of intense mental activity. However, during periods of mental activity the waves usually become asynchronous rather than synchronous so that the voltage falls considerably, despite increased cortical activity, as illustrated in Figure 12–4.

CLINICAL USE OF THE ELECTROENCEPHALOGRAM

One of the most important uses of the EEG is to diagnose different types of epilepsy and to find the focus in the brain causing the epilepsy. This is discussed further below. But, in addition, the EEG can be used to localize brain tumors or other space-occupying lesions of the brain and to diagnose certain types of psychopathic disturbances.

There are two means by which brain tumors can be localized. Some brain tumors are so large that they block electrical activity from a given portion of the cerebral cortex, and when this occurs the voltage of the brain waves is considerably reduced in the region of the tumor. However, more frequently a brain tumor compresses the surrounding neuronal tissue and thereby causes abnormal electrical excitation of these surrounding areas; this in turn leads to synchronous discharges of very high voltage waves in the EEG, as shown in the middle two records of Figure 12–6. Localization of the origin of these spikes on the surface of the scalp is a valuable means for locating the brain tumor.

The upper part of Figure 12–6 shows the placement of 16 different electrodes on the scalp, and the lower part of the figure shows the brain waves from four of these electrodes marked in the figure by X's. Note that in two of these, intense brain waves are recorded and, furthermore, that the two waves are essentially of reverse polarity to each other. This reverse polarity means that the origin of the spikes is somewhere in the area *between* the two respective electrodes. Thus, the excessively excitable area of the brain has been located, and this is a lead to the location of the brain tumor.

Use of brain waves in diagnosing psychopathic abnormalities is generally not very satisfactory because only a few of these cause distinct brain wave patterns. Yet by observing combinations of different types of basic rhythms, reactions of the rhythms to attention, changes of the rhythms with forced breathing to cause alkalosis, the appearance of particular characteristics in the brain waves (such as "spin-

dles" of alpha waves), and so forth, an experienced electroencephalographer can detect at least certain types of psychopathic disturbances. For instance, it was pointed out above that theta waves are frequently found in persons with brain abnormalities.

EPILEPSY

Epilepsy is characterized by uncontrolled excessive activity of either a part of the central nervous system or all of it. A person who is predisposed to epilepsy has attacks when the basal level of excitability of his nervous system (or of the part that is susceptible to the epileptic state) rises above a certain critical threshold. But, as long as the degree of excitability is held below this threshold, no attack occurs.

Basically, the two different types of epilepsy are: *generalized epilepsy* and *focal epilepsy*. Generalized epilepsy involves essentially all parts of the brain at once, whereas focal epilepsy involves only a portion—sometimes only a minute focal spot and other times a moderate portion of the brain.

GENERALIZED EPILEPSY

Grand Mal. Grand mal epilepsy is characterized by extreme neuronal discharges originating in the brain stem portion of the reticular activating system. These then spread throughout the entire central nervous system, to the cortex, to the deeper parts of the brain, and even into the spinal cord to cause generalized *tonic convulsions* of the entire body followed toward the end of the attack by alternating muscular contractions called *clonic convulsions*. The

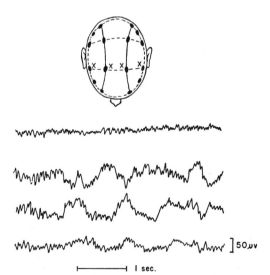

Figure 12–6. Localization of a brain tumor by means of the EEG, illustrating (above) the placement of electrodes and (below) the records from the four electrodes designated by X's.

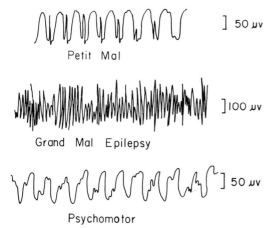

Figure 12–7. Electroencephalograms in different types of epilepsy.

grand mal seizure lasts from a few seconds to as long as three to four minutes and is characterized by post-seizure depression of the entire nervous system; the person remains in stupor for one to many minutes after the attack is over and then often remains severely fatigued for many hours thereafter.

The middle recording of Figure 12–7 illustrates a typical electroencephalogram from almost any region of the cortex during a grand mal attack. This illustrates that high voltage synchronous discharges occur over the entire cortex having almost the same periodicity as the normal alpha waves. Furthermore, the same type of discharge occurs on both sides of the brain at the same time, illustrating that the origin of the abnormality is in the lower centers of the brain that control the activity of the cerebral cortex and not in the cerebral cortex itself.

In experimental animals or even in human beings, grand mal attacks can be initiated by administering neuronal stimulants, such as the well-known drug Metrazol, or they can be caused by insulin hypoglycemia or by the passage of alternating electrical current directly through the brain. Electrical recordings from the thalamus and also from the reticular formation of the brain stem during the grand mal attack show typical high voltage activity in both of these areas similar to that recorded from the cerebral cortex. Furthermore, in an experimental animal, even after transecting the brain stem as low as the mesencephalon, a typical grand mal seizure can still be induced in the portion of the brain stem beneath the transection.

Presumably, therefore, a grand mal attack is caused by intrinsic overexcitability of the neurons that make up the reticular activating structures or from some abnormality of the local neuronal pathways. The synchronous discharges from this region could result from local reverberating circuits.

One might ask: What stops the grand mal attack after a given time? This is believed to result from (1)

fatigue of the neurons involved in precipitating the attack and (2) *active inhibition* by certain structures of the brain. The change from the tonic type of convulsion to the clonic type during the latter part of the grand mal attack has been suggested to result from partial fatigue of the neuronal system so that some of the excited neurons fade out for a moment, then return to activity after a brief rest, only to fatigue a second time and then a third time, and so forth, until the entire seizure is over. The stupor and fatigue that occur after a grand mal seizure is over is believed to result from the intense fatigue of the neurons following their intensive activity during the grand mal attack.

The *active inhibition* that helps to stop the grand mal attack is believed to result from feedback circuits through inhibitory areas of the brain. The grand mal attack undoubtedly excites such areas as the basal ganglia, which in turn emit many inhibitory impulses into the reticular formation of the brain stem. But the nature of such active inhibition is very much a matter of speculation.

Petit Mal Epilepsy. Petit mal epilepsy is closely allied to grand mal epilepsy in that it too almost certainly originates in the brain stem reticular activating system. It is characterized by 5 to 20 seconds of unconsciousness during which the person has several twitchlike contractions of the muscles, usually in the head region—especially blinking of the eyes; this is followed by return of consciousness and resumption of previous activities. The patient may have one such attack in many months, or in rare instances he may have a rapid series of attacks, one following the other. However, the usual course is for the petit mal attacks to appear in late childhood and then to disappear entirely by the age of 30. On occasion, a petit mal epileptic attack will initiate a grand mal attack.

The brain wave pattern in petit mal epilepsy is illustrated by the first record of Figure 12–7, which is typified by a *spike and dome pattern*. The spike portion of this recording is almost identical to the spikes that occur in grand mal epilepsy, but the dome portion is distinctly different. The spike and dome can be recorded over the entire cerebral cortex, illustrating that the seizure originates in the reticular activating system of the brain.

Since petit mal and grand mal epilepsy both originate in essentially the same locus of the brain stem, it is believed that they have the same common cause but that some influence inhibits neuronal activity during the petit mal attack so that it will not progress into the grand mal seizure.

FOCAL EPILEPSY

Focal epilepsy can involve almost any part of the brain, either localized regions of the cerebral cortex or deeper structures of both the cerebrum and brain stem. And almost always, focal epilepsy results from some localized organic lesion of the brain, such as a scar that pulls on the neuronal tissue, a tumor that compresses an area of the brain, or a destroyed area of brain tissue. Lesions such as these can promote extremely rapid discharges in the local neurons, and when the discharge rate rises above approximately 1000 per second, synchronous waves begin to spread over the adjacent cortical regions. These waves presumably result from *localized reverberating circuits* that gradually recruit adjacent areas of the cortex into the discharge zone. The process spreads to adjacent areas at a rate as slow as a few millimeters a minute to as fast as several centimeters per second. When such a wave of excitation spreads over the motor cortex, it causes a progressive "march" of muscular contractions throughout the opposite side of the body, beginning most characteristically in the mouth region and marching progressively downward to the legs, but at other times marching in the opposite direction. This is called *jacksonian epilepsy*.

A focal epileptic attack may remain confined to a single area of the brain, but in many instances the strong signals from the convulsing cortex or other part of the brain excite the brain stem portion of the reticular activating system so greatly that a grand mal epileptic attack ensues as well.

One type of focal epilepsy is the so-called *psychomotor seizure,* which may cause (1) a short period of amnesia, (2) an attack of abnormal rage, (3) sudden anxiety, discomfort, or fear, (4) a moment of incoherent speech or mumbling of some trite phrase, or (5) a motor act to attack someone, to rub the face with the hand, or so forth. Sometimes the person cannot remember his activities during the attack, but at other times he will have been conscious of everything that he had been doing but unable to control it.

The lower tracing of Figure 12–7 illustrates a typical electroencephalogram during a psychomotor attack, showing a low frequency rectangular wave with a frequency between 2 and 4 per second and with superimposed 14 per second waves.

The electroencephalogram can often be used to localize abnormal spiking waves originating in areas of organic brain disease that might predispose to focal epileptic attacks. Once such a focal point is found, surgical excision of the focus frequently prevents future epileptic attacks.

WAKEFULNESS AND SLEEP

The Two Conditions Required for Wakefulness. We have already seen in the discussions earlier in this chapter that wakefulness requires at least a certain level of activity in the reticular activating system. However, there is a second condition also necessary for wakefulness to occur: the nervous activity of the brain must be channeled in the proper directions. For instance, during a grand mal epileptic attack a person's brain is many times as active as it is during normal wakefulness, but nevertheless he is completely unconscious—certainly not a state of wakefulness. Therefore, for the state of wakefulness to occur it is not enough that the brain simply be active.

Sleep is defined as a state of unconsciousness from which a person can be aroused by appropriate sensory or other stimuli. Therefore, the unconsciousness caused by deep anesthesia, by total inactivity of the reticular activating system in diseased states (coma), and by excessive activity of the reticular activating system as occurs in grand mal epilepsy would not be considered to be sleep. However, coma and anesthesia do have many characteristics similar to those of deep sleep.

Two Different Types of Sleep. There are two different ways in which sleep can occur. First, it can result from decreased activity in the reticular activating system; this is called *slow wave sleep* because the brain waves are very slow. Second, sleep can result from abnormal channeling of signals in the brain even though brain activity may not be significantly depressed; this is called *paradoxical sleep* or *desynchronized sleep.*

Most of the sleep during each night is of the slow wave variety; this is the deep, restful type of sleep that the person experiences after having been kept awake for the previous 24 to 48 hours. On the other hand, short episodes of paradoxical sleep usually occur at intervals during each night, and this type of sleep seems to have purposeful functions that will be discussed later.

SLOW WAVE SLEEP

Slow wave sleep is frequently called by different names, such as *deep restful sleep, dreamless sleep, delta wave sleep,* or *normal sleep.* However, we shall see later that paradoxical sleep is also normal and that it has some characteristics of deep sleep.

Electroencephalographic Changes as a Person Falls Asleep. Beginning with wakefulness and proceeding to deep slow wave sleep, the electroencephalogram changes as follows:

1. Alert wakefulness—low voltage, high frequency beta waves showing desynchrony, as illustrated by the second record in Figure 12–3

2. Quiet restfulness—predominance of alpha waves; a type of "synchronized" brain waves

3. Light sleep—slowing of the brain waves to theta or delta low-voltage variety, but interspersed with spindles of alpha waves called *sleep spindles* that last for a few seconds at a time

4. Deep slow wave sleep—high voltage delta waves occurring at a rate of 1 to 2 per second, as illustrated by the fourth record of Figure 12–3.

In paradoxical sleep the brain waves change to still a different pattern, as will be discussed below.

Origin of the Delta Waves in Sleep. When the fiber tracts between the thalamus and the cortex are transected, delta waves are presently generated in the isolated cortex, indicating that this type of wave probably occurs intrinsically in the cortex when it is not being driven from below. Therefore, it is assumed that this is also the origin of the high voltage delta waves during deep slow wave sleep. That is, it is assumed that the degree of activity in the reticular activating system has fallen to a level too low to maintain normal excitabiltiy of the cortex so that the cortex then becomes its own pacemaker.

Characteristics of Deep Slow Wave Sleep. Most of us can understand the characteristics of deep slow wave sleep by referring back to the last time that we were kept awake for more than 24 hours and then remembering the deep sleep that occurred within 30 minutes to an hour after going to sleep. This sleep is dreamless, exceedingly restful, and is associated with a decrease in both peripheral vascular tone and also most of the other vegetative functions of the body as well. There is also a 10 to 30 per cent decrease in blood pressure, respiratory rate, and basal metabolic rate.

PARADOXICAL SLEEP ("REM" SLEEP)

Paradoxical sleep never occurs by itself, but instead is always superimposed onto slow wave sleep. In a normal night of sleep, bouts of paradoxical sleep lasting 5 to 20 minutes appear on the average of every 90 minutes, the first such period occurring 80 to 100 minutes after the person falls asleep. When the person is extremely tired, the duration of each bout of paradoxical sleep is very short, and it may even be absent. On the other hand, as the person has become rested, the duration of the paradoxical bouts greatly increases.

There are several very important characteristics of paradoxical sleep:

1. It is usually associated with active dreaming.

2. The person is even more difficult to arouse than during deep slow wave sleep.

3. The muscle tone throughout the body is

exceedingly depressed, indicating strong activation of the bulboreticular inhibitory system of the lower brain stem.

4. The heart rate and respiration usually become irregular, which is characteristic of the dream state.

5. Despite the extreme inhibition of the peripheral muscles, irregular muscle movements occur. These include, in particular, rapid movements of the eyes; consequently, paradoxical sleep has often been called *REM sleep*, for "rapid eye movements."

6. The electroencephalogram shows a desynchronized pattern of low voltage beta waves similar to those that occur during wakefulness. Therefore, this type of sleep is also frequently called *desynchronized sleep*, meaning desynchronized brain waves.

In summary, paradoxical sleep is a type of sleep in which the brain is probably as active as it is during many states of wakefulness. However, the brain activity is not channeled in the proper direction for the person to be aware of his surroundings and therefore to be awake.

BASIC THEORIES OF SLEEP

Despite the universality of the phenomenon of sleep, physiologists must admit with chagrin that they know very little about the basic mechanism of sleep. However, there are two major schools of thought about the causation of sleep: *The first of these beliefs is that sleep is a passive process,* occurring when the neuronal mechanisms that cause wakefulness become fatigued and therefore succeed to a lower level of activity. *The second theory is that active centers in the brain transmit signals into the reticular activating system to inhibit it and thereby produce sleep.* With either of these theories, it is generally assumed that the usual slow wave type of sleep results from decreased excitability of the reticular activating system, caused passively in the first instance and by active inhibition in the second instance.

The Feedback Theory of Wakefulness and Sleep—a Passive Mechanism of Sleep. From discussions earlier in the chapter we can recall that the reticular activating system can excite the cortex; but, also, the cortex in turn can excite the activating system. Thus, there exists a *positive* "feedback" that helps to keep the ascending reticular activating system active once it becomes excited.

There is also a second positive feedback that probably contributes to maintaining activity in the reticular activating system: The reticular activating system transmits signals not only to the cortex but also to the peripheral musculature. Any peripheral movement in turn transmits somatic sensory signals back into the reticular activating system, and many of these signals also take part in activating it. Thus, this additional positive feedback can help to maintain activity in the system once it begins.

Onset of Wakefulness. Keeping in mind the above two positive feedback mechanisms, we can assume that any arousal signal entering the resting reticular activating system will initiate signals that go both to the cortex and to the peripheral areas of the body. Return signals from both of these areas will further activate the reticular activating system thereby sending out more efferent signals, giving more return signals, and continuing on and on. Thus, once activity is initiated, the level of response will theoretically increase rapidly. This could explain the rapid onset of wakefulness. One of the obvious problems with such a mechanism as this is the possibility that the feedback mechanisms would become overly active and therefore produce a state similar to that of grand mal epilepsy. However, a brief consideration of the theory of positive feedback shows that once the activity reaches a critical level the neuronal discharge rates will begin to saturate so that the feedback gain will decrease to unity. Therefore, the degree of excitation of the reticular activating system will become stable. Furthermore, the level of this excitation plateau, and therefore the level of wakefulness as well, becomes a function of the excitability or fatigue of the neurons in the wakefulness circuit. Thus, this theory has a very solid foundation, and it fits in with the known characteristics of positive feedback.

Onset of Sleep. As neurons become fatigued, the level of positive feedback obviously will decrease in both the cortical and the peripheral circuits. Furthermore, each time one of the millions of parallel neurons in the feedback circuits falls out of activity, lack of this neuron's contribution to the feedback reduces the level of excitability of all the other neurons. Thus, there comes a point when the feedback activity cannot maintain enough excitability in the reticular activating system for the circuits to continue reverberating. Therefore, this could explain the initial slow onset of drowsiness and the final abrupt change from wakefulness to sleep.

Cause of Fatigue of the Neurons. If the passive mechanism for sleep is the correct one, we still need to explain the cause of fatigue of neurons after 16 hours of wakefulness and their recovery of excitability after 8 hours of sleep. We do know that this same phenomenon occurs in the spinal cord and in other areas of the nervous system that are exposed to excessive activity and then to excessive inactivity. For instance, continued facilitation of the spinal cord by fiber tracts from the brain causes decreased excitability of the spinal cord neurons. After the tracts from the brain are cut, the level of excitability of these neurons increases during the first few hours and then increases progressively less rapidly over a period of days and even months. Therefore, it is known that the excitability of neurons changes over a period of hours inversely to their degree of activity. This established fact about neuronal activity fits in well with the passive theory of sleep.

However, it is possible that the local environment of the neurons also changes. Perhaps the neurons secrete some transmitter substance into the local fluids and this in turn causes inhibition after periods of activity, or excitation after periods of inactivity. We will speak more about this shortly.

Active Mechanisms for Causing Sleep. Electrical stimulation under appropriate conditions in widely different areas of the brain can cause sleep. Three of the more important areas for achieving this are:

1. An area in or near the rostral portion of the solitary tracts of the brain stem located bilaterally in the pons.

2. Some areas in the diffuse nuclei of the thalamus.

3. The basal forebrain region between the hypothalamus and the supraorbital areas of the frontal lobes.

Stimulation in these areas at a frequency of 8 to 13 cycles per second (the same frequency as the alpha brain waves) is especially prone to cause sleep, whereas stimulation at other frequencies causes the reverse effect in some instances.

It has also been shown that lesions in the basal forebrain area or bilaterally in the lower pontine reticular substance can cause insomnia—sometimes to the extent that the animal cannot sleep at all, which causes lethal exhaustion within a few days.

Therefore, for obvious reasons, many research workers have come to the conclusion that sleep is caused by increased activity in one or more of these "sleep-producing" centers of the brain. The one most frequently considered to be "the" active sleep center is the bilateral center in the lower brain stem reticular formation near the solitary tracts.

The mechanism of the sleep caused by these sleep-producing centers almost certainly is active inhibition of the reticular activating system.

Mechanism of Paradoxical Sleep. Unfortunately, we do not know the cause of paradoxical sleep. However, the reticular activating system seems to have a periodic excitability cycle occurring once every 90 minutes: first decreased activity, then increased activity, and the system cycling throughout the 24-hour day in this manner. It is on the peaks of these cycles that paradoxical sleep occurs. Indeed, the periodicity of this mechanism has even been demonstrated during wakefulness, with periods of greater and lesser excitability throughout the day.

Thus, for the time being, we can possibly or probably consider paradoxical sleep to be caused by a period of intrinsic activity of the reticular activating system superimposed onto the natural mechanism of sleep—enough of a superimposition to cause dreams but not enough to wake the person. The mechanism seems also to activate the bulboreticular inhibitory area in the lower brain stem, which presumably is the cause of the depressed motor functions of the cord.

What is the purpose of paradoxical sleep? This we do not know, but a purpose speculated (as indeed almost all that we have to say about paradoxical sleep is speculated) would be that it is a periodic test of the intrinsic excitability of the neurons of the system. When this intrinsic excitability is great enough, one could suppose that this test of excitability might cause the person to awaken, but if the level of excitability is below a critical value, the person would pass through this phase of paradoxical sleep and fall back into another cycle of deep slow wave sleep before being tested again 90 minutes later.

Biochemical Theories for the Production of Sleep. Three important findings indicate that the biochemical milieu of the brain stem neurons might change during the wakefulness-sleep cycle, and furthermore, that some sleep-producing substance might be the cause of the cycle.

First, it has been demonstrated that either dialyzed blood or whole cerebrospinal fluid from animals that have been kept awake for several days contains a substance that causes sleep when injected into the ventricular system of an animal. This substance is a *small polypep-tide* with a molecular weight probably less than 500.

Second, it has been found that lesions in the midline area of the brain stem, an area known as the *nuclei of the raphe,* cause insomnia; this condition also causes destruction of a system of neurons that secrete *serotonin* into the reticular activating system. Therefore, it has been suggested that sleep is caused by secretion of serotonin from these neurons; what it is that controls the activity of these neurons is unexplained.

Third, it has been shown that destruction of small bilateral areas in the dorsal part of the upper middle pons, called the *locus ceruleus,* blocks the occurrence of paradoxical sleep. The neurons of these areas secrete norepinephrine. Therefore, it has been suggested that norepinephrine, possibly acting on the reticular activating system, is the factor that causes the paradoxical episodes during sleep. But, here again, the factors that cause the locus ceruleus to turn on and off are completely unknown.

In summary, therefore, changes in the biochemical status of the local neurons in the reticular activating system, or changes in certain specific nuclei, could increase and decrease the activity of this system and thereby could be partially responsible for inducing the states of wakefulness and sleep.

PHYSIOLOGICAL EFFECTS OF SLEEP

Sleep causes two major types of physiological effects: first, effects on the nervous system itself and, second, effects on other structures of the body. The first of these seems to be by far the more important, for any person who has a transected spinal cord in the neck shows no physiological effects in the body beneath the level of transection that can be attributed to a sleep and wakefulness cycle; this lack of sleep and wakefulness causes neither significant harm to the bodily organs nor even any deranged function. On the other hand, lack of sleep certainly does affect the functions of the central nervous system.

Prolonged wakefulness is often associated with progressive malfunction of the mind and behavioral activities of the nervous system. We are all familiar with the increased sluggishness of thought that occurs toward the end of a prolonged wakeful period, but in addition, a person can become irritable or even psychotic following forced wakefulness for prolonged periods of time. Therefore, we can assume that sleep in some way not presently understood restores both normal sensitivities of and normal "balance" between the different parts of the central nervous system. This might be likened to the "rezeroing" of electronic analog computers after prolonged use, for all computers of this type gradually lose their "base line" of operation; it is reasonable to assume that the same effect occurs in the central nervous system, since it, too, is an analog computer (though using a digital method of information transmission). Therefore, in the absence of any definitely demonstrated functional value of sleep, we might postulate, on the basis of known psychological changes that occur with wakefulness and sleep, that sleep performs this rezeroing function for the nervous system. Yet this is but a suggestion based purely on psychological data and on analogy with computers.

Even though, as pointed out above, wakefulness and sleep have not been shown to be necessary for somatic functions of the body, the cycle of enhanced and depressed nervous excitability that follows along with the cycle of wakefulness and sleep does have moderate effects on the peripheral body. For instance, there is enhanced sympathetic activity during wakefulness and also enhanced numbers of impulses to the skeletal musculature to increase muscular tone. Conversely, during sleep sympathetic activity decreases while parasympathetic activity occasionally increases, and the muscular tone becomes almost nil. Therefore, during sleep, arterial blood pressure falls, pulse rate decreases, skin vessels dilate, activity of the gastrointestinal tract sometimes increases, muscles fall into a completely relaxed state, and overall basal metabolic rate of the body falls by about 10 to 20 per cent.

REFERENCES

Andrew, R. J.: Arousal and the causation of behaviour. *Behaviour*, 51:135, 1974.

Ayala, G. F., Dichter, M., Gumnit, B. J., Matsumoto, H., and Spencer, W. A.: Genesis of epileptic interictal spikes. New knowledge of cortical feedback systems suggests a neurophysiological explanation of brief paroxysms. *Brain Res.*, 52:1, 1973.

Barlow, J. S. (ed.): Complementary Electrophysiological Techniques and Methods for Evaluation of the Central Nervous System. Amsterdam, Elsevier Nederland, BV, 1973.

Berger, R. J.: Bioenergetic functions of sleep and activity rhythms and their possible relevance to aging. *Fed. Proc.*, 34:97, 1975.

Brazier, M. A.: Epilepsy: Its Phenomena in Man. New York, Academic Press, 1975.

Clemente, C. D., Purpura, D. P., and Mayer, F. E. (eds.): Sleep and the Maturing Nervous System. New York, Academic Press, Inc., 1972.

Cooper, I. S., Riklan, M., and Snider, R. S. (eds.): The Cerebellum, Epilepsy, and Behavior. New York, Plenum Publishing Corporation, 1974.

Cooper, J. R., Bloom, F. E., and Roth, R. H.: The Biochemical Basis of Neuropharmacology, 2nd Ed. New York, Oxford University Press, 1974.

Costa, E., Gessa, G. L., and Sandler, M. (eds.): Serotonin, New Vistas: Biochemistry and Behavioral and Clinical Studies. New York, Raven Press, 1974.

Eliasson, S. G., Prensky, A. L., and Hardin, W. B., Jr. (eds.): Neurological Pathophysiology. New York, Oxford University Press, 1974.

Freeman, W. J.: Mass Action in the Nervous System: Examination of the Neurophysiological Basis of Adaptive Behavior Through EEG. New York, Academic Press, Inc., 1975.

Freemon, F. R.: Clinical pharmacology of sleep: a critical review of all-night electroencephalographic studies. *Behav. Neuropsychiatry*, 4:49, 1974.

Freemon, F. R.: Sleep Research. Springfield, Ill., Charles C Thomas, Publisher, 1974.

Fried, P. A.: The septum and hyper-reactivity: a review. *Brit. J. Psychol.*, 64:267, 1973.

Greenberg, B., and Pearlman, C.: Cutting the REM nerve: an approach to the adaptive role of REM sleep. *Perspect. Biol. Med.*, 17:513, 1974.

Izquierdo, I., and Nasello, A. G.: Pharmacology of the brain: the hippocampus, learning, and seizures. *Prog. Drug. Res.*, 16:211, 1972.

Jasper, H. H.: Unspecific thalamocortical relations. In Magoun, H. W. (ed.): Handbook of Physiology. Sec. 1, Vol. 2. Baltimore, The Williams & Wilkins Company, 1960, p. 1307.

Johnson, L. C.: Are stages of sleep related to waking behavior? *Amer. Sci.*, 61:326, 1973.

Magoun, H. W.: The Waking Brain, 2nd Ed. Springfield, Ill., Charles C Thomas, Publisher, 1962.

Mills, J. N.: Human circadian rhythms. *Physiol. Rev.*, 46:128, 1966.

Petre-Quadens, O. J., and Schlag, J. D. (eds.): Basic Sleep Mechanisms. New York, Academic Press, Inc., 1974.

Rubin, R. T., Poland, R. E., Rubin, L. E., and Gouin, P. R.: The neuroendocrinology of human sleep. *Life Sci.*, 14:1041, 1974.

Schmidt, R. F. (ed.): Fundamentals of Neurophysiology. Springer-Verlag New York, Inc., 1975.

Shellenberger, M. K., and Walaszek, E. J.: Pharmacology of the central nervous system. *Prog. Neurol. Psychiatry*, 27:67, 1972.

Stenevi, U., Björklund, A., and Moore, R. Y.: Morphological plasticity of central adrenergic neurons. *Brain Behav. Evol.*, 8:110, 1973.

Stern, W. C., and Morgane, P. J.: Theoretical view of REM sleep function: maintenance of catecholamine systems in the central nervous system. *Behav. Biol.*, 11:1, 1974.

Thompson, R. F., and Patterson, M. (eds.): Bioelectric Recording Techniques, Part A. Cellular Processes and Brain Potentials. New York, Academic Press, Inc., 1973.

Wallace, R. K., and Benson, H.: The physiology of meditation. *Sci. Amer.*, 226:84, 1972.

13

The Cerebral Cortex and Intellectual Functions of the Brain

It is ironic that we know least about the mechanisms of the cerebral cortex of all parts of the brain, even though it is by far the largest portion of the nervous system. Yet, we do know the effects of destruction or of specific stimulation of various portions of the cortex, and still more is known from electrical recordings from the cortex or from the surface of the scalp. In the early part of the present chapter the facts known about cortical functions are discussed and then some basic theories of the neuronal mechanisms involved in thought processes, memory, analysis of sensory information, and so forth are presented briefly.

PHYSIOLOGIC ANATOMY OF THE CEREBRAL CORTEX

The functional part of the cerebral cortex is comprised mainly of a thin layer of neurons 2 to 5 mm. in thickness, covering the surface of all the convolutions of the cerebrum and having a total area of about one-quarter of a square meter. The total cerebral cortex contains approximately 10 billion neurons.

Figure 13–1 illustrates the typical structure of the cerebral cortex, showing successive layers of different types of cells. Most of the cells are of three types: *granular, fusiform,* and *pyramidal,* the latter named for their characteristic pyramidal shape. To the right in Figure 13–1 is illustrated the typical organization of nerve fibers within the different layers of the cortex. Note particularly the large number of horizontal fibers extending between adjacent areas of the cortex, but note also the vertical fibers that extend to and from the cortex to lower areas of the brain stem or to distant regions of the cerebral cortex through long association bundles of fibers.

Neurohistologists have divided the cerebral cortex into almost 100 different areas which have slightly different architectural characteristics. Yet in all these different areas there still persist at least crude representations of all the six major layers of the cortex. Furthermore, to the untrained histologist, not more

Figure 13–1. Structure of the cerebral cortex, illustrating: *I,* molecular layer; *II,* external granular layer; *III,* layer of pyramidal cells; *IV,* internal granular layer; *V,* large pyramidal cell layer; *VI,* layer of fusiform or polymorphic cells. (From Ranson and Clark (after Brodmann): Anatomy of the Nervous System, 1959.)

than five major architectural types of cortex can be distinguished as follows: Type 1 contains large numbers of pyramidal cells with few granular cells and, therefore, is often called the *agranular cortex.* At the other extreme, type 5 contains almost no pyramidal cells but is filled with closely packed granule cells and is called the *granular cortex.* Types 2, 3, and 4 have intermediate characteristics containing gradated proportions of pyramidal and agranular cells.

The agranular cortex, which contains large numbers of pyramidal cells, is characteristic of the motor areas of the cerebral cortex; while the granular cortex, containing almost no pyramidal cells, is characteristic of the primary sensory areas. The other three intermediate types of cortex are characteristic of the association areas between the primary sensory and motor regions.

Figure 13–2 shows a map of cortical areas classified on the basis of histological studies by Brodmann. This classification provides a basis for discussion of functional areas of the brain, even though different architectural types of cortex often have similar functions.

Anatomical Relationship of the Cerebral Cortex to the Thalamus and Other Lower Centers. All areas of the cerebral cortex have direct afferent and efferent connections with the thalamus. Figure 13–3 shows the areas of the cerebral cortex connected with specific parts of the thalamus. These connections are in *two* directions, both from the thalamus to the cortex and then from the cortex back to essentially the same area of the thalamus. Furthermore, when the thalamic connections are cut, the functions of the corresponding cortical area become entirely or almost entirely abrogated. Therefore, the cortex operates in close association with the thalamus and can almost be considered both anatomically and functionally a large outgrowth of the thalamus; for this reason the thalamus and the cortex together are called the *thalamocortical system,* as was explained in the previous chapter. Also, all pathways from the

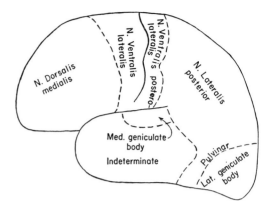

Figure 13–3. Areas of the cerebral cortex that connect with specific portions of the thalamus. (Modified from Elliott: Textbook of the Nervous System. J. B. Lippincott Co.)

sensory organs to the cortex pass through the thalamus, with the single exception of the sensory pathways of the olfactory tract.

FUNCTIONS OF CERTAIN SPECIFIC CORTICAL AREAS

Studies in human beings by neurosurgeons have shown that some specific functions are localized to certain general areas of the cerebral cortex. Figure 13–4 gives a map of some of these areas as determined by Penfield and Rasmussen from electrical stimulation of the cortex or by neurological examination of patients after portions of the cortex had been removed. The

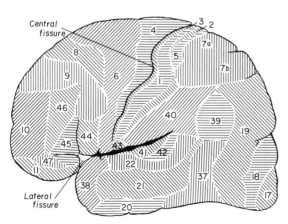

Figure 13–2. Structurally distinctive areas of the human cerebral cortex. (From Brodmann, modified by Buchanan: Functional Neuroanatomy. Lea & Febiger, 1966.)

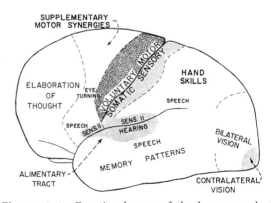

Figure 13–4. Functional areas of the human cerebral cortex as determined by electrical stimulation of the cortex during neurosurgical operations and by neurological examinations of patients with destroyed cortical regions. (From Penfield and Rasmussen: Cerebral Cortex of Man: A Clinical Study of Localization of Function. The Macmillan Co., 1968.)

lightly shaded areas are *primary sensory areas,* while the darkly shaded area is the *voluntary motor area* (also called *primary motor area*) from which muscular movements can be elicited with relatively weak electrical stimuli. These primary sensory and motor areas have highly specific functions, while other areas of the cortex perform more general functions that we call association or cerebration.

SPECIFIC FUNCTIONS OF THE PRIMARY SENSORY AREAS

The primary sensory areas all have certain functions in common. For instance, somatic sensory areas, visual sensory areas, and auditory sensory areas all have spatial localizations of signals from the peripheral receptors (which are discussed in detail in Chapters 7, 18, and 19).

Electrical stimulation of the primary sensory areas in the parietal lobes in awake patients gives relatively uncomplicated sensations. For instance, in the somatic sensory area the patient states that he feels tingling in the skin, numbness, mild "electric" feeling, or, rarely, mild degrees of temperature sensations. And these sensations are localized to discrete areas of the body in accord with the spatial representation in the somatic sensory cortex, as described in Chapter 7. Therefore, it is believed that the primary somatic sensory cortex analyzes only the simple aspects of sensations and that analysis of intricate patterns of sensory experience requires adjacent parts of the parietal lobes called *sensory association areas* to operate in association with this area.

Electrical stimulation of the primary visual cortex in the occipital lobes causes the person to see flashes of light, bright lines, colors, or other simple visions. Here again, the visual images are localized to specific regions of the visual fields in accord with the portion of the primary visual cortex stimulated, as described in Chapter 18. But the visual cortex alone is not capable of complete analysis of complicated visual patterns; for this, the visual cortex must operate in association with adjacent regions of the occipital cortex, the *visual association areas.*

Electrical stimulation of the auditory cortex in the temporal lobes causes a person to hear a simple sound which may be weak or loud, have low or high frequency, or have other uncomplicated characteristics, such as a squeak or even an undulation. But never are words or any other fully intelligible sound heard. Thus, the primary auditory cortex, like the other primary sensory areas, can detect the individual elements of auditory experience but cannot analyze complicated sounds. Therefore, the primary auditory cortex alone is not sufficient to give one even the usual auditory experiences; these can be achieved, however, when the primary area operates together with the *auditory association areas* in adjacent regions of the temporal lobes.

Despite the inability of the primary sensory areas to analyze the incoming sensations fully, when these areas are destroyed, the ability of the person to utilize the respective sensations usually suffers drastically. For instance, loss of the primary visual cortex in one occipital lobe causes a person to become blind in the ipsilateral halves of both retinae, and loss of the primary visual cortices in both hemispheres causes total blindness. Likewise, loss of both primary auditory cortices causes almost total deafness. Loss of the postcentral gyri causes *depression* of somatic sensory sensations—though not total loss—presumably because of additional cortical representation of these sensations in other cortical areas: somatic sensory area II and the motor cortex, for example. (In animals far down the phylogenetic scale, loss of the visual and auditory cortices may have little effect on vision and hearing, and even an anencephalic human infant detects some visual scenes in the absence of the visual cortex, for such a child can observe a moving object and even follow it by movement of its eyes and head.)

Therefore, we can summarize the functions of the primary sensory areas of the human cerebral cortex in the following way: The lower centers of the brain relay a large part of the sensory signals to the cerebral cortex for analysis. In turn, the primary sensory areas transmit the results of their analyses back to the lower centers and to other regions of the cerebral cortex, as is discussed later in the chapter.

THE SENSORY ASSOCIATION AREAS

Around the borders of the primary sensory areas are regions called *sensory association areas* or *secondary sensory areas.* In general, these areas extend 1 to 5 centimeters in one or more directions from the primary sensory areas; each time a primary area receives a sensory signal, secondary signals spread; after a delay of a few milliseconds into the respective association area as well. Part of this spread occurs through subcortical fiber tracts, but a major part also occurs in the thalamus, beginning in the sensory relay nuclei, passing next to corresponding *thalamic association areas,* and then traveling to the association cortex.

The general function of the sensory association areas is to provide a higher level of interpretation of the sensory experiences. The general areas for the interpretative functions for somatic, visual, and auditory experiences are illustrated in Figure 13–5.

Destruction of the sensory association areas greatly reduces the capability of the brain to analyze different characteristics of sensory experiences. For instance, damage in the temporal lobe below and behind the primary auditory area in the "dominant hemisphere" of the brain often causes a person to lose the understanding of words or of other auditory experiences even though he hears them.

Likewise, destruction of areas 18 and 19 of the occipital lobe in the dominant hemisphere or the presence of a brain tumor or other lesion in these areas, which represent the visual association areas, does not cause blindness or prevent normal activation of the primary visual cortex but does greatly reduce the person's ability to interpret what he sees. Such a person often loses his ability to recognize the meanings of words, a condition that is called *word blindness* or *alexia.*

Finally, destruction of the somatic sensory association area in the parietal cortex posterior to primary somatic area I causes the person to lose his spatial perception for location of the different parts of his body. In the case of the

hand that has been "lost," the skills of the hand are greatly reduced. Thus, this area of the cortex seems to be necessary for interpretation of somatic sensory experiences.

The functions of the association areas are described in more detail in Chapter 7 for somatic, in Chapter 18 for visual, and in Chapter 19 for auditory experiences.

INTERPRETATIVE FUNCTION OF THE POSTERIOR TEMPORAL LOBE AND ANGULAR GYRUS REGIONS— THE GENERAL INTERPRETATIVE AREA

The somatic, visual, and auditory association areas, which can actually be called "interpretative areas," all meet one another in the posterior part of the superior temporal lobe and in the anterior part of the angular gyrus, that is, the gyrus at the posterior tip of the lateral fissure where the temporal, parietal, and occipital lobes all come together. This area of confluence of the different sensory interpretative areas plays the greatest single role of any part of the cerebral cortex in the higher levels of brain function that we call *cerebration.* Therefore, this region has frequently been called by different names suggestive of the area having almost global importance: the *general interpretative area,* the *gnostic area,* the *knowing area,* the *tertiary association area,* and so forth.

Following severe damage in the general interpretative area, a person might hear perfectly well and even recognize different words but still might be unable to arrange these words into a coherent thought. Likewise, he may be able to read words from the printed page but be unable to recognize the thought that is conveyed. In addition, he has similar difficulties in understanding the higher levels of meaning of somatic sensory experiences, even though there is no loss of sensation itself.

Electrical stimulation in the temporal lobe, particularly in its posterior part, or in the anterior angular gyrus of the conscious patient occasionally causes a highly complex thought. This is particularly true when the stimulatory electrode is passed deep enough into the brain to approach the corresponding connecting areas of the thalamus. The types of thoughts that might be experienced include memories of complicated visual scenes that one might remember from childhood, auditory hallucinations such as a specific musical piece, or even a discourse by a specific person. For this reason it is believed that complicated memory patterns

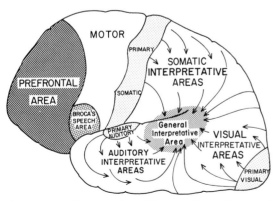

Figure 13–5. Organization of the somatic, auditory, and visual association areas into a general mechanism for interpretation of sensory experience. All of these feed into the *general interpretative area* located in the posterosuperior portion of the temporal lobe and the angular gyrus. Also shown in the figure are the prefrontal area and Broca's speech area.

involving more than one sensory modality are stored at least partially in the temporal lobe and the angular gyrus. This belief is in accord with the importance of the general interpretative area in interpretation of the complicated meanings of different sensory experiences.

Once again we must emphasize the global importance of this area. Loss of it in an adult usually leads to a lifetime thereafter of an almost demented existence.

The Dominant Hemisphere. The interpretative functions of the temporal lobe and angular gyrus are usually highly developed in only one cerebral hemisphere, the *dominant hemisphere*. At birth these regions in both hemispheres have almost the same capability of developing; we know this because removal of either hemisphere in early childhood causes the opposite to develop full dominant characteristics.

A theory that might explain hemispheric dominance in the adult is the following: The attention of the "mind" seems to be directed to one portion of the brain at a time, as was explained in the preceding chapter. Presumably, one angular gyrus region begins to be used to a greater extent than the other, and, thenceforth, because of the tendency to direct one's attention to the better developed region, the rate of learning in the cerebral hemisphere that gains the first start increases rapidly while that in the opposite side remains slight. Therefore, in the normal human being, one side becomes dominant over the other.

In more than 9 out of 10 persons the left temporal lobe and angular gyrus become dominant, and in the remaining one tenth of the population either both sides develop simultaneously to have dual dominance, or, more rarely, the right side alone becomes highly developed.

Usually associated with the dominant temporal lobe and angular gyrus is dominance of certain portions of the somesthetic cortex and motor cortex for control of voluntary motor functions. For instance, as is discussed later in the chapter, the premotor speech area, located far laterally in the intermediate frontal area, is almost always dominant also on the left side of the brain. This speech area causes the formation of words by exciting simultaneously the laryngeal muscles, the respiratory muscles, and the muscles of the mouth.

Though the interpretative areas of the temporal lobe and angular gyrus, as well as many of the motor areas, are highly developed in only a single hemisphere, they are capable of receiving sensory information from both hemispheres and

are also capable of controlling motor activities in both hemispheres, utilizing mainly fiber pathways in the *corpus callosum* for communication between the two hemispheres. This unitary, cross-feeding organization prevents interference between the two sides of the brain; such interference, obviously, could create havoc with both thoughts and motor responses.

Effect of Temporal Lobe and Angular Gyrus Destruction in the Dominant Hemisphere. Destruction of the dominant temporal lobe and angular gyrus in an adult person normally leaves a great void in his intellect because of his inability to interpret the meanings of sensory experiences. Therefore, the neurosurgeon assiduously avoids surgery in this region. The adult can only gradually develop the interpretative functions of the nondominant temporal lobe and angular gyrus, and even then only to a slight extent. Thus, only a small amount of intellect can return. However, if this area is destroyed in a child under six years of age, the opposite side can usually develop to full extent, thus eventually returning the capabilities of the child essentially to normal.

Role of Language in Interpretation and in Intellectual Functions. A major share of our sensory experiences are converted into their language equivalent before being stored in the memory areas of the brain and before being processed for other intellectual purposes. For instance, when we read a book, we do not store the visual images of the words but, instead, store the information in language form. At least the information is converted to language form before its meaning is discerned.

The sensory area of the dominant hemisphere for interpretation of language is closely associated with the primary hearing area located in the auditory association areas of the temporal lobe. This locus probably results from the fact that the first introduction to language is by way of hearing. Later in life, when visual perception of language through the medium of reading develops, the visual information is then presumably channeled into the already developed language regions of the dominant temporal lobe. This probably also explains why the general interpretative area of the brain is more closely allied with the auditory association areas than with other sensory areas of the cortex.

Interpretative Functions that Remain After Destruction of the General Interpretative Area. One of the reasons loss of the general interpretative area is so destructive to the intellectual functions of the body is that most of our intellectual functions operate through the language medium. However, after loss of the general interpretative area, other interpretative functions of the brain still persist, such as capability to react with somatic motor activities in response to visual scenes—that is, ability to associate visual and somatic functions but loss of ability to react verbally. In addition, the temporal lobe of the opposite hemisphere still retains capabilities for associating somatic, visual, and auditory experiences of a nonlanguage nature. Thus, even though we speak of the dominant hemisphere, this dominance is primarily for the language-related intellectual functions, whereas the opposite hemisphere can actually be dominant in some other types of association.

THE PREFRONTAL AREAS

The prefrontal areas are those portions of the frontal lobes that lie anterior to the motor regions, as shown in Figure 13–5. For years, this part of the cortex has been considered to be the locus of the higher intellect of the human being, principally because the main difference between the brain of monkeys and that of man is the great prominence of man's prefrontal areas. Yet efforts to show that the prefrontal cortex is more important in higher intellectual functions than other portions of the cortex have not been successful. Indeed, destruction of the posterior temporal lobe and angular gyrus region in the dominant hemisphere causes infinitely more harm to the intellect than does destruction of both prefrontal areas.

Psychological studies in lower animals have shown that all portions of the cortex not immediately associated with either sensory or motor functions are important in the ability of an animal to learn complicated information—such as a rat's learning to run through a maze—and that all the different areas are approximately equipotent in this regard. Therefore, the importance of the prefrontal areas to the human being is perhaps not that these areas perform some specific function different from those of other cortical areas, but primarily that they supply much additional cortical area in which cerebration can take place.

The prefrontal areas also control some of the autonomic functions of the body by transmitting impulses to the hypothalamus either directly or indirectly through the thalamus. These functions are described in the following two chapters.

Prevention of Distractibility by the Prefrontal Areas.   One of the outstanding characteristics of a person who has lost his prefrontal areas is the ease with which he can be *distracted* from a sequence of thoughts. Likewise, in lower animals whose prefrontal areas have been removed, the ability to concentrate on psychological tests is almost completely lost. The human being without prefrontal areas is still capable of performing many intellectual tasks, such as answering short questions and performing simple arithmetic computations (such as $9 \times 6 = 54$), thus illustrating that the basic intellectual activities of the cerebral cortex are still intact without the prefrontal areas. Yet if concerted *sequences* of cerebral functions are required of the person, he becomes completely disorganized. Therefore, the prefrontal areas seem to be important in keeping the mental functions directed toward goals.

Possible Role of the Prefrontal Lobes for "Immediate Memory."   Some research workers have suggested that the highly distractible nature of a person or animal after the prefrontal lobes have been destroyed results from loss of the ability to retain immediate memory. However, specific psychological tests have proved that prefrontal lobectomized human beings still have almost normal capability for memory provided that the information is presented to the person in such a way that he is not distracted from it while learning. Therefore, it seems that this loss of "immediate memory" results from inability of the brain to classify incoming information and to "code" it for storage in the memory areas. Without this ability to code the information, it is lost immediately from the mind, thus giving the effect of loss of "immediate memory" even though the memory process itself probably is not impaired.

Elaboration of Thought by the Prefrontal Areas.   Another function that has been ascribed to the prefrontal areas by psychologists and neurologists is *elaboration of thought*. This means simply an increase in depth and abstractness of the different thoughts. Psychological tests have shown that prefrontal lobectomized lower animals presented with successive bits of sensory information fail to store these bits in memory—probably because of their inability to code this information, the initial requirement for memory storage, as was discussed above. If the prefrontal areas are intact, many such successive bits of information can be stored in all areas of the brain and can be called forth again and again during the subsequent periods of cerebration. This ability of the prefrontal areas to cause storage—even though it be temporary—of many types of information simultaneously, and then perhaps also to cause recall of this information could well explain the many functions of the brain that we associate with higher intelligence, such as the abilities to (1) plan for the future, (2) delay action in response to incoming sensory signals so that the sensory information can be weighed until the best course of response is decided, (3) consider the consequences of motor actions even before these are performed, (4) solve complicated mathematical, legal, or philosophical problems, (5) correlate all avenues of information in diagnosing rare diseases, and (6) control one's activities in accord with moral laws.

Effects of Destruction of the Prefrontal Areas

The person without prefrontal areas ordinarily acts precipitously in response to incoming sensory signals, such as striking an adversary too large to be beaten instead of pursuing the more judicious course of running away. Also, he is likely to lose many or most of his morals; he has little embarrassment in relation to his excretory, sexual, and social activities; and he is prone to quickly changing moods of sweetness, hate, joy, sadness, exhilaration, and rage. In short, he is a highly *distractible* person with lack of ability to pursue long and complicated thoughts.

THOUGHTS, MEMORY, LEARNING, AND CONSCIOUSNESS

Though all of us know what a *thought* is, any attempt to describe it in abstract terms is almost impossible. The comprehension of a visual scene at a given instant would be a single thought; or overall comprehension of one's surroundings in response to other sensory information would be another thought; projection in one's mind of a mathematical equation is still a third thought. Thus, each instant of awareness could be defined as a thought. And the awareness itself can be defined as *consciousness*.

With the above definitions of thoughts and consciousness in mind, it now becomes easy to define memory and learning. *Memory* is the capability of recalling a thought at least once and usually again and again, and *learning* is the capability of the nervous system to store memories. Therefore, thoughts, consciousness, memory, and learning all go hand in hand and, in so far as the central nervous system is concerned, are almost inseparable.

Our most difficult problem in discussing consciousness, thoughts, memory, and learning is that we do not know the neural mechanism of a thought. We know that destruction of large portions of the cerebral cortex does not prevent a person from having thoughts, but it does reduce his *degree* of awareness of his surroundings. On the other hand, destruction of far smaller portions of the thalamus, or especially of the mesencephalic portion of the reticular activating system can cause tremendously decreased awareness or even complete unconsciousness.

Each thought almost certainly involves simultaneous signals in portions of the cerebral cortex, thalamus, rhinencephalon, and reticular formation of the brain stem. Some crude thoughts probably depend almost entirely on lower centers; the thought of pain is probably a good example, for electrical stimulation of the human cortex rarely elicits anything more than the mildest degrees of pain, while stimulation of certain areas of the hypothalamus and mesencephalon in animals apparently causes excruciating pain. On the other hand, a type of thought pattern that requires mainly the cerebral cortex is that involving vision, because loss of the visual cortex causes complete inability to perceive visual form or color.

Therefore, we might formulate a definition of a thought in terms of neural activity as follows: A thought probably results from the momentary "pattern" of stimulation of many different parts of the nervous system at the same time, probably involving most importantly the cerebral cortex, the thalamus, the rhinencephalon, and the upper reticular formation of the brain stem. The stimulated areas of the rhinencephalon, thalamus, and reticular formation perhaps determine the crude nature of the thought, giving it such qualities as pleasure, displeasure, pain, comfort, crude modalities of sensation, localization to general parts of the body, and other gross characteristics. On the other hand, the stimulated areas of the cortex probably determine the discrete characteristics of the thought (such as specific localization of sensations in the body and of objects in the fields of vision), discrete patterns of sensation (such as the rectangular pattern of a concrete block wall or the texture of a rug), and other individual characteristics that enter into the overall awareness of a particular instant.

MEMORY AND TYPES OF MEMORY

If we accept the above approximation of what constitutes a thought, we can see immediately that the mechanism of memory must be equally as complex as the mechanism of a thought, for, to provide memory, the nervous system must re-create the same spatial and temporal pattern of stimulation in the central nervous system at some future date. Though we cannot explain in detail what a memory is, we do know some of the basic neuronal processes that probably lead to the process of memory.

All of us know that all degrees of memory occur, some memories lasting a few seconds and others lasting hours, days, months, or years. Possibly all of these types of memory are caused by the same mechanism operating to different degrees of fulfillment. Yet, it is also possible that different mechanisms of memory do exist. Indeed, most physiologists classify memory into from two to four different types. For the purpose of the present discussion, we will use the following classification:

1. *Sensory memory*
2. *Short-term memory* or *primary memory*
3. *Long-term memory,* which itself can be divided into *secondary memory* and *tertiary memory*

The basic characteristics of these types of memory are the following:

Sensory Memory. Sensory memory means the ability to retain sensory signals in the sensory areas of the brain for a very short interval of time following the actual sensory experience. Usually these signals remain available for analysis for several hundred milliseconds but are replaced by new sensory signals in less than one second. Nevertheless, during the short interval of time that the instantaneous sensory information remains in the brain it can continue to be used for further processing; most important, it can be "scanned" to pick out the important points. Thus, this is the initial stage of the memory process.

Short-Term Memory (Primary Memory). Short-term memory (or primary memory) is the memory of a few facts, words, numbers, letters, or other bits of information for a few seconds to a minute or more at a time. This is typified by a person's memory of the digits in a telephone number for a short period of time after he has looked up the number in the telephone directory. This type of memory is usually limited to about seven bits of information, and when new bits of information are put into this *short-term store,* some of the older information is displaced. Thus, if a person looks up a second telephone number, the first is usually lost. One of the most important features of short-term memory is that the information in this memory store is instantaneously available so that the

person does not have to search through his mind for it as he does for information that has been put away in the long-term memory stores.

Long-Term Memory. Long-term memory is the storage in the brain of information that can be recalled at some later time—minutes, hours, days, months, or years later. This type of memory has been called *fixed memory, permanent memory,* and by several other names. Long-term memory is also usually divided into two different types, *secondary memory* and *tertiary memory,* the characteristics of which are the following:

A *secondary memory* is a long-term memory that is stored with either a weak or only a moderately strong memory trace. For this reason it is easy to forget and it is sometimes difficult to recall. Furthermore, the time required to search for the information is relatively long. This type of memory can last from several minutes to several years. When the memories are so weak that they will last for only a few minutes to a few days, they are also frequently called *recent memory.*

A *tertiary memory* is a memory that has become so well ingrained in the mind that the memory can usually last the lifetime of the person. Furthermore, the very strong memory traces of this type of memory makes the stored information available within a split second. This type of memory is typified by one's knowledge of his own name, by his ability to recall immediately the numbers from 1 to 10, the letters of the alphabet, and the words that he uses in speech, and also by the memory of his own precise physical structure and of his very familiar immediate surroundings.

PHYSIOLOGICAL BASIS OF MEMORY

Despite the many advances in neurophysiology during the past half century, we still cannot explain what is perhaps the most important function of the brain: its capability for memory. Yet, physiological experiments are beginning to generate conceptual theories of the means by which memory could occur. Some of these are discussed in the following few sections.

Possible Mechanisms for Short-Term Memory. Short-term memory requires a neuronal mechanism that can hold specific information signals for a few seconds to at most a minute or more. Several such mechanisms are the following:

Reverberating Circuit Theory of Short-Term Memory. When a tetanizing electrical stimulus is applied directly to the surface of the cerebral cortex and then is removed after a second or more, the local area excited by this stimulus continues to emit rhythmic action potentials for short periods of time. This effect results from local reverberating circuits, the signals passing through a multistage circuit of neurons in the local area of the cortex itself or perhaps also back and forth between the cortex and the thalamus.

It is postulated that sensory signals reaching the cerebral cortex can set up similar reverberating oscillations and that these could be the basis for short-term memory. Then, as the reverberating circuit fatigues, or as new signals interfere with the reverberations, the short-term memory fades away.

One of the principal observations in support of this theory is that any factor that causes a general disturbance of brain function, such as sudden fright, a very loud noise, or any other sensory experience that attracts the person's undivided attention immediately erases the short-term memory. The memory cannot be recalled when the disturbance is over unless a portion of this memory had already been placed into the long-term memory store, as will be discussed in subsequent sections.

Post-Tetanic Potentiation Theory of Short-Term Memory.   In most parts of the nervous system, including even the anterior motoneurons of the spinal cord, tetanic stimulation of a neuron for a few seconds causes a subsequent increased excitability of the neuron for a few seconds to a few hours.

If during this time the neuron is stimulated again, it responds much more vigorously than normally, a phenomenon called *post-tetanic potentiation*. This is obviously a type of memory that depends on change in the excitability of the involved neurons, and it could be the basis for short-term memory. It is likely that this phenomenon results from some temporary change in the synapses of the neurons.

DC Potential Theory of Short-Term Memory.   Another change that often occurs in neurons following a period of excitation is a prolonged decrease in the membrane potential of the neuron lasting for from seconds to minutes. Because this changes the excitability of the neuron, it could be the basis for short-term memory. Such changes in neuronal potentials are called *DC* potentials or sometimes *electrotonic potentials*. Measurements in the cerebral cortex show that such potentials occur especially in the superficial dendritic layers of the cortex, indicating that the process of short-

term memory could result from changes in dendritic membrane potentials.

Mechanism of Long-Term Memory, Enhancement of Synaptic Transmission Facility

Long-term memory means the ability of the nervous system to recall thoughts long after initial elicitation of the thoughts is over. We know that long-term memory does not depend on continued activity of the nervous system, because the brain can be totally inactivated by cooling, by general anesthesia, by hypoxia, by ischemia, or by any other method and yet memories that have been previously stored are still retained when the brain becomes active once again. Therefore, it is assumed that long-term memory must result from some actual alterations of the synapses, either physical or chemical.

Many different theories have been offered to explain the synaptic changes that cause long-term memory. Among the most important of these are:

1. Anatomical Changes in the Synapses. Cajal, more than half a century ago, discovered that the number of terminal fibrils ending on neuronal cells and dendrites in the cerebral cortex increases with age. Conversely, physiologists have shown that inactivity of regions of the cortex causes thinning of the cortex: for instance, thinning of the primary visual cortex in animals that have lost their eyesight. Also, intense activity of a particular part of the cortex can cause excessive thickening of the cortical shell in that area alone. This has been demonstrated especially in the visual cortex of animals subjected to repeated visual experiences. Finally, some neuroanatomists believe that they can observe electronmicrographic changes in presynaptic terminals that have been subjected to intense and prolonged activity.

All of these observations have led to a widely held belief that fixation of memories in the brain results from physical changes in the synapses themselves: perhaps changes in numbers of presynaptic terminals, perhaps in sizes of the terminals, perhaps in the sizes and conductivities of the dendrites, or perhaps in their chemical compositions. Also, it has been suggested that permanent changes might occur in excitability of the postsynaptic neurons. Such physical changes could cause permanent or semipermanent increase in the degree of facilitation of the synapses, thus allowing signals to pass through the synapses with progressive ease the more often the memory trace is used. This obviously would explain the tendency for memories to become more and more deeply fixed in the nervous system the more often they are recalled or the more often the person repeats the sensory experience that leads to the memory trace.

2. Theoretical Function of RNA in Memory. The discovery that DNA and RNA can act as codes to control reproduction, which in itself is a type of memory from one generation to another, plus the fact that these substances once formed in a cell tend to persist for the lifetime of the cell, has led to the theory that nucleic acids might be involved in memory changes of the neurons, changes that could last for the lifetime of the person. In addition, biochemical studies have shown an increase in RNA in some active neurons. Yet, a mechanism by which RNA could cause facilitation of synaptic transmission has never been found. Therefore, this theory seems to be based mainly on analogy rather than on factual evidence. The only possible supporting evidence is that several research workers have claimed that long-term memory will not occur to a significant extent when the chemical processes for formation of RNA or of protein are blocked. Since these substances are required for anatomical changes in the synapses as well as for RNA synthesis, however, these observations could support almost any type of theory for long-term memory.

3. The Glial Theory and Other Extraneuronal Theories. Anatomists have demonstrated that the structures of glial cells surrounding neurons change markedly under different functional conditions. This obviously has led to the theory that glial changes might increase the facilitation of synapses and, therefore, be the basis of memory. Also, chemists have demonstrated that the quantity and chemical composition of mucopolysaccharides surrounding synapses change under different functional conditions, and this leads to still another theory for memory. However, in both of these instances there has been little more than circumstantial evidence.

Summary. The theory that seems most likely at present for explaining long-term memory is that some actual physical or chemical change occurs in the synaptic knobs themselves or in the postsynaptic neurons, these changes permanently facilitating the transmission of impulses at the synapses. If all the synapses are thus facilitated in a thought circuit, this circuit can be re-excited by any one of many diverse

incoming signals at later dates, thereby causing memory. The overall facilitated circuit is called a *memory engram* or a *memory trace*.

Consolidation of Long-Term Memory

If a memory is to last in the brain so that it can be recalled days later, it must become "consolidated" in the neuronal circuits. This process requires 5 to 10 minutes for minimal consolidation and an hour or more for maximal consolidation. For instance, if a strong sensory impression is made on the brain but is then followed within a minute or so by an electrically induced brain convulsion, the sensory experience will not be remembered at all. Likewise, brain concussion, sudden application of deep general anesthesia, and other effects that temporarily block the dynamic function of the brain can prevent consolidation.

However, if the same sensory stimulus is impressed on the brain and the strong electrical shock is delayed for more than 5 to 10 minutes, at least part of the memory trace will have become established. If the shock is delayed for an hour or more, the memory will have become fully consolidated.

This process of consolidation and the time required for consolidation can probably be explained by the phenomenon of *rehearsal* of the short-term memory as follows:

Role of Rehearsal in Transference of Short-Term Memory into Long-Term Memory. Psychological studies have shown that rehearsal of the same information again and again accelerates and potentiates the degree of transfer of short-term memory into long-term memory, and therefore also accelerates and potentiates the process of consolidation. The brain has a natural tendency to rehearse new-found information, and especially to rehearse new-found information that catches the mind's attention. Therefore, over a period of time the important features of sensory experiences become progressively more and more fixed in the long-term memory stores. This explains why a person can remember small amounts of information studied in depth far better than he can remember large amounts of information studied only superficially. And it also explains why a person who is wide-awake will consolidate memories far better than will a person who is in a state of mental fatigue.

Codifying of Memories During the Process of Consolidation. One of the most important features of the process of consolidation is that memories to be placed permanently into the long-term memory storehouse are first codified into different classes of information. During this process similar information is recalled from the long-term storage bins and is used to help process the new information. The new and old are compared for similarities and for differences, and part of the storage process is to store the information about these similarities and differences rather than simply to store the information unprocessed. Thus, during the process of consolidation, the new memories are not stored randomly in the mind, but instead are stored in direct association with other memories of the same type. This is obviously necessary if one is to be able to scan the memory store at a later date to find the required information.

Transfer of Sensory Memory into Long-Term Memory. Some physiopsychologists believe that sensory memory can be transferred directly into long-term memory without first passing through the stage of short-term memory. This would apply to such information as visual scenes, musical tunes, tactile experiences, and so forth. Here again, the greater the number of times that the person experiences the sensory information, which is a form of rehearsal, the greater also is the degree of consolidation of the memories.

Change of Long-Term Secondary Memory into Long-Term Tertiary Memory—Role of Rehearsal. Rehearsal also plays an extremely important role in changing the weak trace type of long-term memory, called secondary memory, into the strong trace type, called tertiary memory. That is, each time a memory is recalled or each time the same sensory experience is repeated, a more and more indelible memory trace develops in the brain. The memory finally becomes so deeply fixed in the brain that it can be recalled within fractions of a second and it will also last for a lifetime, both of which are the characteristics of long-term tertiary memory.

Role of Specific Parts of the Brain in the Memory Process

Role of the Hippocampus for Rehearsal, Codification, and Consolidation of Memories—Anterograde Amnesia. Persons who have had both hippocampal gyri removed have essentially normal memory for information stored in the brain prior to removal of the hippocampi. However, after loss of these gyri, these persons have very little capability for transferring short-term memory into long-term

memory. That is, they do not have the ability to separate out the important information, to codify it, to rehearse it, and to consolidate it in the long-term memory store. Therefore, these persons develop serious *anterograde amnesia,* meaning simply inability to establish new memories.

Other types of lesions that frequently give anterograde amnesia include lesions of (1) the mammillary bodies, (2) the anterior nuclei of the thalamus, (3) the anterior columns of the fornix, or (4) the dorsal medial nuclei of the thalamus.

Retrograde Amnesia—Possible Relation to Thalamic Lesions. Excessive damage to large portions of the thalamus is incompatible with life. However, lesser thalamic damage will often lead to some degree of retrograde amnesia, which means inability to recall memories from the long-term store even though these memories are still known to be there. In the previous chapter, it was pointed out that the thalamus possibly or probably plays a major role in directing the person's attention to information in different parts of his immediate sensory sphere or of his memory storehouse. Therefore, the thalamus could easily play similar important roles in codifying, storing, and recalling memories.

INTELLECTUAL OPERATIONS OF THE BRAIN

Thus far, we have considered the approximate nature of thoughts and possible mechanisms by which memory and learning can occur. Now we need to consider the mechanisms by which the brain performs complex intellectual operations, such as the analysis of sensory information and the establishment of abstract thoughts. About these mechanisms we know almost nothing, but experiments along these lines have established the following important facts: First, the brain can focus its attention on specific types of information (which was discussed in the preceding chapter). Second, the different qualities of each set of information signals are split away from the central signal and are transmitted to multiple areas of the brain. Third, the brain compares new information with old information in its memory loci. And, fourth, the brain determines patterns of stimulation.

Analysis of Information by Splitting its Qualities. When sensory information enters the nervous system, one of the first steps in its analysis is to transmit the signal to separate parts of the brain that are selectively adapted for detecting specific qualities. For instance, if the hand is placed on a hot stove, (a) pain information is sent through the spinoreticular and spinothalamic tracts into the reticular formation of the brain stem and into certain thalamic and hypothalamic nuclei, (b) tactile information is sent through the dorsal column system to the somesthetic cortex, giving the cortex a detailed description of the part of the hand that is touching the hot stove, and (c) kinesthetic information from the muscles and joints is sent to the cerebellum, the reticular formation, and to higher centers of the brain to give momentary information of the position of the hand. Thus, the different qualities of the overall information are dissected and transmitted to different parts of the brain. It is on the basis of analyses in all these parts of the brain that motor responses to the incoming sensory information are formulated.

One can see that different centers of the brain react to specific qualities of information—the reticular formation and certain regions of the thalamus and hypothalamus to pain, regions of the mesencephalon and hypothalamus to the affective nature of the sensation (that is, whether it is pleasant or unpleasant), the somatic cortex to the localization of sensation, other areas to kinesthetic activities, and others to visual, auditory, gustatory, olfactory, and vestibular information.

Analysis of New Information by Comparison with Memories. We all know that new sensory experiences are immediately compared with previous experiences of the same or similar types. For instance, this is the way we recognize a person whom we know. Yet, it still remains a mystery how we can make these comparisons. One theory suggests that the memory trace might be stored in one layer of the cerebral cortex and that the new incoming sensory experience might be impressed on another layer. If the new pattern of stimulation matches the memory trace, some interaction between the two gives the person a sense of recognition.

Analysis of Patterns. In analyzing information, the brain depends to a great extent on "patterns" of stimulation. For instance, a square is detected as a square regardless of its position or angle of rotation in the visual field. Likewise, a series of parallel bars is detected as parallel bars regardless of their orientation, or a fly is detected as a fly whether it is seen in the peripheral or central field of vision. We can ex-

tend the same logic to the somatic sensory areas, for a person can detect a cube simply by feeling it whether it be in an upright, horizontal, or angulated position. Also, it can be detected even by the feet even though the feet may have never felt a cube before.

It is believed that one of the major methods for analyzing information is to dissect it into its component patterns. For instance, repetitive auditory sensations and visual sensations of a series of lights have at least one characteristic in common: both have the pattern of repetitiveness. Yet we cannot say how patterns of sensations are detected. One theory holds that their detection results from traveling waves passing through the cortex. As these cross the brain they might cause a signal to be transmitted every time they interact with an excited point of the cortex. For instance, if a traveling wave were passing over a visual cortex that is being excited by a regular series of lights, every time this wave should come in contact with an activated point, a signal would theoretically be transmitted away from the cortex to some *analyzer portion* of the brain. The analyzer would receive a train of rhythmic impulses, each impulse denoting a separate light, and this train of impulses could then theoretically give the person the sensation of repetitiveness. Likewise, repetitive sounds entering the ears could transmit a train of impulses to the same analyzer which would also give a sensation of repetitiveness, or movement of the hand over a corrugated surface could give the analyzer the same sensation of repetitiveness.

If we use our imaginations, we can see that only a few different types of analytical patterns can go a long way toward explaining almost all types of sensory impressions.

Processing of Information so that Patterns Can Be Determined. Beautiful examples of the ability of the brain to process information for determination of patterns have been discovered in relation to the visual system. In Chapter 18 we point out that the retina itself processes visual information to a great extent even before it is transmitted into the brain. For instance, the retina is especially responsive to rapidly changing light intensities or to movement of images across the receptors, and the signals sent to the brain are appropriately modified to transmit these qualities. Then, when the image is transmitted through the lateral geniculate body and thence into the primary visual cortex, the visual signals are altered again in such a way that the cortex detects mainly boundaries between light and dark areas. That is, the visual scene is "differentiated'' by this mechanism, bringing out strongly the contrasts of the scene but de-emphasizing the flat areas. This explains why a few lines drawn on a paper can give one the impression of a person's appearance. Certainly the lines do not represent the actual picture of a person, but they do give the visual cortex the same pattern of contrasts that his own visual system would give.

One can see, therefore, that the visual cortex utilizes transformed types of information to point up the most striking characteristics of the visual scene while neglecting unimportant information. Then, the patterns of the visual scene can be extracted from this ''pre-selected'' information.

Conversion of Information in Association Areas of the Brain.   Certain areas of the brain perform specific functions, such as the primary sensory areas and the motor areas. On the other hand, some of the remainder of the brain, the *association areas,* do not necessarily perform functions only associated with a particular modality of sensation or with a specific motor function. These areas often receive information from several sensory inputs and also from other association areas of the brain. Association areas are also located in lower brain regions, such as in the *thalamus* and *caudate nuclei*. Indeed, for every association area in the cortex, there is a reciprocally connected association area of the thalamus. In addition, other areas of the thalamus, such as the centromedial and dorsomedial nuclei, interconnect widely within the thalamus itself and presumably act as association areas between the different thalamic nuclei.

It is in the association areas that information from different sources interact. Thus, the posterior temporal lobe and the angular gyrus of the cerebral cortex, where the temporal, parietal, and occipital lobes all come together, is an association area that receives auditory, visual, and tactile information. Neurophysiological experiments have demonstrated that these interacting types of information can at times inhibit each other and at other times facilitate each other. Yet, how the interactions in the association areas are analyzed beyond this point is still a mystery.

INTELLECTUAL ASPECTS OF MOTOR CONTROL

Control of muscular movements by the cerebral cortex and other areas of the brain was discussed in Chapter 11, but we still need to consider the manner in which the intellectual operations of the brain elicit motor events. Almost all sensory and even abstract experiences of the mind are eventually expressed in some type of motor activity, such as actual muscular movements of a directed nature, tenseness of the muscles, total relaxation of the muscles, attainment of certain postures, tapping of the fingers, grimaces of the face, or speech.

Psychological tests show that the analytical portions of the brain control motor activities in the following sequence of three stages: (1) origin of the thought of the motor activity to be performed, (2) determination of the sequence of movements necessary to perform the overall task, and (3) control of the muscular movements themselves.

Origin of the Thought of a Motor Activity in the General Interpretative Area of the Brain.   A large number of motor movements, which we call subconscious movements, are conceived in the lower regions of the brain, but complex learned tasks can be performed only when the cerebral cortex is present. The most important cortical areas for this purpose are the posterior part of the superior temporal gyrus and the angular gyrus of the dominant hemisphere. The student will immediately recognize this area to be the *general interpretative area* of the brain. Thus, the sensory interactions that take place in this all-important sensory part of the dominant hemisphere not only play a major role in interpreting sensory experiences but also in determining the person's course of motor activities.

Determination of Sequences of Movement.   In our earlier discussion of cortical control of motor activities, it was pointed out that the somatic association area is necessary for performance of complex learned movements; destruction of this area both in animals and human beings causes the motor activities to lose much of their purposefulness. Therefore, it is postulated that once the general interpretative area of the brain has determined the motor activity to be performed, the actual sequences of movement are determined in the somatic association areas as discussed in Chapter 11. Signals are transmitted from here to the motor portion of the brain to control the actual motor movements, as also discussed in Chapter 11.

FUNCTION OF THE BRAIN IN COMMUNICATION

One of the most important differences between the human being and lower animals is the facility with which human beings can communicate with one another. Furthermore, because neurological tests can easily assess the ability of a person to communicate with others, we know perhaps more about the sensory and motor systems related to communication than about any other segment of cortical function. Therefore, we will review rapidly the function of the cortex in communication, and from this one can see immediately how the principles of sensory analysis and motor control that were just discussed apply to this art.

There are two aspects to communication: first, the *sensory aspect,* involving the ears and eyes, and, second, the *motor aspect,* involving vocalization and its control.

Sensory Aspects of Communication. We noted earlier in the chapter that destruction of portions of the *auditory* and *visual association areas* of the cortex can result in inability to understand the spoken word or the written word. These effects are called respectively *auditory receptive aphasia* and *visual receptive aphasia* or, more commonly, *word deafness* and *word blindness* (also called *alexia).* On the other hand, some persons are perfectly capable of understanding either the spoken word or the written word but are unable to interpret their meanings when used to express a thought. This results most frequently when the *angular gyrus* or *posterior portion of the superior temporal gyrus* in the dominant hemisphere is damaged or destroyed. This is considered to be *general sensory aphasia* or *general agnosia.*

Motor Aspects of Communication. *Syntactical Aphasia.* The process of speech involves (a) formation in the mind of thoughts to be expressed and choice of the words to be used and (b) the actual act of vocalization. The formation of thoughts and choice of words is principally the function of the sensory areas of the brain, for we find that a person who has a destructive lesion in the same *posterior temporal lobe and angular gyrus region* that is involved in general sensory aphasia also has inability to formulate intelligible thoughts to be communicated. And at other times the thoughts can be formulated, but the person is unable to put together the appropriate words to express the thought; this results most frequently from destruction of the angular gyrus. These inabilities to formulate thoughts and word sequences are called *syntactical aphasias* or, in honor of the neurologist who first delimited the brain area responsible, *Wernicke's aphasia.*

Motor Aphasia. Often a person is perfectly capable of deciding what he wishes to say, and he is capable of vocalizing, but he simply cannot make his vocal system emit words instead of noises. This effect, called *motor aphasia,* almost always results from damage to *Broca's speech area,* which lies in the *premotor* facial region of the cortex—about 95 per cent of the time in the left hemisphere, as illustrated in Figure 13–5. Therefore, we assume that the *patterns* for control of the larynx, lips, mouth, respiratory system, and other accessory muscles of articulation are all controlled in this area.

Articulation. Finally, we have the act of articulation itself, which means the muscular movements of the mouth, tongue, larynx, and so forth, that are responsible for the actual emission of sound. The facial and laryngeal regions of the motor cortex activate these muscles, and the sensory cortex helps to control the muscle contractions by feedback servomechanisms described in Chapter 11. Destruction of these regions can cause either total or partial inability to speak distinctly.

FUNCTION OF THE CORPUS CALLOSUM AND ANTERIOR COMMISSURE TO TRANSFER THOUGHTS, MEMORIES, AND OTHER INFORMATION TO THE OPPOSITE HEMISPHERE

Fibers in the *corpus callosum* connect the respective cortical areas of the two hemispheres with each other except for the cortices of the anterior portions of the temporal lobes; these temporal cortical areas are interconnected by fibers that pass through the *anterior commissure.* Because of the tremendous number of fibers in the corpus callosum, it was very early believed that this massive structure must have some important function to correlate activities of the two cerebral hemispheres. However, cutting the corpus callosum in experimental animals, or in occasional instances even in the human being, caused no change in the function of the brain that could be discerned by gross observation. Therefore, for a long time the function of the corpus callosum was a mystery.

However, psychological experiments have now demonstrated the function of the corpus callosum and the anterior commissure. This can be explained best by recounting one of the experiments. A monkey is first prepared by cutting the corpus callosum and splitting the optic chiasm longitudinally. Then it is taught to recognize different types of objects with its right eye while its left eye is covered. Then the right eye is covered and the monkey is tested to determine whether or not its left eye can recognize the same object. The answer to this is that the left eye *cannot* recognize the object. Yet, on repeating the same experiment with the optic chiasm still split but the corpus callosum intact, it is found invariably that recognition in one hemisphere of the brain creates recognition also in the opposite hemisphere.

Thus, one of the functions of the corpus callosum and the anterior commissure is to make information stored in the cortex of one hemisphere available to the corresponding cortical area of the opposite hemisphere. Two important examples of such cooperation between the two hemispheres are:

1. Cutting of the corpus callosum blocks transfer of information from the general interpretative area of the dominant hemisphere to the motor cortex on the opposite side of the brain. Therefore, the intellectual functions of the brain, located primarily in the dominant hemisphere, lose much of their control over the right motor cortex and therefore also of the voluntary motor functions of the left hand and arm even though the usual subconscious movements of the left hand and arm are completely normal.

2. Cutting of the corpus callosum prevents transfer of somatic and visual information from the right hemisphere into the general interpretative area of the dominant hemisphere. Therefore, somatic and visual information from the left side of the body frequently fails to reach the general interpretative area of the brain and, therefore, cannot be used for decision-making.

Yet, in one human being recently studied who had been born with congenital absence of the corpus callosum, it was found that most of these associative functions between the hemispheres could be performed. This emphasizes the importance of the lower brain centers, particularly of the reticular formation and of the thalamus, for correlation of activities between the two sides of the brain. Therefore, it should not be thought that the different parts of the cerebral cortex communicate with each other only via subcortical fiber tracts because perhaps equally as much communication occurs by way of the lower centers as well.

REFERENCES

Atkinson, R. C., and Shiffrin, R. M.: The control of short-term memory. *Sci. Amer.*, 225:82, 1971.

Bower, T. G. R.: The object in the world of the infant. *Sci. Amer.*, 225:30, 1971.

Cole, R. A., and Scott, B.: Toward a theory of speech perception. *Psychol. Rev.*, 81:348, 1974.

Corning, W. C., Dyal, J. A., and Willows, A. O. D. (eds.): Invertebrate Learning. Vol. 3. New York, Plenum Publishing Corporation, 1974.

Darley, F. L.: Brain Mechanisms Underlying Speech and Language. New York, Grune & Stratton, Inc., 1967.

Darley, F. L., Aronson, A. E., and Brown, J. R.: Motor Speech Disorders. Philadelphia, W. B. Saunders Company, 1975.

Deutsch, J. A. (ed.): The Physiological Basis of Memory. New York, Academic Press, Inc., 1972.

Dimond, S. J.: The Double Brain. New York, Churchill Livingstone, Div. of Longman, Inc., 1972.

Flanagan, J. L.: The synthesis of speech. *Sci. Amer.*, 226:48, 1972.

Gazzaniga, M. S.: One brain—two minds? *Amer. Sci.*, 60:311, 1972.

Geschwind, N.: Language and the brain. *Sci. Amer.*, 226:76, 1972.

Geschwind, N.: The apraxias: neural mechanisms of disorders of learned movement. *Amer. Sci.*, 63:188, 1975.

Gibbs, M. E., and Mark, R. F.: Inhibition of Memory Formation. New York, Plenum Publishing Corporation, 1973.

Goldensohn, E. S., and Appel, S. H.: Scientific Approaches to Clinical Neurology. Philadelphia, Lea & Febiger, 1975.

Haber, R. N.: How we remember what we see. *Sci. Amer.*, 222:104, 1970.

Hailman, J. P.: How an instinct is learned. *Sci. Amer.*, 221:98, 1969.

Harris, A. J.: Inductive functions of the nervous system. *Ann. Rev. Physiol.*, 36:251, 1974.

Hess, W. R.: The Biology of Mind. Chicago, University of Chicago Press, 1964.

Jakobson, R.: Verbal communication. *Sci. Amer.*, 227:72, 1972.

Jakoubek, B.: Brain Function and Macromolecular Synthesis. New York, Academic Press, Inc., 1974.

Jenkins, J. J., Jimenez-Pabon, E., Shaw, R. E., and Sefer, J. W.: Schuell's Aphasia in Adults. Hagerstown, Md., Harper & Row, Publishers, 1975.

Jyont, R. J., and Goldstein, M. N.: Minor cerebral hemisphere. *Adv. Neurol.*, 7:147, 1975.

Kimura, D.: The asymmetry of the human brain. *Sci. Amer.*, 228:70, 1973.

Kinsbourne, M., and Smith, W. L. (eds.): Hemispheric Disconnection and Cerebral Function. Springfield, Ill., Charles C Thomas, Publisher, 1974.

Luria, A. R.: The functional organization of the brain. *Sci. Amer.*, 222:66, 1970.

McGuigan, F. J., and Schoonover, R. A. (eds.): The Psychophysiology of Thinking; Studies of Covert Processes. New York, Academic Press, Inc., 1973.

Maggio, E.: Psychophysiology of Learning and Memory. Springfield, Ill., Charles C. Thomas, Publisher, 1971.

Mark, R. F.: Memory and Nerve Cell Connections: Criticisms and Contributions from Developmental Neurophysiology. New York, Oxford University Press, 1974.

Mattingly, I. G.: Speech cues and sign stimuli. *Amer. Sci.*, 60:327, 1972.

Nebes, R. D.: Hemispheric specialization in commissurotomized man. *Psychol. Bull.*, 81:1, 1974.

Needham, C. W.: Neurosurgical Syndromes of the Brain. Springfield, Ill., Charles C Thomas, Publisher, 1973.

Ornstein, R. E. (ed.): The Nature of Human Consciousness: a Book of Readings. San Francisco. W. H. Freeman Company, Publishers, 1973.

Penfield, W.: The Excitable Cortex in Conscious Man. Springfield, Ill., Charles C Thomas, Publisher, 1958.

Peters, M., and Ploog, D.: Communication among primates. *Ann. Rev. Physiol.*, 35:221, 1973.

Rosenblatt, J. S.: Learning in newborn kittens. *Sci. Amer.*, 227:18, 1972.

Schultz, A.: A Theory and Consciousness. New York, Philosophical Library, 1973.

Schwartz, M.: Physiological Psychology. New York, Appleton-Century-Crofts, 1973.

Somjen, G. G.: Neurophysiology Studied in Man. (Proceedings of a Symposium held in Paris, 1971.) New York, American Elsevier Publishing Company, 1972.

Stein, D. G., and Rosen, J. J.: Learning and Memory. New York, The Macmillan Company, 1974.

Thompson, R. F.: Introduction to Physiological Psychology. New York, Harper & Row, Publishers, 1975.

Timmons, B. A., and Boudreau, J. P.: Auditory feedback as a major factor in stuttering. *J. Speech Hear. Disord.*, 37:476, 1972.

Tulving, E.: Cue-dependent forgetting. *Amer. Sci.*, 62:74, 1974.

Wassermann, G. D.: Brains and Reasoning; Brain Science as a Basis of Applied and Pure Philosophy. London, Macmillan & Co. Ltd., 1974.

White, M. J.: Hemispheric asymmetries in tachistoscopic information-processing. *Brit. J. Psychol.*, 63:497, 1972.

Wyrwicka, W.: The Mechanisms of Conditioned Behavior. Springfield, Ill., Charles C Thomas, Publisher, 1972.

14

Behavioral Functions of the Brain: The Limbic System, Role of the Hypothalamus, and Control of Vegetative Functions of the Body

Behavior is a function of the entire nervous system, not of any particular portion. Even the discrete cord reflexes are an element of behavior, and the wakefulness and sleep cycle discussed in Chapter 12 is certainly one of the most important of our behavioral patterns. However, in this chapter we will deal with those special types of behavior associated with emotions, subconscious motor and sensory drives, and the intrinsic feelings of pain and pleasure. These functions of the nervous system are performed mainly by subcortical structures located in the basal regions of the brain. However, older portions of the cerebral cortex located on the medial and ventral portions of the cerebral hemispheres also play a role. This overall group of brain structures is frequently called the *limbic system*.

Portions of the limbic system, especially the hypothalamus and related structures, control many of the internal functions of the body, such as body temperature, osmolality of the body fluids, body weight, and so forth; these functions are collectively called *vegetative functions* of the body.

THE LIMBIC SYSTEM

Figure 14–1 illustrates the anatomical structures of the limbic system, showing these to be an interconnected complex of basal brain elements. Located in the midst of all of these is the hypothalamus, which is considered by many anatomists to be a separate structure from the remainder of the limbic system, but which, from a physiological point of view, is considered to be one of the central elements of the system. Therefore, Figure 14–2 illustrates schematically this key position of the hypothalamus in the limbic system and shows that surrounding it are the other subcortical structures of the limbic system, including the *preoptic area*, the *septum*, the *paraolfactory area*, the *epithalamus*, the *anterior nuclei of the thalamus*, *portions of the basal ganglia*, the *hippocampus*, and the *amygdala*. Surrounding the subcortical limbic areas is the *limbic cortex* composed of a ring of cerebral cortex (a) beginning in the *orbitofrontal area* on the ventral surface of the frontal lobes, (b) extending upward in front of and over the corpus callosum onto the medial aspect of the cerebral hemisphere to the *cingulate gyrus*, and finally (c) passing posterior to the corpus callosum and downward onto the ventromedial surface of the temporal lobe to the *hippocampal gyrus, pyriform area,* and *uncus*. Thus, on the medial and ventral surfaces of each cerebral hemisphere is a ring of paleocortex that surrounds a group of deep structures intimately associated with overall behavior and with emotions.

Figure 14–1. Anatomy of the limbic system illustrated by the shaded areas of the figure. (From Warwick and Williams: Gray's Anatomy, 35th Brit. Ed., London, Longman Group Ltd., 1973.)

In the past, many neurophysiologists have lumped the entire limbic system together as a unit structure that controls the different emotional and behavioral patterns of the nervous system. As we learn more about the various portions of this system, it is becoming evident that different areas of the system perform very specific functions.

VEGETATIVE FUNCTIONS OF THE HYPOTHALAMUS

The hypothalamus provides the most important output pathway through which the limbic system controls many major functions of the body, especially the vegetative functions, which are the involuntary functions necessary for living. The different hypothalamic centers are so important in these controls that they represent one of the essential control centers of the body. Some of the specific factors controlled by the hypothalamus are arterial pressure, thirst,

water conservation, body temperature, sexual functions, and many more. To illustrate the organization of the hypothalamus as a functioning unit, we will summarize some of its vegetative functions here.

Figure 14–3 summarizes most of the vegetative functions of the hypothalamus and shows, with the exception of the lateral hypothalamic areas that overlie the areas illustrated, the major nuclei or major areas which when stimulated affect respective vegetative activities. A word of caution must be issued in studying this diagram, however, for the areas that cause specific activities are not nearly so discrete as shown in the figure. The illustrated areas are merely those from which the functions are likely to be elicited. Also, it is not known whether the effects noted in the figure result from activation of specific control nuclei or whether they result merely from activation of fiber tracts leading from control nuclei located elsewhere. For instance, stimulation of the

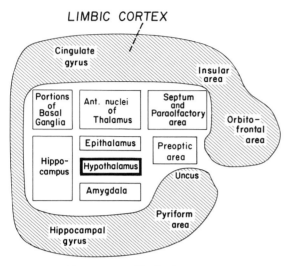

Figure 14–2. The limbic system.

posterior hypothalamus, through which many of the fiber pathways from other portions of the hypothalamus pass, can at times elicit many functions believed to be controlled primarily by other hypothalamic nuclei. With this caution in mind, we can give the following general description to the vegetative control functions of the hypothalamus.

Cardiovascular Regulation. Stimulation of widespread areas throughout the hypothalamus can cause every known type of neurogenic effect in the cardiovascular system, including increased arterial pressure, decreased arterial pressure, increased

heart rate, and decreased heart rate. In general, stimulation in the *posterior* and *lateral hypothalamus* increases the arterial pressure and heart rate, while stimulation in the *preoptic area* often has opposite effects, causing a decrease in both heart rate and arterial pressure. These effects are transmitted mainly through the cardiovascular control centers in the reticular substance of the medulla and pons.

Regulation of Body Temperature. Large areas in the anterior portion of the hypothalamus, especially in the *preoptic area,* are concerned with regulation of body temperature. An increase in temperature of the blood flowing through these areas increases their activity, while a decrease in temperature decreases their activity. In turn, these areas control the mechanisms for increasing or decreasing body temperature, such as sweating and skin temperature.

Regulation of Body Water. The hypothalamus regulates body water in two separate ways, by (1) creating the sensation of thirst, which makes an animal drink water, and (2) controlling the excretion of water into the urine. An area called the *thirst center* is located in the lateral hypothalamus. When the electrolytes inside the neurons of this small center become too concentrated, the animal develops an intense desire to drink water; he will search out the nearest source of water and drink enough to return the electrolyte concentration of the thirst center to normal.

Control of renal excretion of water is vested mainly in the *supraoptic nuclei.* When the body fluids become too concentrated, the neurons of this area become stimulated and secrete a hormone called *antidiuretic hormone.* This hormone is stored in the posterior pituitary gland and when released into the blood acts on the collecting ducts of the kidneys to cause massive reabsorption of water, thereby de-

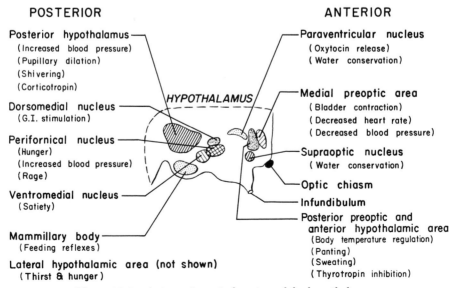

Figure 14–3. Autonomic control centers of the hypothalamus.

creasing the loss of water into the urine. Thus, both the intake and output of body water are controlled.

Regulation of Uterine Contractility and of Milk Ejection by the Breasts. Stimulation of the paraventricular nuclei causes its neuronal cells to secrete the hormone *oxytocin*. This in turn causes increased contractility of the uterus and also contraction of the myoepithelial cells that surround the alveoli of the breasts, which then causes the alveoli to empty the milk through the nipples. At the end of pregnancy especially large quantities of oxytocin are secreted, and this secretion helps to promote labor contractions that expel the baby. Also, when a baby suckles the mother's breast oxytocin is released, and this release performs the necessary function of expelling the milk through the nipple so that the baby can nourish itself. When this mechanism fails, the mother becomes unable to feed her baby.

Gastrointestinal and Feeding Regulation. Excitation of several areas of the hypothalamus causes an animal to experience extreme hunger, a voracious appetite, and an intense desire to search for food. The two areas that, when excited, are most associated with hunger are the *perifornical nucleus* and the *lateral hypothalamic area*. On the other hand, damage to these areas of the hypothalamus causes the animal to lose desire for food, sometimes causing starvation.

A center that opposes the desire for food, called the *satiety center,* is located in the *ventromedial nucleus*. When this center is stimulated, an animal that is eating food suddenly stops eating and shows complete indifference to the food. On the other hand, if this area is destroyed, the animal cannot be satiated, but instead, his hypothalamic hunger centers become overactive so that he has a voracious appetite, often resulting in tremendous obesity.

Another area of the hypothalamus that enters into the overall control of gastrointestinal activity is the *dorsomedial nucleus* which, when stimulated, increases the degree of peristalsis in the gut and also increases glandular secretion. Also, the *mammillary body* enters into many feeding reflexes, such as licking the lips and swallowing.

Hypothalamic Control of the Anterior Pituitary Gland. Stimulation of certain areas of the hypothalamus also causes the anterior pituitary gland to secrete its hormones. This subject is a key element in the study of endocrinology. Although we will not discuss it in detail here, briefly, the basic mechanism of the control of the anterior pituitary is the following:

The anterior pituitary receives its blood supply mainly from veins that flow into the anterior pituitary sinuses from the lower part of the hypothalamus. As the blood courses through the hypothalamus before reaching the anterior pituitary, *neurosecretory substances* are secreted into the blood by various hypothalamic nuclei. They are then transported in the blood to the pituitary tissues where they act on the glandular cells to cause release of the anterior pituitary hormones.

thalamus has been said to cause secretion of specific hormones: (1) preoptic and anterior hypothalamic nuclei, thyrotropin; (2) posterior hypothalamus and median eminence of the infundibulum, corticotropin; (3) median eminence, follicle-stimulating hormone; and (4) anterior hypothalamus, luteinizing hormone.

Summary. A number of discrete areas of the hypothalamus have now been found that control specific vegetative functions. However, these areas are still poorly delimited, so much so that the above separation of different areas for different hypothalamic functions is partially artificial.

ROLE OF THE RETICULAR FORMATION IN BEHAVIORAL FUNCTIONS OF THE BRAIN

At this point we need to recognize that many of the behavioral functions elicited from the hypothalamus and from other limbic structures are mediated through the reticular formation of the brain stem. It was pointed out in Chapters 10 and 12 that stimulation of the excitatory portion of the reticular formation can cause high degrees of somatic excitability; in Chapter 15 we will see that most of the signals for control of the autonomic nervous system either originate in or are transmitted from higher centers through nuclei located in the brain stem reticular formation.

Therefore, from a physiological point of view the reticular formation is a very important part of the limbic system even though anatomically it is considered to be a separate entity. A very important route of communication between the limbic system and the reticular formation is the *medial forebrain bundle* that extends from the septal and orbitofrontal cortical regions downward through the hypothalamus to the reticular formation. This bundle carries fibers in both directions, forming a trunk-line communication system. A second route of communication is through short pathways among the reticular formation, the thalamus, the hypothalamus, and most of the other contiguous areas of the basal brain.

BEHAVIORAL FUNCTIONS OF THE LIMBIC SYSTEM

PLEASURE AND PAIN; REWARD AND PUNISHMENT

In recent years, it has been learned that many hypothalamic and other limbic structures are particularly concerned with the affective nature of sensory sensations—that is, with whether the sensations are *pleasant* or *painful*. These affective qualities are also called *reward* and *punishment* or *satisfaction* and *aversion*. Electrical stimulation of certain regions pleases or satisfies the animal, whereas electrical stimulation of other regions causes extreme pain, fear, defense, escape reactions, and all the other elements of punishment. Obviously, these two oppositely responding systems greatly affect the behavior of the animal.

Reward Centers. Figure 14–4 illustrates a technique that has been used for localizing the specific reward and punishment areas of the brain. In this figure a lever is placed at the side of the cage and is arranged so that depressing the lever makes electrical contact with a stimulator. Electrodes are placed successively at different areas in the brain so that the animal can stimulate the area by pressing the lever. If stimulating the particular area gives the animal a sense of reward, then he will press the lever again and again, sometimes as much as 7000 times per hour. Furthermore, when offered the choice of eating some delectable food as opposed to the opportunity to stimulate the reward center, he often chooses the electrical stimulation.

By using this procedure, the major reward centers have been found to be located in the septum and hypothalamus, primarily *along the*

Figure 14–4. Technique for localizing reward and punishment centers in the brain of a monkey.

course of the medial forebrain bundle and *in the ventromedial nuclei of the hypothalamus*. Less potent reward centers, which are probably secondary to the major ones in the septum and hypothalamus, are found in the amygdala, certain areas of the thalamus and basal ganglia, and finally extending downward into the basal tegmentum of the mesencephalon.

Punishment Centers. The apparatus illustrated in Figure 14–4 can also be connected so that pressing the lever turns off rather than turns on an electrical stimulus. In this case, the animal will not turn the stimulus off when the electrode is in one of the reward areas, but when it is in certain other areas he immediately learns to turn it off. Stimulation in these areas causes the animal to show all the signs of pain, displeasure, and punishment. Furthermore, prolonged stimulation for 24 hours or more causes the animal to become severely sick and actually leads to death.

By means of this technique, the principal centers for pain, punishment, and escape tendencies have been found in the *central gray area surrounding the aqueduct of Sylvius in the mesencephalon* and extending upward into the *periventricular structures of the hypothalamus and thalamus*. The *perifornical nucleus* of the hypothalamus is the most reactive of all the hypothalamic areas.

It is particularly interesting that stimulation in the pain and punishment centers can frequently inhibit the reward and pleasure centers completely, illustrating that pain can take precedence over pleasure and reward.

Importance of Reward and Punishment in Behavior. Almost everything that we do depends on reward and punishment. If we are doing something that is rewarding, we continue to do it; if it is punishing, we cease to do it. Therefore, the reward and punishment centers undoubtedly constitute one of the most important of all the controllers of our bodily activities, our motivations, and so forth.

Importance of Reward and Punishment in Learning and Memory—Habituation or Reinforcement. Animal experiments have shown that a sensory experience causing neither reward nor punishment is remembered hardly at all. Electrical recordings have shown that new and novel sensory stimuli always excite the cerebral cortex. But repetition of the stimulus over and over leads to almost complete extinction of the cortical response if the sensory experience does not elicit either a sense of reward or punishment. Thus, the animal becomes *habituated* to the sensory stimulus, and thereafter ignores this stimulus.

If the stimulus causes either reward or punishment rather than indifference, however, the cortical response becomes progressively more and more intense with repetitive stimulation instead of fading away, and the response is said to be *reinforced*. Thus, an animal builds up strong memory traces for sensations that are either rewarding or punishing but, on the other hand, develops complete habituation to indifferent sensory stimuli. Therefore, it is evident that the reward and punishment centers of the midbrain have much to do with selecting the information that we learn.

Effect of Tranquilizers on the Reward and Punishment Centers. Administration of a tranquilizer, such as chlorpromazine, inhibits both the reward and punishment centers, thereby greatly decreasing the affective reactivity of the animal. Therefore, it is presumed that tranquilizers function in psychotic states by suppressing many of the important behavioral areas of the hypothalamus and its associated regions of the brain.

THE AFFECTIVE-DEFENSIVE PATTERN— RAGE

An emotional pattern that involves the hypothalamus and has been well characterized by Hess is the affective-defensive pattern. This can be described as follows:

Stimulation of the punishment centers of the brain, especially the *perifornical nuclei of the hypothalamus,* which are also the hypothalamic regions that give the most intense sensation of punishment, causes the animal to (1) develop a defense posture, (2) extend its claws, (3) lift its tail, (4) hiss, (5) spit, (6) growl, and (7) develop pilo-erection, wide-open eyes, and dilated pupils. Furthermore, even the slightest provocation causes an immediate savage attack. This is approximately the behavior that one would expect from an animal being severely punished, and it is a pattern of behavior that is called *rage*.

Stimulation of the more rostral areas of the punishment areas—in the midline preoptic areas—causes mainly fear and anxiety, associated with a tendency for the animal to run away.

All aspects of the rage phenomenon can still be elicited after decortication of an animal; most aspects can be evoked even after the thalamus is removed but with the hypothalamus intact, except that *spontaneous* rage is more likely to occur if the thalamus is intact. Also, a still more primitive pattern of rage can occur even in animals whose brain stems are sectioned below the hypothalamus but above the mesencephalon. In these animals, extremely noxious somatic sensory stimuli will cause the animal to grimace, to develop a defense posture, and to become generally excited. Therefore, much if not most of the rage pattern is mediated through the brain stem reticular formation.

Docility and Tameness. Exactly the opposite emotional behavioral patterns occur when the reward centers are stimulated: docility and tameness.

FUNCTION OF THE HYPOTHALAMUS AND ADJACENT AREAS IN SLEEP, WAKEFULNESS, ALERTNESS, AND EXCITEMENT

Stimulation of regions of the hypothalamus dorsal to the mammillary bodies greatly excites the reticular activating system and therefore causes wakefulness, alertness, and excitement. In addition, the sympathetic nervous system becomes excited in general, increasing the arterial pressure, causing pupillary dilatation, and enhancing other activities associated with sympathetic activity.

On the other hand, stimulation in the septum, in a few areas of the lateral or anterior hypothalamus, or in isolated points of the thalamic portions of the reticular activating system often inhibits the mesencephalic portion of the reticular activating system, causing somnolence and sometimes actual sleep. Thus, the hypothalamus and other limbic structures indirectly contribute much to the control of the degree of excitement and alertness.

PSYCHOSOMATIC EFFECTS OF THE HYPOTHALAMUS AND RETICULAR ACTIVATING SYSTEM

We are all familiar with the fact that abnormal function in the central nervous system can frequently lead to serious dysfunction of the different somatic organs of the body. This is also true in experimental animals, for, as pointed out above, prolonged electrical stimulation in the punishment regions of the brain can actually lead to severe sickness of the animal, culminating in death within 24 to 48 hours. We need, therefore, to understand briefly the mechanisms by which stimulatory effects in the brain can affect the peripheral organs. Ordinarily, this occurs through three routes: (1) through the motor nerves to the skeletal muscles throughout the body, (2) through the autonomic nerves to the different internal organs of the body, and (3) through the hormones secreted by the pituitary gland in response to nervous activity in the hypothalamus.

Psychosomatic Disorders Transmitted Through the Skeletal Nervous System. Abnormal psychic states can greatly alter the degree of nervous stimulation to the skeletal musculature throughout the body and thereby increase or decrease the skeletal muscular tone. During states of attention the general skeletal muscular tone as well as sympathetic tone normally increases, whereas during somnolent states skeletal muscular and sympathetic activity both decrease greatly. In neurotic and psychotic states, such as anxiety, tension, and mania, generalized overactivity of both the muscles and sympathetic system often occur throughout the body. This in turn results in intense feedback from the muscle proprioceptors to the reticular activating system, and the epinephrine circulating in the blood as a result of the sympathetic activity perhaps also excites the reticular activating system, both of which undoubtedly help to maintain an extreme degree of wakefulness and alertness that characterizes these emotional states. Unfortunately, though, the wakefulness prevents adequate sleep and also leads to progressive bodily fatigue but still inability to go to sleep.

Transmission of Psychosomatic Effects Through the Autonomic Nervous System. Many psychosomatic abnormalities result from hyperactivity of either the sympathetic or parasympathetic system. In general, hyperactivity of the sympathetic system occurs in widespread areas of the body at the same time rather than in focal areas, and the usual effects are (1) increased heart rate—sometimes with palpitation of the heart, (2) increased arterial pressure, (3) constipation, and (4) increased metabolic rate. On the other hand, parasympathetic signals are likely to be much more focal. For instance, stimulation of specific areas in the dorsal motor nuclei of the vagus nerves can cause more or less specifically (1) increased or decreased heart rate and palpitation of the heart, (2) esophageal spasm, (3) increased peristalsis in the upper gastrointestinal tract, or (4) increased hyperacidity of the stomach with resultant development of peptic ulcer. Stimulation of the sacral region of the parasympathetic system, on the other hand, is likely to cause extreme colonic glandular secretion and peristalsis with resulting diarrhea. One can readily see, then, that emotional patterns controlling the sympathetic and parasympathetic centers of the hypothalamus can cause wide varieties of peripheral psychosomatic effects.

Psychosomatic Effects Transmitted Through the Anterior Pituitary Gland. Electrical stimulation of the posterior hypothalamus increases the secretion of corticotropin by the anterior pituitary gland (as explained earlier in the chapter) and therefore indirectly increases the output of adrenocortical hormones. One of the effects of this is a gradual increase in stomach hyperacidity because of the effect of glucocorticoids on stomach secretion. Over a prolonged period of time this obviously could lead to peptic ulcer, which is a well-known effect of hypersecretion by the adrenal cortex. Likewise, activity in the anterior hypothalamus increases the pituitary secretion of thyrotropin, which in turn increases the output of thyroxine and leads to an elevated basal metabolic rate. It is well known that different types of emotional disturbances can lead to thyrotoxicosis (excess secretion of thyroid hormone), this presumably resulting from overactivity in the anterior hypothalamus.

From these examples, therefore, it is evident that many types of psychosomatic diseases of the body can be caused by abnormal control of anterior pituitary secretion.

FUNCTIONS OF OTHER PARTS OF THE LIMBIC SYSTEM

A large portion of the signals originating in other parts of the limbic system besides the hypothalamus are funneled through the hypothalamus, giving rise to various vegetative or behavioral effects that we know to result when the hypothalamus is stimulated. Other signals are funneled into the reticular activating system to control the degree of wakefulness, alertness, and attention. And still other behavioral signals are transmitted directly from the limbic structures into nonlimbic portions of the cerebral cortex to affect such diverse activities of the cortex as its analytical functions, its sensory functions, and even at times its motor functions.

Yet, unfortunately, the effects caused by many of the different limbic structures are mainly subjective, which prevents adequate experimental study in animals. Therefore, our knowledge of the functions of many of the limbic structures is very poor indeed. About the best that we can do at present is to catalogue some of the overt effects known to occur when these parts of the limbic system are stimulated.

FUNCTIONS OF THE AMYGDALA

The amygdala is a complex of nuclei located immediately beneath the medial surface of the cerebral cortex in the pole of each temporal lobe. In lower animals, this complex is concerned primarily with association of olfactory stimuli with stimuli from other parts of the brain. Indeed, it is pointed out in Chapter 20 that one of the major divisions of the olfactory tract leads directly to a portion of the amygdala called the *corticomedial nuclei* that lie immediately beneath the cortex in the pyriform area of the temporal lobe. However, in the human being, another portion of the amygdala, the *basolateral nuclei,* has become much more highly developed than the olfactory portion and plays very important roles in many behavioral activities not generally associated with olfactory stimuli.

The amygdala receives impulses from all portions of the limbic cortex, from the orbital surfaces of the frontal lobes, from the cingulate gyrus, and from the hippocampal gyrus. In turn, it transmits signals (a) back into these same cortical areas, (b) into the hippocampus, (c) into the septum, (d) the thalamus, and (e) especially into the hypothalamus.

Effects of Stimulating the Amygdala. In general, stimulation in the amygdala can cause almost all the same effects as those elicited by stimulation of the hypothalamus, plus still other effects. The effects that are mediated through the hypothalamus include (1) increases or decreases in arterial pressure, (2) increases or decreases in heart rate, (3) increases or decreases in gastrointestinal motility and secretion, (4) defecation and micturition, (5) pupillary dilatation or, rarely, constriction, (6) pilo-erection, (7) secretion of the various anterior pituitary hormones, including especially the gonadotropins and corticotropin.

Aside from these effects mediated through the hypothalamus, amygdala stimulation can also cause different types of involuntary movement. These include (1) tonic movements, such as raising the head or bending the body, (2) circling movements, (3) occasionally clonic, rhythmic movements, and (4) different types of movements associated with olfaction and eating, such as licking, chewing, and swallowing. And stimulation can alter respiration or at other times stop all movements of an animal, freezing the animal in its present postural state, a phenomenon called the *arrest reaction*.

In addition, stimulation of certain amygdaloid nuclei can rarely cause a pattern of rage, escape, punishment, and pain similar to the affective-defense pattern elicited from the hypothalamus as described above. And stimulation of other nuclei can give reactions of reward and pleasure.

Finally, excitation of still other portions of the amygdala can cause sexual activities that include erection, copulatory movements, ejaculation, ovulation, uterine activity, and premature labor.

In short, stimulation of appropriate portions of the amygdaloid nuclei can give almost any pattern of behavior. It is believed that the normal function of the amygdaloid nuclei is to help control the overall pattern of behavior demanded for each occasion.

FUNCTIONS OF THE HIPPOCAMPUS

The hippocampus is an elongated structure composed of a modified type of cerebral cortex. It folds inward to form the ventral surface of the inferior horn of the lateral ventricle. One end of the hippocampus abuts against the amygdaloid nuclei, and it also fuses along one of its borders with the hippocampal gyrus, which is the cortex of the ventromedial surface of the temporal lobe. The hippocampus has numerous connections with almost all parts of the limbic system, including especially the amygdala, hippocampal gyrus, cingulate gyrus, hypothalamus, and other areas closely related to the hypothalamus.

Unfortunately, as is true of most limbic structures, we know very little about the overall function of the hippocampus and, therefore, for the present can only describe some overt effects that occur when this area is stimulated or destroyed.

Stimulation of different regions of the hippocampus can cause *involuntary tonic or clonic movements* in different parts of the body. At times it causes *rage or other emotional reactions*. And stimulation sometimes causes different types of *sexual phenomena*. One of the most remarkable effects of stimulation in conscious man is immediate *loss of contact* with any person with whom he might be talking; indicating that the hippocampus can play a role in determining a person's attention.

A special feature of the hippocampus is that weak electrical stimuli can cause local epileptic seizures in this region. These seizures cause various psychomotor effects including olfactory, visual, auditory, tactile, and other types of hallucinations that are uncontrollable even though the person has not lost consciousness and even though he knows the hallucinations to be unreal. One of the reasons for this hyperexcitability of the hippocampus is probably that it is composed of a different type of cortex from that elsewhere in the cerebrum, having only three layers instead of the six layers found elsewhere.

Theoretical Function of the Hippocampus. Almost any type of sensory experience causes instantaneous activation of different parts of the hippocampus, and the hippocampus in turn distributes many outgoing signals to the hypothalamus and other parts of the limbic system through the *fornix*. Thus, one of the major sources of input signals to the hypothalamus and other limbic structures is the hippocampus. On the basis of this, it is often stated that the primary role of the hippocampus is to provide a channel through which different incoming sensory signals can excite appropriate limbic reactions.

Function of the Hippocampus in Learning. Earlier in the chapter (and also in the previous chapter) it was pointed out that reward and punishment centers play a major role in determining which information will be stored in memory. A person becomes rapidly habituated to indifferent stimuli but learns assiduously any sensory experience that causes either pain or pleasure. Yet what is the route by which reward and punishment centers receive their original information? It has been suggested that the hippocampus plays the role of associating the affective characteristics of different sensory signals and then in turn transmitting the correlated information into the reward or punishment areas of the hypothalamus and other limbic centers to help control the information that a person will learn. In fact, when the hippocampus has been removed bilaterally, a person develops anterograde amnesia, which means that it is difficult or almost impossible for him to store new memories. This is especially true for verbal information, perhaps because the temporal lobes are particularly concerned with this type of information.

FUNCTION OF THE HIPPOCAMPAL, CINGULATE, AND ORBITOFRONTAL CORTEX

Probably the most poorly understood portion of the entire limbic system is the ring of cerebral cortex, called the *limbic cortex,* that surrounds the subcortical limbic structures. The limbic cortex is among the oldest of all parts of the cerebral cortex. In lower animals it plays a major role in various olfactory, gustatory, and feeding phenomena. However, in the human being, these functions of the limbic cortex are of minor importance. Instead, the limbic cortex of the human being is believed to be the cerebral association cortex for control of the lower centers that have to do primarily with behavior. For instance, the hippocampal gyrus has close interconnections with the hippocampus and thence through the fornix with almost all areas of the limbic system, especially with the hypothalamus. The cingulate gyrus likewise connects directly with the hippocampus and also with all other limbic areas. Finally, the orbitofrontal cortex interconnects profusely with the septal area, hypothalamus, preoptic area, and other associated regions.

Effect of Stimulation. Stimulation of the different regions of the limbic cortex has failed to give any real idea of their functions, because the effects are just as diverse as those already recounted for stimulation of the hypothalamus, amygdala, or hippocampus, including such effects as (a) inhibition or acceleration of respiration, (b) facilitation or inhibition of spontaneous or cortical induced movements, (c) facilitation of clonic or tonic movements of the body, (d) vocalization, (e) chewing, (f) licking, (g) swallowing, (h) cardiovascular effects, such as increases or decreases in arterial pressure and increases or decreases in heart rate, (i) gastric effects, such as increases or decreases in gastrointestinal motility, (j) increases or decreases in gastrointestinal secretions, and (k) affective reactions including rage, docility, excitement, alertness, etc.

Effect of Ablation of Different Portions of the Limbic Cortex. Ablation experiments also have failed to give much idea of limbic cortical function, because the effects observed by different experimenters have often been quite different from each other. Also, the effects of ablation have sometimes been so inconsequential that no changes have been observed in the animal's behavior. However, the following general effects have been observed following ablation of certain specific areas.

Ablation of the Anterior Portion of the Cingulate Gyri. Bilateral removal of the anterior portion of cingulate gyri causes increased tameness of an animal to the extent that he no longer has fear of a man even though this fear might have existed preoperatively. Furthermore, previous rage reactions are suppressed, and the animal seems to lack "social consciousness."

Ablation of the Posterior Orbital Cortex. Bilateral removal of the posterior portion of the fronto-orbital cortex often causes an animal to develop insomnia and an intense degree of motor restlessness, becoming unable to sit still, but instead moving continually.

Ablation of the Anterior Temporal Region–The Klüver-Bucy Syndrome. When the anterior temporal cortex is removed, many important subcortical structures are also frequently damaged or removed, including especially the amygdala. Therefore, it is doubtful that what has been learned from anterior temporal ablation is of particular value in determining the function of the temporal limbic *cortex.* However, removal of the entire anterior tip of the temporal lobe in the dominant hemisphere of a monkey, and sometimes in man, causes intense changes in behavior, including (1) excessive tendency to examine objects, (2) loss of fear, (3) decreased aggressiveness, (4) tameness, (5) changes in dietary habits such that a herbivorous animal sometimes even becomes carnivorous, and (6) sometimes psychic blindness. This combination of effects is called the Klüver-Bucy syndrome.

In cats, opposite effects are sometimes observed, such as extreme savagery and rage. Yet, in other cats, removal of the anterior temporal poles causes extreme docility. Since different experimenters remove or damage different amounts of tissue in their experiments, these results show primarily that the anterior temporal poles, including the sublying amygdala, can have diverse effects on behavior, depending on the precise areas destroyed. This is to be expected because of the great diversity of effects that can be caused by stimulation of different areas of the amygdala and other closely associated regions.

Overall Function of the Hippocampal Gyrus, Cingulate Gyrus, and Orbitofrontal Cortex. After the above discussion, we find ourselves immediately perplexed regarding the function of the cortical regions of the limbic system. The reason for this probably is that these regions are actually association areas that correlate information from many sources but cause no direct, overt effects that can be observed objectively. Thus, in the insular and anterior temporal cortex we find gustatory and olfactory associations in particular. In the hippocampal gyrus, there is a tendency for complex auditory associations. In the cingulate cortex, there is some reason to believe that sensorimotor associations occur. And, finally, the orbitofrontal cortex presumably aids in the analytical functions of the prefrontal lobes.

Therefore, until further information is available, it is perhaps best to state that the cortical regions of the limbic system occupy intermediate associative positions between the functions of the remainder of the cerebral cortex and the functions of the lower centers for control of behavioral patterns.

REFERENCES

Clemente, C. D., and Chase, M. H.: Neurological substrates of aggressive behavior. Ann. Rev. Physiol., 35:329, 1973.

Cooper, J. B., Bloom, F. E., and Roth, R. H.: The Biochemical Basis of Neuropharmacology, 2nd Ed. New York, Oxford University Press, 1974.

Davidson, J. M., and Levine, S.: Endocrine regulation of behavior. Ann. Rev. Physiol., 34:375, 1972.

Defeudis, F. V.: Central Cholinergic Systems and Behavior. New York, Academic Press, Inc., 1974.

DiCara, L. (ed.): Limbic and Autonomic Nervous Systems Research. New York, Plenum Publishing Corporation, 1975.

Estes, W. K.: Reinforcement in human behavior. Amer. Sci., 60:723, 1972.

Frohman, L. A.: The hypothalamus and metabolic control. Pathobiol. Ann., 1:353, 1971.

Gazzaniga, M. S., and Blakemore, C.: Handbook of Psychobiology. New York, Academic Press, Inc, 1975.

Grenell, R. G., and Gabay, S. (eds.): Biological Foundations of Psychiatry. New York, Raven Press, 1975.

Gunderson, E. K. E., and Rahe, R. H. (eds.): Life Stress and Illness. Springfield, Ill., Charles C Thomas, Publisher, 1974.

Herd, J. A.: Physiology of strong emotions. Physiologist, 15:5, 1972.

Hollister, L. E.: Clinical Use of Psychotherapeutic Drugs. Springfield, Ill., Charles C Thomas, Publisher, 1974.

Hyvarinen, J.: CNS: afferent mechanism with emphasis on physiological and behavioral correlations. Ann. Rev. Physiol., 35:243, 1973.

Isaacson, R. L.: The Limbic System. New York, Plenum Publishing Corporation, 1974.

Kiev, A. (ed.): Somatic Manifestations of Depressive Disorders. New York, American Elsevier Publishing Co., Inc., 1975.

Lester, D.: A Physiological Basis for Personality Traits. Springfield, Ill., Charles C Thomas, Publisher, 1974.

Levi, L. (ed.): Emotions: Their Parameters and Measurement. New York, Raven Press, 1975.

Levine, S.: Stress and behavior. Sci. Amer., 224:26, 1971.

Luborsky, L.: New directions in research on neurotic and psychosomatic symptoms. Amer. Sci., 58:661, 1970.

Mandell, A. J. (ed.): Neurobiological Mechanisms of Adaptation and Behavior. (Advances in Biochemical Psychopharmacology. Vol. 13.) New York, Raven Press, 1975.

Millon, T.: Medical Behavioral Science. Philadelphia, W. B. Saunders Company, 1975.

Olds, J.: Hypothalamic substrates of reward. Physiol. Rev., 42:554, 1962.

Rolls, E. T.: The Brain and Reward. Oxford, Pergamon Press, 1975.

Sabelli, H. C. (ed.): Chemical Modulation of Brain Function. New York, Raven Press, 1973.

Schally, A. V., Kastin, A. J., and Arimura, A.: The hypothalamus and reproduction. Amer. J. Obstet. Gynecol., 114:423, 1972.

Smythies, J. R.: Brain Mechanisms and Behavior. New York, Academic Press, Inc., 1970.

Stearns, F. R.: Anger: Psychology, Physiology, Pathology. Springfield, Ill., Charles C Thomas, Publisher, 1972.

Strumwasser, F.: Neural and humoral factors in the temporal organization of behavior. Physiologist, 16:9, 1973.

Thomas, A., Chess, S., and Birch, H. G.: The origin of personality. Sci. Amer., 223:102, 1970.

Usdin, E. (ed.): Neuropsychopharmacology of Monoamines and Their Regulatory Enzymes. New York, Raven Press, 1975.

Wayner, M. J.: Specificity of behavioral regulation. Physiol. Behav., 12:851, 1974.

Weil, J. L.: A Neurophysiological Model of Emotional and Intentional Behavior. Springfield, Ill., Charles C Thomas, Publisher, 1974.

Widroe, H. J. (ed.): Human Behavior and Brain Function. Springfield, Ill., Charles C Thomas, Publisher, 1975.

Winter, A. (ed.): The Surgical Control of Behavior. Springfield, Ill., Charles C Thomas, Publisher, 1971.

Zimmermann, E., and George, R. (eds.): Narcotics and the Hypothalamus. (Kroc Foundation Series. Vol. 2.) New York, Raven Press, 1974.

15

The Autonomic Nervous System; The Adrenal Medulla

The portion of the nervous system that controls the visceral functions of the body is called the *autonomic nervous system*. This system helps to control arterial pressure, gastrointestinal motility and secretion, urinary output, sweating, body temperature, and many other activities, some of which are controlled almost entirely by the autonomic nervous system and some only partially.

GENERAL ORGANIZATION OF THE AUTONOMIC NERVOUS SYSTEM

The autonomic nervous system is activated mainly by centers located in the *spinal cord, brain stem,* and *hypothalamus.* Also, portions of the cerebral cortex can transmit impulses to the lower centers and in this way influence autonomic control. Often the autonomic nervous system operates by means of *visceral reflexes.* That is, sensory signals from parts of the body send impulses into the centers of the cord, brain stem, or hypothalamus, and these in turn transmit appropriate reflex responses back to the visceral organs to control their activities.

The autonomic impulses are transmitted to the body through two major subdivisions called the *sympathetic* and *parasympathetic systems,* the characteristics and functions of which follow.

PHYSIOLOGIC ANATOMY OF THE SYMPATHETIC NERVOUS SYSTEM

Figure 15–1 illustrates the general organization of the sympathetic nervous system, showing one of the two *sympathetic chains* to the side of the spinal column and nerves extending to the different internal organs. The sympathetic nerves originate in the spinal cord between the segments T-1 and L-2. They begin in the *sympathetic motoneurons* of the *intermediolateral horns* of the spinal gray matter.

Preganglionic and Postganglionic Sympathetic Neurons. The sympathetic nerves are different from skeletal motor nerves in the following way: Each motor pathway to a skeletal muscle is comprised of a single fiber originating in the cord. Each sympathetic pathway is comprised of a *preganglionic neuron* and a *postganglionic neuron.* The cell body of the preganglionic neuron lies in the intermediolateral horn of the spinal cord, and its fiber passes, as illustrated in Figure 15–2, through an *anterior root* of the cord into a *spinal nerve.* From here, the preganglionic fiber leaves the spinal nerve immediately and passes through the *white ramus* to a *ganglion* of the *sympathetic chain.* Here the fiber either synapses immediately with postganglionic neurons or often passes on through the chain into one of its radiating nerves to synapse with postganglionic neurons in an outlying sympathetic ganglion. The fiber of each postganglionic neuron than travels to its destination in one of the organs.

Sympathetic Nerve Fibers in the Skeletal Nerves. Many of the fibers from the postganglionic neurons in the sympathetic chain pass back into the spinal nerves through *gray rami* (see Fig. 15–2) at all levels of the cord. These pathways are made up of type C fibers that extend to all parts of the body in the skeletal nerves. They control the blood vessels, sweat glands, and pilo-erector muscles of the hairs. Approximately 8 per cent of the fibers in the average skeletal nerve are sympathetic fibers, a fact that indicates their importance.

Segmental Distribution of Sympathetic Nerves. The sympathetic pathways originating in the different segments of the spinal cord are not necessarily distributed to the same part of the body as the spinal nerve fibers from the same segments. Instead, the

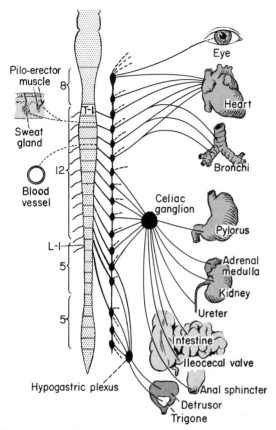

Figure 15–1. The sympathetic nervous system. Dashed lines represent postganglionic fibers in the gray rami leading into the spinal nerves for distribution to blood vessels, sweat glands, and pilo-erector muscles.

that secrete epinephrine and norepinephrine. These secretory cells are embryologically derived from nervous tissue and are analogous to postganglionic neurons; indeed, they even have rudimentary nerve fibers.

PHYSIOLOGIC ANATOMY OF THE PARASYMPATHETIC NERVOUS SYSTEM

The parasympathetic nervous system is illustrated in Figure 15–3, showing that parasympathetic fibers leave the central nervous system through several of the cranial nerves, the second and third sacral spinal nerves, and occasionally the first and fourth sacral nerves. About 75 per cent of all parasympathetic nerve fibers are in the vagus nerves, passing to the entire thoracic and abdominal regions of the body. However, the vagus nerve is not entirely parasympathetic in function because it also carries some voluntary skeletal nerve fibers from the nucleus ambiguous to the laryngeal and pharyngeal muscles and some afferent nerve fibers from the baroreceptors of the arteries and from stretch receptors of the lungs to the medulla. Nevertheless, when a physiologist speaks of the parasympathetic nervous system, in the back of his mind he thinks mainly of the two vagus nerves. The vagus nerves supply parasympathetic nerves to the heart, the lungs, the esophagus, the stomach, the small intestine, the proximal half of the colon, the liver, the gallbladder, the pancreas, and the upper portions of the ureters.

Parasympathetic fibers in the *third nerve* flow to the pupillary sphincters and ciliary muscles of the eye. Fibers from the *seventh nerve* pass to the lacrimal, nasal, and submaxillary glands, and fibers from the *ninth nerve* pass to the parotid gland.

sympathetic fibers from T-1 generally pass up the sympathetic chain into the head; from T-2 into the neck; T-3, T-4, T-5, and T-6 into the thorax; T-7, T-8, T-9, T-10, and T-11 into the abdomen; T-12, L-1, and L-2 into the legs. This distribution is only approximate and overlaps greatly.

The distribution of sympathetic nerves to each organ is determined partly by the position in the embryo at which the organ originates. For instance, the heart receives many sympathetic nerves from the neck portion of the sympathetic chain because the heart originates in the neck of the embryo. Likewise, the abdominal organs receive their sympathetic innervation from the lower thoracic segments because the primitive gut originates in the lower thoracic area.

Special Nature of the Sympathetic Nerve Endings in the Adrenal Medullae. Preganglionic sympathetic nerve fibers pass, without synapsing, all the way from the intermediolateral horn cells of the spinal cord, through the sympathetic chains, through the splanchnic nerves, and finally into the adrenal medullae. There they end directly on special cells

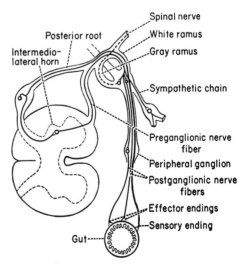

Figure 15–2. Nerve connections between the spinal cord, sympathetic chain, spinal nerves, and peripheral sympathetic nerves.

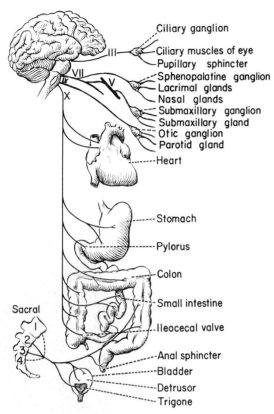

Figure 15–3. The parasympathetic nervous system.

The sacral parasympathetic fibers congregate in the form of the *nervi erigentes,* which leave the sacral plexus on each side of the cord and distribute their peripheral fibers to the descending colon, rectum, bladder and lower portions of the ureters. Also, this sacral group of parasympathetics supplies fibers to the external genitalia to cause various sexual reactions.

Preganglionic and Postganglionic Parasympathetic Neurons. The parasympathetic system, like the sympathetic, has both preganglionic and postganglionic neurons, but, except in the case of a few cranial parasympathetic nerves, the preganglionic fibers pass uninterrupted to the organ that is to be excited by parasympathetic impulses. In the wall of the organ are located the *postganglionic neurons* of the parasympathetic system. The preganglionic fibers synapse with these; and then short postganglionic fibers, 1 millimeter to several centimeters in length, leave the neurons to spread in the substance of the organ. This location of the parasympathetic postganglionic neurons in the visceral organ itself is quite different from the arrangement of the sympathetic ganglia, for the cell bodies of the sympathetic postganglionic neurons are always located in ganglia of the sympathetic chain or in various other discrete ganglia in the abdomen or thorax rather than in the excited organ itself.

BASIC CHARACTERISTICS OF SYMPATHETIC AND PARASYMPATHETIC FUNCTION

CHOLINERGIC AND ADRENERGIC FIBERS—SECRETION OF ACETYLCHOLINE OR NOREPINEPHRINE BY THE POSTGANGLIONIC NEURONS

It will be recalled from Chapter 3 that skeletal nerve endings secrete acetylcholine. This is also true of the *preganglionic neurons* of both the sympathetic and parasympathetic system, and it is true, too, of the *parasympathetic postganglionic neurons*. Therefore, all these fibers are said to be *cholinergic because they secrete acetylcholine at their nerve endings.*

A few of the postganglionic endings of the sympathetic nervous system also secrete acetylcholine, and these fibers, too, are cholinergic; but by far the majority of the sympathetic postganglionic endings secrete *norepinephrine*. These fibers are said to be *adrenergic,* a term derived from *noradrenalin,* which is the English name for norepinephrine. Thus, there is a basic functional difference between the respective postganglionic neurons of the parasympathetic and sympathetic systems, one secreting acetylcholine and the other principally norepinephrine. The chemical structures of these substances are the following:

$$CH_3-\underset{\underset{O}{\|}}{C}-O-CH_2-CH_2-\overset{+}{\underset{\underset{CH_3}{|}}{N}}\overset{CH_3}{\underset{CH_3}{}}$$

Acetylcholine

Norepinephrine

The acetylcholine and norepinephrine secreted by the postganglionic neurons act on the different organs to cause the respective parasympathetic or sympathetic effects. Therefore, these substances are called *parasympathetic* and *sympathetic mediators,* respectively, or sometimes *cholinergic* and *adrenergic* mediators.

Mechanism of Secretion of Acetylcholine and Norepinephrine by Autonomic Nerve Endings. Secretion of the transmitter substances acetylcholine and norepinephrine by autonomic nerve endings occurs in the same way as secretion at other synapses, as described previously for the central nervous system in Chapter 4 and for the neuromuscular junction in Chapter 3. Briefly, the nerve endings of both the sympathetic and parasympathetic systems contain large numbers of small transmitter vesicles about 300 to 600 Ångstroms in diameter. The vesicles in the cholinergic nerve endings contain acetylcholine and in electronmicrographs have a clear appearance. The vesicles in the adrenergic nerve endings contain norepinephrine and are granular in appearance.

Some of the autonomic nerve endings are similar to but much smaller in size than those of the skeletal muscle neuromuscular junction; this is especially true of the endings on some types of smooth muscle cells, as was explained in Chapter 3. However, most of the terminal filaments merely touch the effector cells of the organs that they innervate as they pass by; in some instances they terminate in connective tissue located adjacent to the cells that are to be stimulated. Where these filaments pass over the effector cells, they usually have bulbous enlargements called *varicosities,* and it is in these varicosities that the transmitter vesicles of acetylcholine and norepinephrine are found. Also in the varicosities are large numbers of mitochondria to supply the ATP required to energize acetylcholine and norepinephrine synthesis.

When an action potential spreads over the terminal fibers, the depolarization process increases the permeability of the fiber membrane to calcium ions, thus allowing these to diffuse in moderate numbers into the nerve terminals. There they interact with the vesicles adjacent to the membrane, causing them in some way not yet understood to fuse with the nerve membrane and to empty their contents to the exterior. Thus, the transmitter substance is secreted.

Synthesis of Acetylcholine, its Destruction After Secretion, and Duration of Action. Acetylcholine is continually synthesized in the terminal endings of cholinergic nerve fibers. Most of this synthesis probably occurs in the axoplasm and the acetylcholine is then transported to the interior of the vesicles, though it is possible that some of it is also synthesized in the vesicles themselves. The basic chemical reaction of this synthesis is the following:

$$\text{Acetyl-CoA} + \text{Choline} \xrightarrow[\text{acetylase}]{\text{choline}} \text{Acetylcholine}$$

Once the acetylcholine has been secreted by the cholinergic nerve ending, most of it is split into acetate ion and choline by the enzyme *cholinesterase* that is present both in the terminal nerve ending itself and on the surface of the receptor organ. Thus, this is the same mechanism of acetylcholine destruction as

occurs at the neuromuscular junctions of skeletal nerve fibers. The choline that is formed is in turn transported back into the terminal nerve ending where it is used again for synthesis of new acetylcholine. Though most of the acetylcholine is usually destroyed within a fraction of a second after its secretion, it sometimes persists for as long as several seconds, and a small amount also diffuses into the surrounding fluids. These fluids contain a different type of cholinesterase called *serum cholinesterase* that destroys the remaining acetylcholine within another few seconds. Therefore, the action of acetylcholine released by cholinergic nerve fibers usually lasts for a few seconds at most and more often for only a fraction of a second.

Synthesis of Norepinephrine, Its Removal, and Duration of Action. Synthesis of norepinephrine begins in the axoplasm of the terminal nerve endings of adrenergic nerve fibers but is completed inside the vesicles. The basic steps are the following:

1. Tyrosine $\xrightarrow{\text{hydroxylation}}$ DOPA

2. DOPA $\xrightarrow{\text{decarboxylation}}$ Dopamine

3. Transport of dopamine into the vesicles

4. Dopamine $\xrightarrow{\text{hydroxylation}}$ Norepinephrine

In the adrenal medulla this reaction goes still one step further to form epinephrine as follows:

5. Norepinephrine $\xrightarrow{\text{methylation}}$ Epinephrine

Following secretion of norepinephrine by the terminal nerve endings, it is removed from the secretory site in three different ways: (1) re-uptake into the adrenergic nerve endings themselves by an active transport process—accounting for removal of 50 to 80 per cent of the secreted norepinephrine; (2) diffusion away from the nerve endings into the surrounding body fluids and thence into the blood—accounting for removal of most of the remainder of the norepinephrine; and (3) destruction by enzymes to a slight extent (one of these enzymes is *monamine oxidase,* which is found in the nerve endings themselves, and another is *catechol-O-methyl transferase,* which is present diffusely in all tissues).

Ordinarily, the norepinephrine secreted directly in a tissue by adrenergic nerve endings remains active for only a few seconds, illustrating that its re-uptake and diffusion away from the tissue is rapid. However, the norepinephrine and epinephrine secreted into the blood by the adrenal medullae remain active until they diffuse into some tissue where they are destroyed by catechol-O-methyl transferase; this occurs mainly in the liver. Therefore, when secreted into the blood, both norepinephrine and epinephrine remain very active for 10 to 30 seconds, followed by decreasing activity thereafter for one to several minutes.

RECEPTOR SUBSTANCES OF THE EFFECTOR ORGANS

The acetylcholine, norepinephrine, and epinephrine secreted by the autonomic nervous system all stimulate the effector organs by first reacting with receptor substances in the effector cells. The receptor is believed in most instances to be in the cell membrane and is probably a protein or a lipoprotein. The most likely mechanism for function of the receptor is that the transmitter substance first binds with the receptor and this causes a basic change in the molecular structure of the receptor compound. Because the receptor is an integral part of the cell membrane, this structural change often alters the permeability of the cell membrane to various ions—for instance, to allow rapid influx of sodium, chloride, or calcium ions into the cell or to allow rapid efflux of potassium ions out of the cell. These ionic changes then usually alter the membrane potential, sometimes eliciting action potentials (as occurs in smooth muscle cells) and at other times causing electrotonic effects on the cells (as occurs on glandular cells) to produce the responses. The ions themselves have direct effects on the receptor cells, such as the effect of calcium ions to promote smooth muscle contraction.

Another way that the receptor can function, besides changing the membrane permeability, is to activate an enzyme in the cell membrane—this enzyme in turn promoting chemical reactions within the cell. For instance, epinephrine increases the activity of *adenyl cyclase* in some cell membranes, and this effect causes the formation of cyclic AMP inside the cell; the cyclic AMP then initiates many intracellular activities.

The Acetylcholine Receptors—"Muscarinic" and "Nicotinic" Receptors. Acetylcholine activates at least two different types of receptors. These are called *muscarinic* and *nicotinic* receptors. The reason for these names is that muscarine, a poison from toadstools, also activates the muscarinic receptors but will not activate the nicotinic receptors, whereas nicotine will activate the other receptors; finally, acetylcholine activates both of them.

The muscarinic receptors are found in all the effector cells stimulated by the postganglionic neurons of the parasympathetic nervous system as well as those stimulated by the cholinergic nerve endings of the sympathetic system.

The nicotinic receptors are found in the membranes of sympathetic and parasympathetic postganglionic neurons and in the membranes of skeletal muscle fibers at the neuromuscular junction (discussed in Chapter 3).

An understanding of the two different types of receptors is especially important because specific drugs are frequently used in the practice of medicine to stimulate or to block one or the other of the two types of receptors.

The Adrenergic Receptors—"Alpha" and "Beta" Receptors. Research experiments using different drugs (called *sympathomimetic drugs*) to mimic the action of norepinephrine on sympathetic effector organs have shown that there are at least two—and perhaps more—different types of adrenergic receptors. At present these are generally classified as *alpha receptors* and *beta receptors*. Norepinephrine and epinephrine, both of which are secreted by the adrenal medulla, have somewhat different effects in exciting these two receptors. Norepinephrine excites mainly alpha receptors but excites the beta receptors to a slight extent as well. On the other hand, epinephrine excites both types of receptors approximately equally. Therefore, the relative effects of norepinephrine and epinephrine on different effector organs is determined by the types of receptors in the organs. Obviously, if they are all beta receptors, epinephrine will be the more effective excitant.

Table 15–1 gives the distribution of alpha and beta receptors in some of the organs and systems controlled by the sympathetics. Note that certain alpha functions are excitatory while others are inhibitory. Likewise, certain beta functions are excitatory and others are inhibitory. Therefore, alpha and beta receptors are not necessarily associated with excitation or inhibition but simply with the affinity of the hormone for the receptors in a given effector organ.

A synthetic hormone closely similar to epi-

Table 15–1. Relationships of Adrenergic Receptors to Function

Alpha Receptor	Beta Receptor
Vasoconstriction	Vasodilatation
Iris dilatation	Cardioacceleration
Intestinal relaxation	Increased myocardial strength
Pilomotor contraction	Myometrial relaxation
	Intestinal relaxation
	Uterus relaxation
	Bronchodilatation
	Calorigenesis
	Muscle glycogenolysis
	Lipolysis

nephrine and norepinephrine, *isopropyl norepinephrine,* has an extremely strong action on beta receptors but almost no action on alpha receptors. Later in the chapter we will discuss various drugs that can mimic the adrenergic actions of epinephrine and norepinephrine or that will block specifically the alpha or beta receptors.

EXCITATORY AND INHIBITORY ACTIONS OF SYMPATHETIC AND PARASYMPATHETIC STIMULATION

Table 15–2 gives the effect on different visceral functions of the body caused by stimulating the parasympathetic and sympathetic nerves. From this table it can be seen that *sympathetic stimulation causes excitatory effects in some organs but inhibitory effects in others. Likewise, parasympathetic stimulation causes excitation in some organs but inhibition in others.* Also, when sympathetic stimulation excites a particular organ, parasympathetic stimulation often inhibits it, illustrating that the two systems occasionally act reciprocally to each other. However, most organs are dominantly controlled by one or the other of the two systems, so that, except in a few instances, the two systems do not actively oppose each other.

There is no generalization one can use to explain whether sympathetic or parasympathetic stimulation will cause excitation or inhibition of a particular organ. Therefore, to understand sympathetic and parasympathetic function, one must learn the functions of these two nervous systems as listed in Table 15–2. Some of these

TABLE 15–2.   **Autonomic Effects on Various Organs of the Body**

Organ	*Effect of Sympathetic Stimulation*	*Effect of Parasympathetic Stimulation*
Eye: Pupil	Dilated	Contracted
Ciliary muscle	None	Excited
Glands: Nasal	Vasoconstriction	Stimulation of thin, copious
Lacrimal		secretion containing many enzymes
Parotid		
Submaxillary		
Gastric		
Pancreatic		
Sweat glands	Copious sweating (cholinergic)	None
Apocrine glands	Thick, odoriferous secretion	None
Heart: Muscle	Increased rate	Slowed rate
	Increased force of contraction	Decreased force of atrial contraction
Coronaries	Vasodilated	Constricted
Lungs: Bronchi	Dilated	Constricted
Blood vessels	Mildly constricted	None
Gut: Lumen	Decreased peristalsis and tone	Increased peristalsis and tone
Sphincter	Increased tone	Decreased tone
Liver	Glucose released	None
Gallbladder and bile ducts	Inhibited	Excited
Kidney	Decreased output	None
Ureter	Inhibited	Excited
Bladder: Detrusor	Inhibited	Excited
Trigone	Excited	Inhibited
Penis	Ejaculation	Erection
Systemic blood vessels:		
Abdominal	Constricted	None
Muscle	Constricted (adrenergic)	None
	Dilated (cholinergic)	
Skin	Constricted (adrenergic)	Dilated
	Dilated (cholinergic)	
Blood: Coagulation	Increased	None
Glucose	Increased	None
Basal metabolism	Increased up to 100%	None
Adrenal cortical secretion	Increased	None
Mental activity	Increased	None
Piloerector muscles	Excited	None
Skeletal muscle	Increased glycogenolysis	None
	Increased strength	

functions need to be clarified in still greater detail as follows:

EFFECTS OF SYMPATHETIC AND PARASYMPATHETIC STIMULATION ON SPECIFIC ORGANS

The Eye. Two functions of the eye are controlled by the autonomic nervous system: These are the pupillary opening and the focus of the lens. Sympathetic stimulation contracts the meridional *fibers of the iris* and, therefore, dilates the pupil, whereas parasympathetic stimulation contracts the *circular muscle of the iris* to constrict the pupil. The parasympathetics that control the pupil are reflexly stimulated when excess light enters the eyes; this reflex reduces the pupillary opening and decreases the amount of light that strikes the retina. On the other hand, the sympathetics become stimulated during periods of excitement and, therefore, increase the pupillary opening at these times.

Focusing of the lens is controlled entirely by the parasympathetic nervous system. The lens is normally held in a flattened state by tension of its radial ligaments. Parasympathetic excitation contracts the *ciliary muscle,* which releases this tension and allows the lens to become more convex. This causes the eye to focus on objects near at hand. The focusing mechanism is discussed in Chapters 16 and 18 in relation to function of the eyes.

The Glands of the Body. The *nasal, lacrimal, salivary,* and many *gastrointestinal glands* are all strongly stimulated by the parasympathetic nervous system, resulting in copious quantities of secretion. The glands of the alimentary tract most strongly stimulated by the parasympathetics are those of the upper tract, especially those of the mouth and stomach. The glands of the small and large intestines are controlled principally by local factors in the intestinal tract itself and not by the autonomic nerves.

Sympathetic stimulation has a slight direct effect on glandular cells in causing formation of a concentrated secretion. However, it also causes vasoconstriction of the blood vessels supplying the glands and in this way often reduces their rates of secretion.

The *sweat glands* secrete large quantities of sweat when the sympathetic nerves are stimulated, but no effect is caused by stimulating the parasympathetic nerves. However, the sympathetic fibers to most sweat glands are *cholinergic,* in contrast to most other sympathetic fibers, which are adrenergic. Furthermore, the sweat glands are stimulated primarily by centers in the hypothalamus that are usually considered to be parasympathetic centers. Therefore, sweating could be called a parasympathetic function.

The *apocrine glands* secrete a thick, odoriferous secretion as a result of sympathetic stimulation, but they do not react to parasympathetic stimulation. Furthermore, the apocrine glands, despite their close embryological relationship to sweat glands, are controlled by adrenergic fibers rather than by cholinergic fibers and are controlled by the sympathetic centers of the central nervous system rather than by the parasympathetic centers.

The Gastrointestinal System. The gastrointestinal system has its own intrinsic set of nerves known as the *intramural plexus.* However, both parasympathetic and sympathetic stimulation can affect gastrointestinal activity—parasympathetic especially. Parasympathetic stimulation, in general, increases the overall degree of activity of the gastrointestinal tract by promoting peristalsis, thus allowing rapid propulsion of contents along the tract. This propulsive effect is associated with simultaneous increases in rates of secretion by many of the gastrointestinal glands, which was described above.

Normal function of the gastrointestinal tract is not very dependent on sympathetic stimulation. However, in some diseases, strong sympathetic stimulation inhibits peristalsis and increases the tone of the sphincters. The net result is greatly slowed propulsion of food through the tract.

The Heart. In general, sympathetic stimulation increases the overall activity of the heart. This is accomplished by increasing both the rate and force of the heartbeat. Parasympathetic stimulation causes mainly the opposite effects, decreasing the overall activity of the heart. To express these effects in another way, sympathetic stimulation increases the effectiveness of the heart as a pump, whereas parasympathetic stimulation decreases its effectiveness. However, sympathetic stimulation unfortunately also greatly increases the metabolism of the heart while parasympathetic stimulation decreases its metabolism and allows the heart a certain degree of rest.

Systemic Blood Vessels. Most blood vessels, especially those of the abdominal viscera and the skin of the limbs, are constricted by sympathetic stimulation. Parasympathetic stimulation generally has almost no effects on blood vessels but does dilate vessels in certain restricted areas such as in the blush area of the face.

Effect of Sympathetic and Parasympathetic Stimulation on Arterial Pressure. The arterial pressure in the circulatory system is caused by propulsion of blood by the heart and by resistance to flow of this blood through the vascular system. In general, sympathetic stimulation increases both propulsion by the heart and resistance to flow, which can cause the pressure to increase greatly.

On the other hand, parasympathetic stimulation decreases the pumping effectiveness of the heart, which lowers the pressure a moderate amount, though not nearly so much as the sympathetics can increase the pressure.

The Lungs. In general, the structures in the lungs do not have extensive sympathetic or parasympathetic innervation. Therefore, all effects of stimulation are mild. Sympathetic stimulation can mildly dilate the bronchi and mildly constrict the blood vessels. On the contrary, parasympathetic stimulation can cause mild constriction of the bronchi and can perhaps mildly dilate the vessels.

Effects of Sympathetic and Parasympathetic Stimulation on Other Functions of the Body. Because of the great importance of the sympathetic and parasympathetic control systems, these are discussed many times in this text in relation to a myriad of body functions that are not considered in detail here. In general, most of the entodermal structures, such as the ducts of the liver, the gallbladder, the ureter, and the bladder, are inhibited by sympathetic stimulation but excited by parasympathetic stimulation. Sympathetic stimulation also has metabolic effects, causing release of glucose from the liver, increase in blood glucose concentration, increase in glycogenolysis in muscle, increase in muscle strength, increase in basal metabolic rate, and increase in mental activity. Finally, the sympathetics and parasympathetics are involved in regulating the male and female sexual acts, which are essential for fertilization of the ovum.

FUNCTION OF THE ADRENAL MEDULLAE

Stimulation of the sympathetic nerves to the adrenal medullae causes large quantities of epinephrine and norepinephrine to be released into the circulating blood, and these two hormones in turn are carried in the blood to all tissues of the body. On the average, approximately 80 per cent of the secretion is epinephrine and 20 per cent norepinephrine, though the relative proportions of these change considerably under different physiological conditions.

The circulating norepinephrine has almost the same effects on the different organs as those caused by direct sympathetic stimulation, except that *the effects last about 10 times as long* because norepinephrine is removed from the blood slowly. For instance, norepinephrine causes constriction of essentially all the blood vessels of the body; it causes increased activity of the heart, inhibition of the gastrointestinal tract, dilation of the pupil of the eye, and so forth.

Epinephrine, also, causes almost the same effects as those caused by norepinephrine, but the effects differ in the following respects: First, epinephrine has a greater effect on cardiac activity than norepinephrine. Second, epinephrine causes only weak constriction of the blood vessels of the muscles in comparison with a much stronger constriction that results from norepinephrine. Since the muscle vessels represent a major segment of all vessels of the body, this difference is of special importance because

norepinephrine greatly increases the total peripheral resistance and thereby greatly elevates arterial pressure, whereas epinephrine raises the arterial pressure to a less extent but increases the cardiac output considerably because of its effect on the heart and veins.

A third difference between the action of epinephrine and norepinephrine relates to their effects on tissue metabolism. Epinephrine probably has several times as great a metabolic effect as norepinephrine. Indeed, the epinephrine secreted by the adrenal medullae increases the metabolic rate of the body often to as much as 100 per cent above normal, in this way increasing the activity and excitability of the whole body. It also increases the rate of other metabolic activities, such as glycogenolysis in the liver and muscle and glucose release into the blood.

In summary, stimulation of the adrenal medullae causes the release of hormones that have almost the same effects throughout the body as direct sympathetic stimulation, except that the effects are greatly prolonged. The only significant differences are caused by the epinephrine in the secretion, which increases the rate of metabolism and cardiac output to a greater extent than is caused by direct sympathetic stimulation.

Value of the Adrenal Medullae to the Function of the Sympathetic Nervous System. Usually, when any part of the sympathetic nervous system is stimulated, the entire system, or at least major portions of it, is stimulated at the same time. Therefore, norepinephrine and epinephrine are almost always released by the adrenal medullae at the same time that the different organs are being stimulated directly by the sympathetic nerves. Therefore, the organs are actually stimulated in two different ways simultaneously, directly by the sympathetic nerves and indirectly by the medullary hormones. The two means of stimulation support each other, and either can usually substitute for the other. For instance, destruction of the direct sympathetic pathways to the organs does not abrogate excitation of the organs because norepinephrine and epinephrine are still released into the circulating fluids and indirectly cause stimulation. Likewise, total loss of the two adrenal medullae usually has little significant effect on the operation of the sympathetic nervous system because the direct pathways can still perform almost all the necessary duties. Thus, the dual mechanism of sympathetic stimulation provides a safety factor, one mechanism substituting for the other when the second is missing.

Another important value of the adrenal medullae is the capability of epinephrine and norepinephrine to stimulate structures of the body that are not innervated by direct sympathetic fibers. For instance, the metabolic rate of every cell of the body is increased by these hormones, especially by epinephrine, even though only a small proportion of all the cells in the body are innervated by sympathetic fibers.

RELATIONSHIP OF STIMULUS RATE TO DEGREE OF SYMPATHETIC AND PARASYMPATHETIC EFFECT

A special difference between the autonomic nervous system and the skeletal nervous system is the low frequency of stimulation required for full activation of autonomic effectors. In general, only one impulse every second or so suffices to maintain normal sympathetic or parasympathetic effect, and full activation occurs when the nerve fibers discharge 10 to 30 times per second. This compares with full activation in the skeletal nervous system at about 75 to 200 impulses per second.

SYMPATHETIC AND PARASYMPATHETIC "TONE"

The sympathetic and parasympathetic systems are continually active, and the basal rates of activity are known, respectively, as *sympathetic tone* or *parasympathetic tone.*

The value of tone is that it allows a single nervous system to increase or to decrease the activity of a stimulated organ. For instance, sympathetic tone normally keeps almost all the blood vessels of the body constricted to approximately half their maximum diameter. By increasing the degree of sympathetic stimulation, the vessels can be constricted even more; but, on the other hand, by inhibiting the normal tone, the vessels can be dilated. If it were not for the continual sympathetic tone, the sympathetic system could cause only vasoconstriction, never vasodilatation.

Another interesting example of tone is that of the parasympathetics in the gastrointestinal tract. Surgical removal of the parasympathetic supply to the gut by cutting the vagi can cause serious and prolonged gastric and intestinal "atony," thus illustrating that in normal function the parasympathetic tone to the gut is strong. This tone can be decreased by the brain, thereby inhibiting gastrointestinal motility, or, on the other hand, it can be increased, thereby promoting increased gastrointestinal activity.

Tone Caused by Basal Secretion of Norepinephrine and Epinephrine by the Adrenal Medullae. The normal resting rate of secretion by the adrenal medullae is about 0.2 μgm./kg./min. of epinephrine and about 0.05 μgm./kg./min. of norepinephrine. These quantities are considerable—indeed, enough to maintain the blood pressure almost up to the normal value even if all direct sympathetic pathways to the cardiovascular system are removed. Therefore, it is obvious that much of the overall tone of the sympathetic nervous system results from basal secretion of epinephrine and norepinephrine in addition to that which results from direct sympathetic stimulation.

Effect of Loss of Sympathetic or Parasympathetic Tone Following Denervation. Immediately after a sympathetic or parasympathetic nerve is cut, the innervated organ loses its sympathetic or parasympathetic tone. In the case of the blood vessels, for instance, cutting the sympathetic nerves results immediately in almost maximal vasodilatation. However, over several days or weeks, the *intrinsic tone* in the smooth muscle of the vessels increases, usually restoring almost normal vasoconstriction.

Essentially the same events occur in most effector organs whenever sympathetic or parasympathetic tone is lost. That is, intrinsic compensation soon develops to return the function of the organ almost to its normal basal level. However, in the parasympathetic system the compensation sometimes requires many months. For instance, loss of parasympathetic tone to the heart increases the heart rate from 90 to 160 beats per minute in a dog, and this will still be about 120 six months later.

DENERVATION SUPERSENSITIVITY OF SYMPATHETIC AND PARASYMPATHETIC ORGANS FOLLOWING DENERVATION

During the first week or so after a sympathetic or parasympathetic nerve is destroyed, the innervated organ becomes more and more sensitive to injected norepinephrine or acetylcholine, respectively. This effect is illustrated in Figure 15–4; the blood flow in the forearm before removal of the sympathetics was 200 ml. per minute, and a test dose of norepinephrine caused only a slight depression in flow. Then the stellate ganglion was removed, and normal sympathetic tone was lost. At first, the blood flow rose markedly

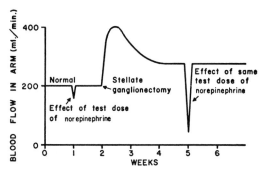

Figure 15–4. Effect of sympathectomy on blood flow in the arm, and the effect of a test dose of norepinephrine before and after sympathectomy, showing sensitization of the vasculature to norepinephrine.

because of the lost vascular tone, but over a period of days to weeks the blood flow returned almost to normal because of progressive increase in intrinsic tone of the vascular musculature itself, thus compensating for the loss of sympathetic tone. Another test dose of norepinephrine was then administered and the blood flow decreased much more than before, illustrating that the blood vessels had become about two to four times as responsive to norepinephrine as previously. This phenomenon is called *denervation supersensitivity.* It occurs in both sympathetic and parasympathetic organs and to a far greater extent in some organs than in others, often increasing the response as much as 10-fold.

Mechansim of Denervation Supersensitivity. The precise cause of denervation supersensitivity is not known, although several suggestions have been made. In the case of the sympathetic nervous system, it is supposed that destruction of the nerve endings prevents removal of norepinephrine or epinephrine by the process of re-uptake into the nerve endings. Likewise, the monamine oxidase that is found in the nerve endings is not available to help destroy the norepinephrine or epinephrine. Therefore, these two hormones can act strongly and for prolonged periods of time on the receptor organs.

In the case of acetylcholine supersensitivity, it is possible that loss of cholinesterase, particularly that which is attached to the nerve endings themselves, causes part of the supersensitivity. On the other hand, it is also possible that some functional system of the receptor cells themselves increases in activity when the cells are not continually bombarded by nerve stimuli.

THE AUTONOMIC REFLEXES

It is mainly by means of autonomic reflexes that the autonomic nervous system regulates visceral functions. Throughout this text the functions of these reflexes are discussed in detail in relation to individual organs, but, to illustrate their importance, a few are presented here briefly.

Cardiovascular Autonomic Reflexes. Several reflexes in the cardiovascular system help to control the arterial blood pressure, cardiac output, and heart rate. One of these is the *baroreceptor reflex,* which is one of the most important of the cardiovascular reflexes. Briefly, stretch receptors called *baroreceptors* are located in the walls of the major arteries, including the carotid arteries and the aorta. When these become stretched by high pressure, signals are transmitted to the brain stem, where they inhibit the sympathetic centers. This results in decreased sympathetic impulses to the heart and blood vessels, which allows the arterial pressure to fall back toward normal.

The Gastrointestinal Autonomic Reflexes. The uppermost part of the gastrointestinal tract and the rectum are controlled principally by autonomic reflexes. For instance, the smell of appetizing food initiates signals from the nose to the vagal, glossopharyngeal, and salivary nuclei of the brain stem. These in turn transmit signals through the parasympathetic nerves to the secretory glands of the mouth and stomach, causing secretion of digestive juices even before food enters the mouth. And when fecal matter fills the rectum at the other end of the alimentary canal, sensory impulses initiated by stretching the rectum are sent to the sacral portion of the spinal cord, and a reflex signal is retransmitted through the parasympathetics to the distal parts of the colon; these result in strong peristaltic contractions that empty the bowel.

Other Autonomic Reflexes. Emptying of the bladder is also controlled in the same way as emptying of the rectum; stretching the bladder sends impulses to the sacral cord, and this in turn causes contraction of the bladder as well as relaxation of the urinary sphincters, thereby promoting micturition.

Also important are the sexual reflexes which are initiated both by psychic stimuli from the brain and stimuli from the sexual organs. Impulses from these sources converge on the sacral cord and, in the male, result, first, in erection, mainly a parasympathetic function, and then in ejaculation, a sympathetic function.

Other autonomic reflexes include reflex contributions to the regulation of pancreatic secretion, gallbladder emptying, urinary excretion, sweating, blood glucose concentration, and many other visceral functions, all of which are essential to continued existence and well-being of the body.

MASS DISCHARGE OF THE SYMPATHETIC SYSTEM VERSUS DISCRETE CHARACTERISTICS OF PARASYMPATHETIC REFLEXES

In general, large portions of the sympathetic nervous system often become stimulated simultaneously, a phenomenon called *mass discharge*. This characteristic of sympathetic action is in keeping with the usually diffuse nature of sympathetic function, such as overall regulation of arterial pressure or of metabolic rate.

However, in a few instances sympathetic activity does occur in isolated portions of the system. The most important of these are: (1) In the process of heat regulation, the sympathetics control sweating and blood flow in the skin without affecting other organs innervated by the sympathetics. (2) During muscular activity in some animals, cholinergic vasodilator fibers of the skeletal muscles are stimulated independently of all the remainder of the sympathetic system. (3) Many "local reflexes" involving the spinal cord but not the higher nervous centers affect local areas. For instance, heating a local skin area causes local vasodilatation and enhanced local sweating, while cooling causes the opposite effects.

In contrast to the sympathetic system, most reflexes of the parasympathetic system are very specific. For instance, parasympathetic cardiovascular reflexes usually act only on the heart to increase or decrease its rate of beating. Likewise, parasympathetic reflexes frequently cause secretion only in the mouth or, in other instances, secretion only by the stomach glands. Finally, the rectal emptying reflex does not affect other parts of the bowel to a major extent.

Yet there is often association between closely allied parasympathetic functions. For instance, though salivary secretion can occur independently of gastric secretion, these two often also occur together, and pancreatic secretion frequently occurs at the same time. Also, the rectal emptying reflex often initiates a bladder emptying reflex, resulting in simultaneous emptying of both the bladder and rectum. Conversely, the bladder emptying reflex can help to initiate rectal emptying.

"ALARM" OR "STRESS" FUNCTION OF THE SYMPATHETIC NERVOUS SYSTEM

From the above discussions of the sympathetic nervous system, one can already see that mass sympathetic discharge increases in many ways the capability of the body to perform vigorous muscle activity. Let us quickly summarize these ways:

1. increased arterial pressure
2. increased blood flow to active muscles concurrent with decreased blood flow to organs that are not needed for rapid activity
3. increased rates of cellular metabolism throughout the body
4. increased blood glucose concentration
5. increased glycolysis in muscle
6. increased muscle strength
7. increased mental activity
8. increased rate of blood coagulation

The sum of these effects permits the person to perform far more strenuous physical activity than would otherwise be possible. Since it is physical *stress* that usually excites the sympathetic system, it is frequently said that the purpose of the sympathetic system is to provide extra activation of the body in states of stress: this is often called the sympathetic stress *reaction*.

The sympathetic system is also strongly activated in many emotional states. For instance, in the state of *rage*, which is elicited mainly by stimulating the hypothalamus, signals are transmitted downward through the reticular formation and spinal cord to cause massive sympathetic discharge, and all of the sympathetic events listed above ensue immediately. This is called the sympathetic *alarm reaction*. It is also frequently called the *fight or flight reaction* because an animal in this state decides almost instantly whether to stand and fight or to run. In either event, the sympathetic alarm reaction makes its subsequent activities extremely vigorous.

MEDULLARY, PONTINE, AND MESENCEPHALIC CONTROL OF THE AUTONOMIC NERVOUS SYSTEM

Many areas in the reticular substance of the medulla, pons, and mesencephalon, as well as many special nuclei, (see Fig. 15–5) control different autonomic functions such as arterial pressure, heart rate, glandular secretion in the upper part of the gastrointestinal tract, gastrointestinal peristalsis, the degree of contraction of the urinary bladder, and many others. The con-

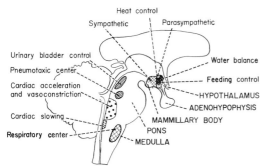

Figure 15–5. Autonomic control centers of the brain stem.

trol of each of these is discussed in detail at appropriate points in this text. Suffice it to point out here that the most important factors controlled in the lower brain stem are arterial pressure, heart rate, and respiration. Indeed, transection of the brain stem at the midpontile level allows normal basal control of arterial pressure to continue as before but prevents its modulation by higher nervous centers, particularly the hypothalamus. On the other hand, transection immediately below the medulla causes the arterial pressure to fall to about one-half normal. Closely associated with the cardiovascular regulatory centers in the medulla is the medullary center for regulation of respiration, a center that causes breathing. Though this is not considered to be an autonomic function, it is one of the *involuntary* functions of the body.

Control of Lower Brain Stem Autonomic Centers by Higher Areas. Signals from the hypothalamus and even from the cerebrum can affect the activities of almost all the lower brain stem autonomic control centers. For instance, stimulation in appropriate areas of the hypothalamus can activate the medullary cardiovascular control centers strongly enough to increase the arterial pressure to more than double normal. Likewise, higher centers can transmit signals into the lower centers to control body temperature, increase or decrease salivation and gastrointestinal activity, or to cause urinary bladder contraction. Therefore, to a great extent the autonomic centers in the lower brain stem are relay stations for control activities initiated at higher levels of the brain.

In the previous chapter it was also pointed out that many of the behavioral responses of an animal are mediated through the hypothalamus, reticular formation, and the autonomic nervous system. Indeed, the higher areas of the brain can alter the function of the whole autonomic nervous system or of portions of it strongly enough to cause severe autonomic-induced dis-

ease, such as peptic ulcer, constipation, heart palpitation, and even heart attacks.

PHARMACOLOGY OF THE AUTONOMIC NERVOUS SYSTEM

DRUGS THAT ACT ON ADRENERGIC EFFECTOR ORGANS—THE SYMPATHOMIMETIC DRUGS

From the foregoing discussion, it is obvious that intravenous injection of norepinephrine causes essentially the same effects throughout the body as sympathetic stimulation. Therefore, norepinephrine is called a *sympathomimetic*, or *adrenergic*, *drug*. Other sympathomimetic drugs include *epinephrine*, *phenylephrine*, *methoxamine*, and many others. These differ from each other in the degree to which they stimulate different sympathetic effector organs and in their duration of action. Norepinephrine and epinephrine have actions as short as one to three minutes, while the actions of most other commonly used sympathomimetic drugs last 30 minutes to 2 hours.

Drugs that Cause Release of Norepinephrine from Nerve Endings. Certain drugs have a sympathomimetic action in an indirect manner rather than by directly exciting adrenergic effector organs. These drugs include ephedrine, tyramine, and amphetamine. Their effect is to cause release of norepinephrine from its storage vesicles in the sympathetic nerve endings. The norepinephrine in turn causes the sympathetic effects.

Drugs that Block Adrenergic Activity. Adrenergic activity can be blocked at several different points in the stimulatory process as follows:

1. The synthesis and storage of norepinephrine in the sympathetic nerve endings can be prevented. The best known drug that causes this effect is *reserpine*.

2. Release of norepinephrine from the sympathetic endings can be blocked. This is caused by *guanethidine*.

3. The *alpha* receptors can be blocked. Two drugs that cause this effect are *phenoxybenzamine* and *phentolamine*.

4. The beta receptors can be blocked. A drug that does this is *propanolol*.

5. Sympathetic activity can be blocked by drugs that block transmission of nerve impulses through the autonomic ganglia. These are discussed in the following section, but the most important drug for blockade of both sympathetic and parasympathetic transmission through the ganglia is *hexamethonium*.

DRUGS THAT ACT ON CHOLINERGIC EFFECTOR ORGANS

Parasympathomimetic Drugs (Muscarinic Drugs). Acetylcholine injected intravenously usually does not cause exactly the same effects throughout the body as parasympathetic stimulation because the acetylcholine is destroyed by cholinesterase in the blood and body fluids before it can reach all the effector organs. Yet a number of other drugs that are not so rapidly destroyed can produce typical parasympathetic effects, and these are called parasympathomimetic drugs.

Three commonly used parasympathomimetic drugs are *pilocarpine, methacholine,* and *carbamylcholine.* Although these drugs have almost the same effects on the different effector organs as does parasympathetic stimulation, there are slight variations. For instance, carbamylcholine is especially active on the bladder and gastrointestinal tract, while methacholine is especially active on the cardiovascular system and eyes.

Parasympathomimetic drugs act on the effector organs of cholinergic *sympathetic* fibers also. For instance, these drugs cause profuse sweating. Also, they cause vascular dilatation, this effect occurring even in vessels not innervated by cholinergic fibers.

Drugs that Have a Parasympathetic Potentiating Effect. Some drugs do not have a direct effect on parasympathetic effector organs but do potentiate the effects of the naturally secreted acetylcholine at the parasympathetic endings. These are the same drugs as those listed in Chapter 3 that potentiate the effect of acetylcholine at the neuromuscular junction—that is, *neostigmine, physostigmine,* and *diisopropyl fluorophosphate.* These inhibit cholinesterase, thus preventing rapid destruction of the acetylcholine liberated by the parasympathetic nerve endings. As a consequence, the quantity of acetylcholine acting on the effector organs progressively increases with successive stimuli, and the degree of action also increases.

Drugs that Block Cholinergic Activity at Effector Organs. *Atropine* and similar drugs, such as *homatropine* and *scopolamine,* block the action of acetylcholine on cholinergic effector organs. However, these drugs do not affect the nicotinic action of acetylcholine on the postganglionic neurons or on skeletal muscle.

DRUGS THAT STIMULATE THE POSTGANGLIONIC NEURONS— "NICOTINIC DRUGS"

The preganglionic neurons of both the parasympathetic and sympathetic nervous systems secrete acetylcholine at their endings, and the acetylcholine in turn stimulates the postganglionic neurons. Therefore, injected acetylcholine can also stimulate the postganglionic neurons of both systems, thereby causing both sympathetic and parasympathetic effects in the body. *Nicotine* is a drug that can also stimulate postganglionic neurons in the same manner as acetylcholine because the neuronal membranes contain *nicotinic receptors,* but it cannot directly stimulate the autonomic effector organs, which have

muscarinic receptors as explained earlier in the chapter. Therefore, drugs that cause autonomic effects by stimulating the postganglionic neurons are frequently called nicotinic drugs. Some drugs, such as *acetylcholine* itself, *carbamylcholine* and *methacholine,* have both nicotinic and muscarinic actions, whereas pilocarpine has only muscarinic actions.

Nicotine excites both the sympathetic and parasympathetic systems at the same time, resulting in strong sympathetic vasoconstriction in the abdominal organs and limbs, but at the same time resulting in parasympathetic effects, such as increased gastrointestinal activity and, sometimes, slowing of the heart.

Ganglionic Blocking Drugs. Many important drugs block impulse transmission from the preganglionic neurons to the postganglionic neurons, including *tetraethyl ammonium ion, hexamethonium ion,* and *pentolinium.* These inhibit impulse transmission in both the sympathetic and parasympathetic systems simultaneously. They are often used for blocking sympathetic activity but rarely for blocking parasympathetic activity because the sympathetic blockade usually far overshadows the effects of parasympathetic blockade. The ganglionic blocking drugs have been especially important in reducing arterial pressure in patients with hypertension.

REFERENCES

Axelsson, J.: Catecholamine functions. *Ann. Rev. Physiol.,* 33:1, 1971.
Banks, P., and Mayor, D.: Intra-axonal transport in noradrenergic neurons in the sympathetic nervous system. *Biochem. Soc. Symp.,* 36:133, 1972.
Bennett, M. R.: Autonomic Neuromuscular Transmission. Physiological Society Monograph, 1972.
Bhagat, B. D.: Recent Advances in Adrenergic Mechanisms. Springfield, Ill., Charles C Thomas, Publisher, 1971.
Carrier, O., Jr.: Pharmacology of the Peripheral Autonomic Nervous System. Chicago, Year Book Medical Publishers, 1972.
Costa, E., and Sandler, M. (eds.): Monoamine Oxidases—New Vistas. (Advances in Biochemical Psychopharmacology. Vol. 5.) New York, Raven Press, 1972.
Dahlström, A.: Aminergic transmission. Introduction and short review. *Brain Res.,* 62:441, 1973.
De Potter, W. P., Chubb, I. W., and De Schaepdryver, A. F.: Pharmacological aspects of peripheral noradrenergic transmission. *Arch. Int. Pharmacodyn. Ther.,* 196(Suppl. 196):258, 1972.
DiCara, L. V.: Learning in the autonomic nervous system. *Sci. Amer.,* 222:30, 1970.
Fonnum, F.: Recent developments in biochemical investigations of cholinergic transmission. *Brain Res.,* 62:497, 1973.
Gebber, G. L., and Snyder, D. W.: Hypothalamic control of baroreceptor reflexes. *Amer. J. Physiol.,* 218:124, 1970.
Geffen, L. B., and Livett, B. G.: Synaptic vesicles in sympathetic neurons. *Physiol. Rev.,* 51:98, 1971.
Guyton, A. C., and Gillespie, W. M., Jr.: Constant infusion of epinephrine: rate of epinephrine secretion and destruction in the body. *Amer. J. Physiol.,* 165:319, 1951.
Guyton, A. C., and Reeder, R. C.: Quantitative studies on the autonomic actions of curare. *J. Pharmacol. Exp. Ther.,* 98:188, 1950.
Häggendal, J.: Some aspects of the release of the adrenergic transmitter. *J. Neural Transm.,* Suppl. 11:135, 1974.
Hess, W. R.: The Functional Organization of the Diencephalon. New York, Grune & Stratton, Inc., 1958.

Hingerty, D., and O'Boyle, A.: Clinical Chemistry of the Adrenal Medulla. Springfield, Ill., Charles C Thomas, Publisher, 1972.

Jenkinson, D. H.: Classification and properties of peripheral adrenergic receptors. *Brit. Med. Bull., 29*:142, 1973.

Joó, F.: On the problem of the origin of nerve terminals in the sympathetic ganglia. *J. Neural Transm., Suppl. 11*:285, 1974.

Koizumi, K., and Brooks, C. M.: The integration of autonomic system reactions: a discussion of autonomic reflexes, their control and their association with somatic reactions. *Ergeb. Physiol., 67*:1, 1972.

McGeer, P. L., and McGeer, E. G.: Neurotransmitter synthetic enzymes. *Prog. Neurobiol., 2*:69, 1973.

Molinoff, P. B., Nelson, D. L., and Orcutt, J. C.: Dopamine-beta-hydroxylase and the regulation of the noradrenergic neuron. *Adv. Biochem. Psychopharmacol., 12*:95, 1974.

Nickerson, M.: Adrenergic receptors. *Circ. Res., 32(Suppl. 1)*:53, 1973.

Paton, D. M. (ed.): The Mechanism of Neuronal and Extraneuronal Transport of Catecholamines. New York, Raven Press, 1975.

Réthelyi, M.: Spinal transmission of autonomic processes. *J. Neural. Transm., Suppl. 11*:195, 1974.

Robinson, G. A., and Sutherland, E. W.: On the relation of cyclic AMP to adrenergic receptors and sympathin. *Adv. Cytopharmacol., 1*:263, 1971.

Sato, A., and Schmidt, R. F.: Somatosympathetic reflexes: afferent fibers, central pathways, and discharge characteristics. *Physiol. Rev., 53*:916, 1973.

Silver, A.: The Biology of Cholinesterases. New York, American Elsevier Publishing Co., Inc., 1974.

Smith, A. D.: Cellular control of the uptake, storage, and release of noradrenaline in sympathetic nerves. *Biochem. Soc. Symp. 36*:103, 1972.

Steer, M. L., Atlas, D., and Levitzki, A.: Inter-relations between beta-adrenergic receptors, adenylate cyclase, and calcium. *New Engl. J. Med., 292*:409, 1975.

Taxi, J.: Dynamics of transmissional ultrastructures in sympathetic neurones on the rat. *J. Neural Transm., Suppl. 11*:103, 1974.

von Euler, U. S.: Noradrenaline. Springfield, Illinois, Charles C Thomas, Publisher, 1956.

Winkler, H., Schneider, F. H., Rufener, C., Nakane, P. K., and Hörtnagl, H.: Membranes of adrenal medulla: their role in exocytosis. *Adv. Cytopharmacol., 2*:127, 1974.

PART III
THE SPECIAL SENSES

16

The Eye:
I. Optics of Vision

PHYSICAL PRINCIPLES OF OPTICS

Before it is possible to understand the optical systems of the eye, the student must be thoroughly familiar with the basic physical principles of optics, including the physics of refraction, and have a knowledge of focusing, depth of focus, and so forth. Therefore, in the present study of the optics of the eye, a brief review of these physical principles is first presented, and then the optics of the eye are discussed.

REFRACTION OF LIGHT

The Refractive Index of a Transparent Substance. Light rays travel through a vacuum at a velocity of approximately 300,000 kilometers per second and practically as fast through air and other gaseous media but much slower through transparent solids and liquids. The refractive index of a transparent substance is the *ratio* of the velocity of light in air to that in the substance. Obviously, the refractive index of air itself is 1.00.

If light travels through a particular type of glass at a velocity of 200,000 kilometers per second, the refractive index of this glass is 300,000 divided by 200,000, or 1.50.

Refraction of Light Rays at an Interface Between Two Media with Different Refractive Indices. When light waves traveling forward in a beam, as shown in the upper part of Figure 16–1, strike an interface that is perpendicular to the beam, the waves enter the second refractive medium without deviating in their course. The only effect that occurs is decreased velocity of transmission. On the other hand, if, as illustrated in the lower part of Figure 16–1, the light waves strike an angulated interface, the light waves bend if the refractive indices of the two media are different from each other. In this particular figure the light waves are leaving air, which has a refractive index of 1.00, and are entering a block of glass having a refractive index of 1.50. When the beam first strikes the angulated interface, the lower edge of the beam enters the glass ahead of the upper edge. The wave front in the upper portion of the beam continues to travel at a velocity of 300,000 kilometers per second while that which has entered the glass travels at a velocity of 200,000 kilometers per second. This causes the upper portion of the wave front to move ahead of the lower portion so that it is no longer vertical but is angulated to the right. Because *the direction in which light travels is always perpendicular to the wave front,* the direction of travel of the light beam now bends downward.

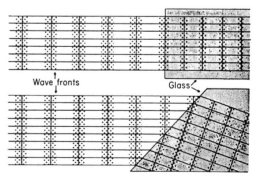

Figure 16–1. Wave fronts entering (*top*) a glass surface perpendicular to the light rays and (*bottom*) a glass surface angulated to the light rays. This figure illustrates that the distance between waves after they enter the glass is shortened to approximately two-thirds that in air. It also illustrates that light rays striking an angulated glass surface are refracted.

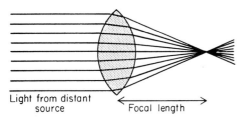

Figure 16–2. Bending of light rays at each surface of a convex spherical lens, showing that parallel light rays are focused to a point focus.

The bending of light rays at an angulated interface is known as *refraction*. Note particularly that the degree of refraction increases as a function of (1) the ratio of the two refractive indices of the two transparent media and (2) the degree of angulation between the interface and the wave front of the beam.

APPLICATION OF REFRACTIVE PRINCIPLES TO LENSES

The Convex Lens. Figure 16–2 shows parallel light rays entering a convex lens. The light rays passing through the center of the lens strike the lens exactly perpendicular to the lens surfaces and therefore pass through the lens without being refracted at all. Toward either edge of the lens, however, the light rays strike a progressively more angulated interface. Therefore, the outer rays bend more and more toward the center.

When the rays have passed through the glass, the outer rays bend still more toward the center. Thus, parallel light rays entering an appropriately formed convex lens come to a single point focus at some distance beyond the lens.

The Concave Lens. Figure 16–3 shows the effect of a concave lens on parallel light rays. The rays that enter the very center of the lens strike an interface that is absolutely perpendicular to the beam and, therefore, do not refract at all. The rays at the edge of the lens enter the lens ahead of the rays toward the center. This is opposite to the effect in the convex lens, and it causes the peripheral light rays to *diverge* away from the light rays that pass through the center of the lens.

Thus, the concave lens *diverges* light rays, whereas the convex lens *converges* light rays.

Spherical versus Cylindrical Lenses. Figure 16–4 illustrates both a convex *spherical* lens and a convex *cylindrical* lens. Note that the convex cylindrical lens bends light rays from the two sides of the lens but not from either the top or the bottom. Therefore, parallel light rays are bent to a focal *line*. On the other hand, light rays that pass through the spherical lens are refracted at all edges of the lens toward the central ray, and all the rays come to a focal *point*.

The cylindrical lens is well illustrated by a test tube full of water. If the test tube is placed in a beam of sunlight and a piece of paper is brought progressively closer to the tube, a certain distance will be found at which the light rays come to a focal line. On the other hand, the spherical lens is illustrated by an ordinary magnifying glass. If such a lens is placed in a beam of sunlight and a piece of paper is brought progressively closer to the lens, the light rays will impinge on a common focal point at an appropriate distance.

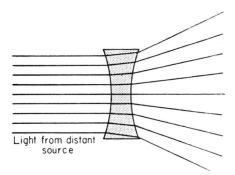

Figure 16–3. Bending of light rays at each surface of a concave spherical lens, illustrating that parallel light rays are diverged by a concave lens.

Figure 16–4. *Top:* Point focus of parallel light rays by a spherical convex lens. *Bottom:* Line focus of parallel light rays by a cylindrical convex lens.

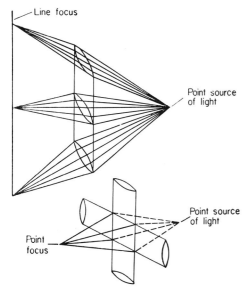

Figure 16–5. Two cylindrical convex lenses at right angles to each other, illustrating that one lens converges light rays in one plane and the other lens converges light rays in the plane at right angles. The two lenses combined give the same point focus as that obtained with a spherical convex lens.

Concave cylindrical lenses *diverge* light rays in only one plane in the same manner that convex cylindrical lenses converge light rays in one plane.

Figure 16–5 shows two convex cylindrical lenses at right angles to each other. The vertical cylindrical lens causes convergence of the light rays that pass through the two sides of the lens. The horizontal lens converges the top and bottom rays. Thus, all the light rays come to a single point focus. In other words, *two cylindrical lenses crossed at right angles to each other perform the same function as one spherical lens of the same refractive power.*

FOCUSING BY CONVEX LENSES

The distance from a convex lens at which parallel rays converge to a common focal point is the *focal length* of the lens. The diagram at the top of Figure 16–6 illustrates this focusing of parallel light rays. In the middle diagram of Figure 16–6, the light rays that enter the convex lens are not parallel but are diverging because the origin of the light is a point source not far away from the lens itself. The rays striking the center of the lens are perpendicular to the lens surface and pass through the lens without any refraction. In the discussion above it was shown that the degree of bending of light rays is a function of (a) the ratio of refractive indices at the interface and (b) the angle of incidence of the light rays. Therefore, the edges of the convex lens bend the diverging rays approximately the same amount as they do parallel rays because the greater refraction at one interface is ap-

proximately balanced by less refraction at the other interface. However, because these rays are already diverging, even though they are bent the same extent as parallel rays, it can be seen from the diagram that they do not come to a point focus at the same distance away from the lens as do the parallel rays. In other words, when rays of light that are already diverging enter a convex lens, the distance of focus on the other side of the lens is farther from the lens than is the case when the entering rays are parallel to each other.

In the lower diagram of Figure 16–6 are shown light rays that also are diverging toward a convex lens that has far greater curvature than that of the upper two lenses of the figure. In this diagram the distance from the lens at which the light rays come to a focus is exactly the same as that from the lens in the first diagram, in which the lens was convex but the light rays entering it were parallel. This illustrates that both parallel rays and diverging rays can be focused at the same distance behind a lens provided that the lens changes its convexity. It is obvious that the nearer the point source of light is to the lens, the greater is the divergence of the light rays and the greater must be the curvature of the lens to cause focusing at the same distance.

The relationship of focal length of the lens, distance of the point source of light, and distance of focus is expressed by the following formula:

$$\frac{1}{f} = \frac{1}{a} + \frac{1}{b}$$

in which *f* is the focal length of the lens, *a* the distance of the point source of light from the lens, and *b* the distance of focus from the lens.

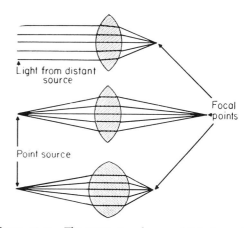

Figure 16–6. The upper two lenses of this figure have the same strength, but the light rays entering the top lens are parallel, while those entering the second lens are diverging; the effect of parallel versus diverging rays on the focal distance is illustrated. The bottom lens has far more refractive power than either of the other two lenses, illustrating that the stronger the lens the nearer to the lens is the point focus.

FORMATION OF AN IMAGE BY A CONVEX LENS

The upper drawing of Figure 16–7 illustrates a convex lens with two point sources of light to the left. Because light rays from any point source pass through the center of a convex lens without being refracted in either direction, the light rays from both point sources of light are shown to pass straight through the lens center. Furthermore, the other light rays from each point source of light, passing through the upper and side edges of the lens, all come to point focus behind the lens *directly in line with each respective point source of light and the center of the lens.*

Any object in front of the lens is in reality a mosaic of point sources of light. Some of these points are very bright, some are very weak, and they vary in color. The light rays from each point source of light that enter the very center of the convex lens pass directly through this lens without any of the rays bending. Furthermore, the light rays that enter the edges of the lens finally come to focal points behind the lens in line with the rays that pass through the center. Therefore, every point source of light on the object comes to a separate point focus on the opposite side of the lens. If all portions of the object are the same distance in front of the lens, all the focal points behind the lens will fall in a common plane a certain distance behind the lens. If a white piece of paper is placed at this distance, one can see an image of the object, as is illustrated in the lower portion of Figure 16–7. However, this image is upside down with respect to the original object, and the two lateral sides of the image are reversed with respect to the original. This is the method by which the lens of a camera focuses light rays on the camera film.

MEASUREMENT OF THE REFRACTIVE POWER OF A LENS—THE DIOPTER

The more a lens bends light rays, the greater is its "refractive power." This refractive power is measured in terms of *diopters.* The refractive power of a

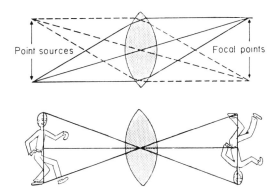

Figure 16–7. The top drawing illustrates two point sources of light focused at two separate points on the opposite side of the lens. The lower drawing illustrates formation of an image by a convex spherical lens.

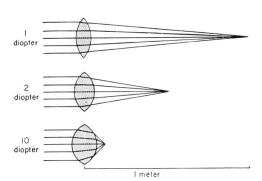

Figure 16–8. Effect of lens strength on the focal distance.

convex lens is equal to 1 meter divided by its focal length. Thus a spherical lens has a refractive power of +1 diopter when it is capable of converging parallel light rays to a focal point 1 meter beyond the lens, as illustrated in Figure 16–8. If the lens is capable of bending parallel light rays twice as much as a lens with a power of +1 diopter, it is said to have a strength of +2 diopters, and, obviously, the light rays come to a focal point 0.5 meter beyond the lens. A lens capable of converging parallel light rays to a focal point only 10 cm. beyond the lens has a refractive power of +10 diopters.

The refractive power of concave lenses cannot be stated in terms of the focal distance beyond the lens because the light rays diverge rather than focus to a point. Therefore, the power of a concave lens is stated in terms of its ability to diverge light rays in comparison with the ability of convex lenses to converge light rays. That is, if a concave lens diverges light rays the same amount that a 1 diopter convex lens converges them, the concave lens is said to have a dioptric strength of −1. Likewise, if the concave lens diverges the light rays as much as a +10 diopter lens converges them, it is said to have a strength of −10 diopters.

Note particularly that concave lenses can "neutralize" the refractive power of convex lenses. Thus, placing a 1 diopter concave lens immediately in front of a 1 diopter convex lens results in a lens system with zero refractive power.

The strengths of cylindrical lenses are computed in the same manner as the strengths of spherical lenses. If a cylindrical lens focuses parallel light rays to a line focus 1 meter beyond the lens, it has a strength of +1 diopter. On the other hand, if a cylindrical lens of a concave type *diverges* light rays as much as a +1 diopter cylindrical lens *converges* them, it has a strength of −1 diopter.

THE OPTICS OF THE EYE

THE EYE AS A CAMERA

The eye, as illustrated in Figure 16–9 is optically equivalent to the usual photographic cam-

Figure 16–9. The eye as a camera. The numbers are the refractive indices.

era, for it has a lens system, a variable aperture system, and a retina that corresponds to the film. The lens system of the eye is composed of (1) the interface between air and the anterior surface of the cornea, (2) the interface between the posterior surface of the cornea and the aqueous humor, (3) the interface between the aqueous humor and the anterior surface of the lens, and (4) the interface between the posterior surface of the lens and the vitreous humor. The refractive index of air is 1; the cornea, 1.38; the aqueous humor, 1.33; the lens (on the average), 1.40; and the vitreous humor, 1.34.

The Reduced Eye. If all the refractive surfaces of the eye are algebraically added together and then considered to be one single lens, the optics of the normal eye may be simplified and represented schematically as a "reduced eye." This is useful in simple calculations. In the reduced eye, a single lens is considered to exist with its central point 17 mm. in front of the retina and to have a total refractive power of approximtely 59 diopters when the lens is accommodated for distant vision.

The anterior surface of the cornea provides about 48 diopters of the eye's total dioptric strength for three reasons: (1) the refractive index of the cornea is markedly different from that of air; (2) the surface of the cornea is further away from the retina than are the surfaces of the eye lens; and (3) the curvature of the cornea is reasonably great.

The posterior surface of the cornea is concave and actually acts as a concave lens, but, because the difference in refractive index of the cornea and the aqueous humor is slight, this posterior surface of the cornea has a refractive power of only about −4 diopters, which neutralizes only a small part of the refractive power of the other refractive surfaces of the eye.

The total refractive power of the crystalline lens of the eye when it is surrounded by fluid on each side is only 15 diopters of the total refrac-tive power of the eye's lens system. If this lens were removed from the eye and then surrounded by air, its refractive power would be about 150 diopters. Thus, it can be seen that the lens inside the eye is not nearly so powerful as it is outside the eye. The reason for this is that the fluids surrounding the lens have refractive indices not greatly different from the refractive index of the lens itself, the smallness of the differences greatly decreasing the amount of light refraction at the lens interfaces. But the importance of the crystalline lens is that its curvature and therefore also its strength can change to provide accommodation, which will be discussed later in the chapter.

Formation of an Image on the Retina. In exactly the same manner that a glass lens can focus an image on a sheet of paper, the lens system of the eye can also focus an image on the retina. The image is inverted and reversed with respect to the object. However, the mind perceives objects in the upright position despite the upside down orientation on the retina because the brain is trained to consider an inverted image as the normal.

THE MECHANISM OF ACCOMMODATION

The refractive power of the crystalline lens of the eye can be voluntarily increased from 15 diopters to approximately 29 diopters in young children; this is a total "accommodation" of 14 diopters. To do this, the shape of the lens is changed from that of a moderately convex lens to that of a very convex lens. The mechanism of this is the following:

Normally, the lens is composed of a strong elastic capsule filled with viscous proteinaceous, but transparent fibers. When the lens is in a relaxed state, with no tension on its capsule, it assumes a spherical shape, owing entirely to the elasticity of the lens capsule. However, as illustrated in Figure 16–10, approximately 70 ligaments attach radially around the lens, pulling the lens edges toward the edge of the choroid. These ligaments are constantly tensed by the elastic pull of their attachments to the choroid, and the tension on the ligaments causes the lens to remain relatively flat under normal resting conditions of the eye. At the insertions of the ligaments in the choroid is the ciliary muscle, which has two sets of smooth muscle fibers, the *meridional fibers* and the *circular fibers*. The meridional fibers extend from the corneoscleral junction to the insertions of the ligaments in the choroid approximately 2 to

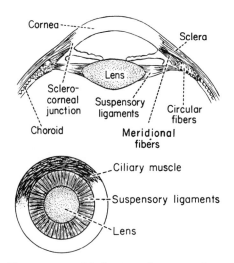

Figure 16–10. Mechanism of accommodation.

3 mm. behind the corneoscleral junction. When these muscle fibers contract, the insertions of the ligaments are pulled forward, thereby releasing a certain amount of tension on the crystalline lens. The circular fibers are arranged circularly all the way around the eye so that when they contract a sphincter-like action occurs, decreasing the diameter of the circle of ligament attachments and allowing the ligaments to pull less on the lens capsule.

Thus, contraction of both sets of smooth muscle fibers in the ciliary muscle relaxes the ligaments to the lens capsule, and the lens assumes a more spherical shape, like that of a balloon, because of elasticity of its capsule. When the ciliary muscle is completely relaxed, the dioptric strength of the lens is as weak as it can become. On the other hand, when the ciliary muscle contracts as strongly as possible, the dioptric strength of the lens becomes maximal.

Autonomic Control of Accommodation. The ciliary muscle is controlled mainly by the parasympathetic nervous system but also to a slight extent by the sympathetic system, as will be discussed in Chapter 18. Stimulation of the parasympathetic fibers to the eye contracts the ciliary muscle, which in turn relaxes the ligaments of the lens and increases its refractive power. With an increased refractive power, the eye is capable of focusing on objects that are nearer to it than is an eye with less refractive power. Consequently, as a distant object moves toward the eye, the number of parasympathetic impulses impinging on the ciliary muscle must be progressively increased for the eye to keep the object constantly in focus. Sympathetic stimulation has a weak effect in relaxing the ciliary muscle and therefore in focusing the eye for far vision.

Presbyopia. As a person grows older, his lens loses its elastic nature and becomes a relatively solid mass, probably because of progressive denaturation of the proteins. Therefore, the ability of the lens to assume a spherical shape progressively decreases, and the power of accommodation decreases from approximately 14 diopters shortly after birth to approximately 2 diopters at the age of 45 to 50. Thereafter, the lens of the eye may be considered to be almost totally nonaccommodating, which condition is known as "presbyopia."

Once a person has reached the state of presbyopia, each eye remains focused permanently at an almost constant distance; this distance depends on the physical characteristics of each individual's eyes. Obviously, the eyes can no longer accommodate for both near and far vision. Therefore, for an older person to see clearly both in the distance and nearby, he must wear bifocal glasses with the upper segment focused for far-seeing and the lower segment focused for near-seeing.

THE PUPILLARY APERTURE

A major function of the iris is to increase the amount of light that enters the eye during darkness and to decrease the light that enters the eye in bright light. The reflexes for controlling this mechanism will be considered in the discussion of the neurology of the eye in Chapter 18. The amount of light that enters the eye through the pupil is proportional to the area of the pupil or to the *square of the diameter* of the pupil. The pupil of the human eye can become as small as approximately 1.5 mm. and as large as 8 mm. in diameter. Therefore, the quantity of light entering the eye may vary approximately 30 times as a result of changes in pupillary aperture size.

Depth of Focus of the Lens System of the Eye. Figure 16–11 illustrates two separate eyes that are exactly alike except that the diameters of the pupillary apertures are different. In the upper eye the pupillary aperture is small, and in the lower eye the aperture is large. In front of each of these two eyes are two small point sources of light, and light from each passes through the pupillary aperture and focuses on the retina. Consequently, in both eyes the retina sees two spots of light in perfect focus. It is evident from the diagrams, however, that if the

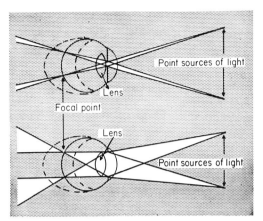

Figure 16–11. Effect of small and large pupillary apertures on the depth of focus.

retina is moved forward or backward to an out-of-focus position, the size of each spot will not change much in the upper eye, but in the lower eye the size of each spot will increase greatly, and it becomes a "blur circle." In other words, the upper lens system has far greater *depth of focus* than the bottom lens system. When a lens system has great depth of focus, the retina can be considerably displaced from the focal plane and still discern the various points of an image rather distinctly; whereas, when a lens system has a shallow depth of focus, moving the retina only slightly away from the focal plane causes extreme blurring of the image.

The greatest possible depth of focus occurs when the pupil is extremely small. The reason for this is that with a very small aperture the eye acts more or less as a pinhole camera. It will be recalled from the study of physics that light rays coming from an object and passing through a pinhole are in focus on any surface at all distances beyond the pinhole. In other words, the depth of focus of a pinhole camera is infinite.

"NORMAL" ABERRATIONS OF VISION

Spherical Aberration. The crystalline lens of the eye is not nearly so regularly formed as lenses made by good opticians. Indeed, the light rays passing through the peripheral edges of the eye lens are not brought to really sharp focus with the other light rays, as illustrated in Figure 16–12. This effect is known as "spherical aberration," and the lens system of the human eye is quite subject to such an error. Therefore, increasing the aperture of the pupil progressively decreases the sharpness of focus. This partially explains why visual acuity is decreased at

low illumination levels which cause the pupil to dilate.

Chromatic Aberration. The lens of the eye is also subject to "chromatic aberration," which is illustrated in Figure 16–13. This means that the refractive power of the lens is different for the different colors, so that different colors focus at different distances behind the lens. Furthermore, the greater the aperture of the lens, the greater are the errors of chromatic aberration, for those light rays passing through the center of the lens are proportionately less affected than are the rays passing through the periphery of the lens.

Diffractive Errors of the Eye. Still another error in the optical system of all eyes is "diffraction" of light rays. Diffraction means bending of light rays as they pass over sharp edges; this obviously occurs as the rays pass over the edges of the pupil. Diffractive errors become especially important when the pupil becomes very small, because "interference" patterns then appear on the retina. A thorough consideration of diffraction at this point is impossible, and this phenomenon is simply noted to explain that as the pupil becomes 1.5 mm. in size the sharpness of vision becomes less than when the pupil is approximately 2.5 mm. in size despite the fact that the depth of focus is better the smaller the pupillary diameter.

Cataracts. Cataracts are an especially common eye abnormality that occurs in older people. A cataract is a cloudy or opaque area in the lens. In the early stage of cataract formation the proteins in the lens fibers immediately beneath the capsule become denatured. Later, these same proteins coagulate to form opaque areas in place of the normal transparent protein fibers of the lens. Finally, in still later stages, calcium is often deposited in the coagulated proteins, thus further increasing the opacity.

When a cataract has obscured light transmission so greatly that it seriously impairs vision, the condition can be corrected by surgical removal of the entire lens. When this is done, however, the eye loses a large portion of its refractive power, which must be replaced by a powerful convex lens (about +15 diopters) in front of the eye, as will be explained in the following sections.

ERRORS OF REFRACTION

Emmetropia. As shown in Figure 16–14, the eye is considered to be normal or "emmetropic" if, when

Figure 16–12. Spherical aberration.

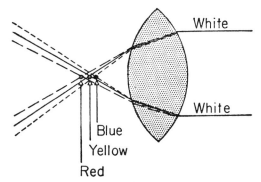

Figure 16–13. Chromatic aberration.

the ciliary muscle is completely relaxed, parallel light rays from distant objects are in sharp focus on the retina. This means that the emmetropic eye can, with its ciliary muscle completely relaxed, see all distant objects clearly, but to focus objects at close range it must contract its ciliary muscle and thereby provide various degrees of accommodation.

Hypermetropia (Hyperopia). Hypermetropia, which is also known as "far-sightedness," is due either to an eyeball that is too short or to a lens system that is too weak when the ciliary muscle is completely relaxed. In this condition, parallel light rays are not bent sufficiently by the lens system to come to a focus by the time they reach the retina. In order to overcome this abnormality, the ciliary muscle may contract to increase the strength of the lens. Therefore, the far-sighted person is capable, by using his mechanism of accommodation, of focusing distant objects on his retina. If he has used only a small amount of strength in his ciliary muscle to accommo-

date for the distant objects, then he still has much accommodative power left, and objects closer and closer to the eye can also be focused sharply until the ciliary muscle has contracted to its limit. The distance of the object away from the eye at this point is known as the "near point" of vision.

In old age, when the lens becomes presbyopic, the far-sighted person often is not able to accommodate his lens sufficiently to focus even distant objects, much less to focus near objects.

Myopia. In myopia, or "near-sightedness," even when the ciliary muscle is completely relaxed, the strength of the lens is still so great that light rays coming from distant objects are focused in front of the retina. This is usually due to too long an eyeball but it can occasionally result from too much power of the lens system of the eye.

No mechanism exists by which the eye can decrease the strength of its lens beyond that which exists when the ciliary muscle is completely relaxed. Therefore, the myopic person has no mechanism by which he can ever focus distant objects sharply on his retina. However, as an object comes nearer and nearer to his eye it finally comes near enough that its image is focused on the retina. Then, when the object comes still closer to the eye, the person can use his mechanism of accommodation to keep the image focused clearly. Therefore, a myopic person has a definite limiting "far point" for acute vision as well as a "near point"; when an object comes inside the "far point," he can use his mechanism of accommodation to keep the object in focus until the object reaches the "near point."

Correction of Myopia and Hypermetropia by Use of Lenses. It will be recalled that light rays passing through a concave lens diverge. Therefore, if the refractive surfaces of the eye have too much refractive power, as in myopia, some of this excessive refractive power can be neutralized by placing in front of the eye a concave spherical lens, which will diverge rays. On the other hand, in a person who has hypermetropia—that is, one who has too weak a lens for the distance of the retina away from the lens—the abnormal vision can be corrected by adding refractive power with a convex lens in front of the eye. These corrections are illustrated in Figure 16–15. One usually determines the strength of the concave or convex lens needed for clear vision by "trial and error"—that is, by trying first a strong lens and then a stronger or weaker lens until the one that gives the best visual acuity is found.

Astigmatism. Astigmatism is a refractive error of the lens system of the eye caused usually by an oblong shape of the cornea or, rarely, by an oblong shape of the lens. A lens surface like the side of an egg lying edgewise to the incoming light would be an example of an astigmatic lens. The degree of curvature in a plane through the long axis of the egg is not nearly so great as the degree of curvature in a plane through the short axis. The same is true of an astigmatic lens. Because the curvature of the astigmatic lens along one plane is less than the curvature along

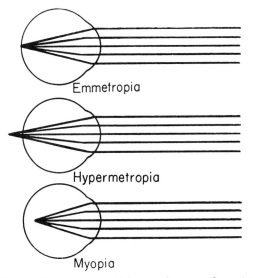

Figure 16–14. Parallel light rays focus on the retina in emmetropia, behind the retina in hypermetropia, and in front of the retina in myopia.

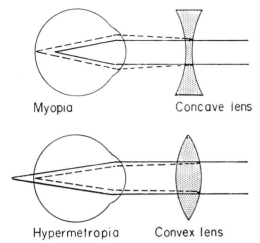

Figure 16–15. Correction of myopia with a concave lens and correction of hypermetropia with a convex lens.

the other plane, light rays striking the peripheral portions of the lens in one plane are not bent nearly so much as are rays striking the peripheral portions of the other plane.

This is illustrated in Figure 16–16, which shows what happens to rays of light emanating from a point source and passing through an oblong astigmatic lens. The light rays in the vertical plane, which is indicated by plane BD, are refracted greatly by the astigmatic lens because of the greater curvature in the vertical direction than in the horizontal direction. However, the light rays in the horizontal plane, indicated by plane AC, are bent not nearly so much as the light rays in the vertical plane. It is obvious, therefore, that the light rays passing through an astigmatic lens do not all come to a common focal point because the light rays passing through one plane of the lens focus far in front of those passing through the other plane.

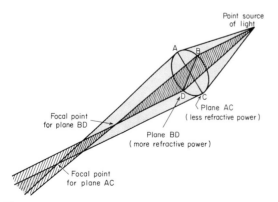

Figure 16–16. Astigmatism, illustrating that light rays focus at one focal distance in one focal plane and at another focal distance in the plane at right angles.

Placing an appropriate *spherical* lens in front of an astigmatic eye can bring the light rays that pass through *one plane* of the lens into focus on the retina, but spherical lenses can never bring *all* the light rays into complete focus at the same time. This is the reason why astigmatism is a very undesirable refractive error of the eyes. Furthermore, the accommodative powers of the eyes cannot compensate for astigmatism for the same reasons that spherical lenses placed in front of the eyes cannot correct the condition.

Correction of Astigmatism with a Cylindrical Lens. In correcting astigmatism with lenses it must always be remembered that two cylindrical lenses of equal strength may be crossed at right angles to give the same refractive effects as a spherical lens of the same strength. However, if one of the crossed cylindrical lenses has a different strength from that of the second lens, the light rays in one plane may not be brought to a common focal point with the light rays in the opposite plane. This is the situation that one usually finds in the astigmatic eye. In other words, one may consider an astigmatic eye as having a lens system made up of two cylindrical lenses of slightly different strengths. Another way of looking at the astigmatic lens system of the eye is that this system is a spherical lens with a superimposed cylindrical lens.

To correct the focusing of an astigmatic lens system, it is necessary to determine both the *strength* of the cylindrical lens needed to neutralize the excess cylindrical power of the eye lens and the *axis* of this abnormal cylindrical lens.

There are several methods for determining the axis of the abnormal cylindrical component of the lens system of an eye. One of these methods is based on the use of parallel black bars, as shown in Figure 16–17. Some of these parallel bars are vertical, some horizontal, and some at various angles to the vertical and horizontal axes. After placing, by trial and error, various spherical lenses in front of the astigmatic eye, a strength of lens will usually be found that will cause sharp focus of one set of these parallel bars on the retina of the astigmatic eye. If there is no accompanying myopia or hypermetropia, the spherical lens may not be necessary.

It can be shown from the physical principles of optics discussed earlier in this chapter that the axis of the *out-of-focus* cylindrical component of the optical system is parallel to the black bars that are fuzzy in appearance. Once this axis is found, the examiner tries progressively stronger and weaker positive or negative cylindrical lenses, the axes of which are placed parallel to the out-of-focus bars until the patient sees all the crossed bars with equal clarity. When this has been accomplished, the examiner directs the optician to grind a special lens having both the spherical correction plus the cylindrical correction at the appropriate axis.

Correction of Optical Abnormalities by Use of Contact Lenses. In recent years, either glass or plastic contact lenses have been used to fit snugly against the anterior surface of the cornea. These

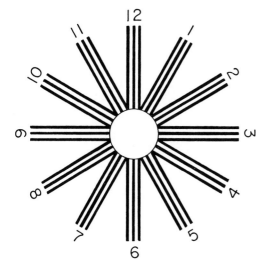

Figure 16–17. Chart composed of parallel black bars for determining the axis (meridian) of astigmatism.

lenses are held in place by a thin layer of tears that fill the space between the contact lens and the anterior surface.

A special feature of the contact lens is that it nullifies almost entirely the refraction that normally occurs at the anterior surface of the cornea. The reason for this is that the tears between the contact lens and the cornea have a refractive index almost equal to that of the cornea so that no longer does the anterior surface of the cornea play a significant role in the eye's optical system. Instead, the anterior surface of the contact lens now plays the major role and its posterior surface a minor role, the refraction of this lens now substituting for the cornea's usual refraction. This is especially important in persons whose eye refractive errors are caused by an abnormally shaped cornea, such as persons who have an odd-shaped, bulging cornea—a condition called *keratoconus*. Without the contact lens the bulging cornea causes such severe abnormality of vision that almost no glasses can correct the vision satisfactorily; when a contact lens is used, however, the corneal refraction is neutralized, and normal refraction by the contact lens is substituted in its place.

The contact lens has several other advantages as well, including (1) the lens turns with the eye and gives a broader field of clear vision than do usual glasses, and (2) the contact lens has little effect on the size of the object that the person sees through the lens; on the other hand, lenses placed several centimeters in front of the eye do affect the size of the image even though they do correct the focus.

SIZE OF THE IMAGE ON THE RETINA AND VISUAL ACUITY

If the distance from an object to the eye lens is 17 meters and the distance from the center of

the lens to the image is 17 millimeters, the ratio of the object size to image size is 1000 to 1. Therefore, an object 17 meters in front of the eye and 1 meter in size produces an image on the retina 1 millimeter in size.

Theoretically, a point of light from a distant point source, when focused on the retina, should be infinitely small. However, since the lens system of the eye is not perfect, such a retinal spot ordinarily has a total diameter of about 11 microns even with maximum resolution of the optical system. However, it is brightest in its very center and shades off gradually toward the edges.

The average diameter of cones *in the fovea* of the retina, the central part of the retina where vision is most highly developed, is approximately 1.5 microns, which is one-seventh the diameter of the spot of light. Nevertheless, since the spot of light has a bright center point and shaded edges, a person can distinguish two separate points if their centers lie approximately 2 microns apart on the retina, which is slightly greater than the width of a foveal cone. This discrimination between points is illustrated in Figure 16–18.

The maximum visual acuity of the human eye for discriminating between point sources of light is 26 seconds. That is, when light rays from two separate points strike the eye with an angle of at least 26 seconds between them, they can usually be recognized as two points instead of one. This means that a person with maximal acuity looking at two bright pinpoint spots of light 10 meters away can barely distinguish the spots as separate entities when they are 1 millimeter apart.

The fovea is only a fraction of a millimeter in diameter, which means that maximum visual acuity occurs in only 3 degrees of the visual field. Outside this foveal area the visual acuity

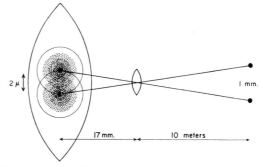

Figure 16–18. Maximal visual acuity for two point sources of light.

is reduced 5- to 10-fold, and it becomes progressively poorer as the periphery is approached. This is caused by the connection of many rods and cones to the same nerve fiber, as discussed in Chapter 18.

Clinical Method for Stating Visual Acuity. Usually the test chart for testing eyes is placed 20 feet away from the tested person, and if the person can see the letters of the size that he should be able to see at 20 feet, he is said to have 20/20 vision: that is, normal vision. If he can see only letters that he should be able to see at 200 feet, he is said to have 20/200 vision. On the other hand, if he can see at 20 feet letters that he should be able to see only at 15 feet, he is said to have 20/15 vision. In other words, the clinical method for expressing visual acuity is to use a mathematical fraction that expresses the ratio of two distances, which is also the ratio of one's visual acuity to that of the normal person.

DETERMINATION OF DISTANCE OF AN OBJECT FROM THE EYE— DEPTH PERCEPTION

There are three major means by which the visual apparatus normally perceives distance, a phenomenon that is known as depth perception. These are (1) relative sizes of objects, (2) moving parallax, and (3) stereopsis.

Determination of Distance by Relative Sizes. If a person knows that a man is six feet tall and then he sees this man even with only one eye, he can determine how far away the man is simply by the size of the man's image on his retina. He does not consciously think about the size of this image, but his brain has learned to determine automatically from the image sizes the distances of objects from the eye when the dimensions of these objects are already known.

Determination of Distance by Moving Parallax. Another important means by which the eyes determine distance is that of moving parallax. If a person looks off into the distance with his eyes completely still, he perceives no moving parallax, but, when he moves his head to one side or the other, the images of objects close to him move rapidly across his retinae while the images of distant objects remain rather stationary. For instance, if he moves his head 1 inch and an object is only 1 inch in front of his eye, the image moves almost all the way across his retinae, whereas the image of an object 200 feet away from his eyes does not move perceptibly. Thus, by this mechanism of moving paral-

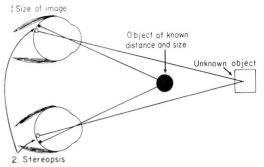

Figure 16–19. Perception of distance (1) by the size of the image on the retina and (2) as a result of stereopsis.

lax, one can tell the *relative distances* of different objects even though only one eye is used.

Determination of Distance by Stereopsis. Another method by which one perceives parallax is that of binocular vision. Because one eye is a little more than 2 inches to one side of the other eye, the images on the two retinae are different one from the other—that is, an object that is 1 inch in front of the bridge of the nose forms an image on the temporal portion of the retina of each eye, whereas a small object 20 feet in front of the nose has its image at closely corresponding points in the middle of the eye. This type of parallax is illustrated in Figure 16–19, which shows the images of a black spot and a square actually reversed on the retinae because they are at different distances in front of the eyes. This gives a type of parallax that is present all the time when both eyes are being used. It is almost entirely this binocular parallax (or stereopsis) that gives a person with two eyes far greater ability to judge relative distances *when objects are nearby* than a person who has only one eye. However, stereopsis is virtually useless for depth perception at distances beyond 200 feet.

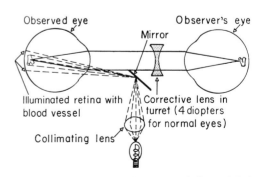

Figure 16–20. The optical system of the ophthalmoscope.

OPTICAL INSTRUMENTS

THE OPHTHALMOSCOPE

The ophthalmoscope is an instrument designed so that an observer can look through it into another person's eye and see the retina with clarity. Though the ophthalmoscope appears to be a relatively complicated instrument, its principles are simple. The basic portions of such an instrument are illustrated in Figure 16–20 and may be explained as follows:

If a bright spot of light is on the retina of an emmetropic eye, light rays from the spot diverge toward the lens system of the eye, and, after they pass through the lens system, they are parallel with each other because the retina is located in the focal plane of the lens. When these parallel rays pass into an emmetropic eye of another person, they focus to a point on the retina of the second person because his retina is in the focal plane of his lens. Therefore, any spot of light on the retina of the observed eye comes to a focal spot on the retina of the observing eye. Likewise, when the bright spot of light is moved to different portions of the observed retina, the focal spot on the retina of the observer also moves approximately an equal amount. Thus, if the retina of one person is made to emit light, the image of his retina will be focused on the retina of the observer provided that the two eyes are simply looking into each other. These principles, of course, apply only to completely emmetropic eyes.

To make an ophthalmoscope, one need only devise a means for illuminating the retina to be examined. Then, the reflected light from that retina can be seen by the observer simply by putting the two eyes close to each other. To illuminate the retina of the observed eye, an angulated mirror or a segment of a prism is placed in front of the observed eye in such a manner that light from a bulb is reflected into the observed eye. Thus, the retina is illuminated through the pupil, and the observer sees into the subject's pupil by looking over the edge of the mirror or prism, or preferably *through* an appropriately designed prism so that the light will not have to enter the pupil at an angle.

It was noted above that these principles apply only to persons with completely emmetropic eyes. If the refractive power of either eye is abnormal, it is necessary to correct this refractive power in order for the observer to see a sharp image of the observed retina. Therefore, the usual ophthalmoscope has a series of about 20 lenses mounted on a turret so that the turret can be rotated from one lens to another, and the correction for abnormal refractive power of either or both eyes can be made at the same time by selecting a single lens of appropriate strength. In normal young persons, when the two eyes come close together, a natural accommodative reflex occurs that causes approximately +2 diopters increase in the strength of the lens of each eye. To correct for this, it is necessary that the lens turret be rotated to approximately −4 diopters correction.

(1) Glows on this side in myopia

I diopter lens

(2) Glows on this side in hypermetropia

(3) Glows over entire pupil in emmetropia

Figure 16–21. The retinoscope.

THE RETINOSCOPE

The retinoscope, illustrated in Figure 16–21, is an instrument that can be used to determine the refractive power of an eye even though the subject cannot converse with the observer. Such a procedure is valuable for fitting glasses to an infant.

To use the retinoscope, one places a bright spot of light behind and to one side of the observed eye, and stands 1 meter away, looking through a hole in the middle of a mirror. The observer then rotates this mirror from side to side, casting a reflected beam of light into the pupil of the observed eye while the subject keeps his gaze intently on the observer's eye. If the observed eye is normal, when this beam of light travels across the pupil the entire pupil suddenly glows red. If the eye has abnormal refractive powers, the red glow appears either on the side of the pupil into which the light first shines or on the opposite side of the pupil—one or the other. *In hyperopia the first glow appears on the side of the pupil from which the light beam is being moved. In myopia the first glow appears on the opposite side of the pupil.* The cause of this difference is that the lens of the hyperopic eye is too weak and that of the myopic eye too strong to focus the light from the edge of the pupil on the retina exactly in line with the observer's eye. For a fuller understanding of this effect, however, the student is referred to texts on physiologic optics.

One can fit glasses to a patient by placing selected lenses in front of the observed eye one at a time until the glow suddenly covers the pupil over its entire extent rather than spreading from one side of the pupil to the other. However, it should be noted that in retinoscopy one tests an eye that is focused on the observer's eye at 1 meter's distance. This must be taken into consideration in prescribing glasses; 1 diopter strength must be subtracted for far vision.

REFERENCES

Armington, J. C.: Vision. *Ann. Rev. Physiol.*, 27:163, 1965.

Bodis-Wollner, I.: On dissociated visual functions. *Mt. Sinai J. Med. N.Y.*, 41:38, 1974.

Campbell, C. J., Koester, C. J., Rittler, M. C., and Tackaberry R. B.: Physiological Optics. Hagerstown, Md., Harper & Row, Publishers, 1974.

Clayton, R. M.: Problems of differentiation in the vertebrate lens. *Curr. Top. Dev. Biol.*, 5:115, 1970.

Davson, H.: The Physiology of the Eye, 3rd Ed. New York, Academic Press, Inc., 1972.

Davson, H., and Graham, L. T., Jr.: The Eye. Vols. 1–6. New York, Academic Press, Inc. 1969–1974.

Duke-Elder, S., and Perkins, E. S. (eds.): The Transparency of the Cornea. Springfield, Ill., Charles C Thomas, Publisher, 1960.

Follmann, P.: Dynamography. *Ophthalmologica*, 169:192, 1974.

Linksz, A.: Physiology of the Eye. Vol. 1. Optics. New York, Grune & Stratton, Inc., 1950.

Paterson, C. A.: Extracellular space of the crystalline lens. *Amer. J. Physiol.*, 218:797, 1970.

Polyak, S.: The Vertebrate Visual System. Chicago, University of Chicago Press, 1957.

Rabbetts, R. B.: A comparison of astigmatism and cyclophoria in distance and near vision. *Brit. J. Physiol. Opt.*, 27:161, 1973.

Ruben, M.: Textbook of Contact Lens Practice. Baltimore, The Williams & Wilkins Company, 1973.

Sekuler, R.: Spatial vision. *Ann. Rev. Psychol.*, 25:195, 1974.

Siegel, I. M.: Optics and visual physiology. *Arch. Ophthalmol.*, 90:327, 1973.

Sloane, A. E.: Manual of Refraction. Boston, Little, Brown and Company, 1961.

Toates, F. M.: Accommodation function of the human eye. *Physiol. Rev.*, 52:828, 1972.

Tommila, V.: Stereoscopic and binocular vision. *Ophthalmologica*, 169:90, 1974.

Trevor-Roper, P.: The Eye and Its Disorders. Philadelphia, J. B. Lippincott Company, 1974.

Whitteridge, D.: Binocular vision and cortical function. *Proc. R. Soc. Med.*, 65:947, 1972.

Witkovsky, P.: Peripheral mechanisms of vision. *Ann. Rev. Physiol.*, 33:257, 1971.

17

The Eye:
II. Receptor Functions of the Retina

The retina is the light-sensitive portion of the eye, containing the cones, which are mainly responsible for color vision, and the rods, which are mainly responsible for vision in the dark. When the rods and cones are excited, signals are transmitted through successive neurons in the retina itself and finally into the optic nerve fibers and cerebral cortex. The purpose of the present chapter is to explain specifically the mechanisms by which the rods and cones detect both white and colored light.

ANATOMY AND FUNCTION OF THE STRUCTURAL ELEMENTS OF THE RETINA

The Layers of the Retina. Figure 17–1 shows the functional components of the retina arranged in layers from the outside to the inside as follows: (1) pigment layer, (2) layer of rods and cones projecting into the pigment, (3) outer lining membrane, (4) outer nuclear layer, (5) outer plexiform layer, (6) inner nuclear layer, (7) inner plexiform layer, (8) ganglionic layer, (9) layer of optic nerve fibers, and (10) inner limiting membrane.

After light passes through the lens system of the eye and then through the vitreous humor, it enters the retina from the bottom (see Figure 17–1): that is, it passes through the ganglion cells, the plexiform layer, the nuclear layer, and the limiting membranes before it finally reaches the layer of rods and cones located all the way on the opposite side of the retina. This distance is a thickness of several hundred microns; visual acuity is obviously decreased by this

passage through such nonhomogeneous tissue. However, in the central region of the retina, as will be discussed below, the initial layers are pulled aside to prevent this loss of acuity.

The Foveal Region of the Retina and its Importance in Acute Vision. A minute area in the center of the retina, illustrated in Figure 17–2, called the *macula* and occupying a total area of less than 1 square millimeter is especially capable of acute and detailed vision. This area is composed entirely of cones, but the cones are very much elongated and

Figure 17–1. Plan of the retinal neurons. (From Polyak: The Retina. University of Chicago Press.)

Figure 17–2. Photomicrograph of the macula and of the fovea in its center. Note that the inner layers of the retina are pulled to the side to decrease the interference with light transmission. (From Bloom and Fawcett: A Textbook of Histology, 10th Ed., 1975; courtesy of H. Mizoguchi.)

have a diameter of only 1.5 microns in contradistinction to the very large cones located farther peripherally in the retina. The central portion of the macula, only 0.4 mm. in diameter, is called the *fovea;* in this region the blood vessels, the ganglion cells, the inner nuclear layer of cells, and the plexiform layers are all displaced to one side rather than resting directly on top of the cones. This allows light to pass unimpeded to the cones rather than through several layers of retina, which aids immensely in the acuity of visual perception by this region of the retina.

The Rods and Cones. Figure 17–3 is a diagrammatic representation of a photoreceptor (either a rod or a cone) though the cones may be distinguished by having a conical upper end. In general, the rods are narrower and longer than the cones, but this is not always the case. In the peripheral portions of the retina the rods are 2 to 5 microns in diameter whereas the cones are 5 to 8 microns in diameter; in the central part of the retina, in the fovea, the cones have a diameter of only 1.5 microns.

To the right in Figure 17–3 are illustrated the four major functional segments of either a rod or a cone: (1) the outer segment, (2) the inner segment, (3) the nucleus, and (4) the synaptic body. It is in the outer segment that the light-sensitive photochemical is found. In the case of the rods, this is *rhodopsin,* and in the cones it is one of several photochemicals almost exactly the same as rhodopsin except for a difference in spectral sensitivity. The cross-marks in the outer segment represent discs formed by infoldings of the cell membrane. These act as shelves to which the photosensitive pigments are attached. In this outer segment the concentration of the photosensitive pigments is approximately 40 per cent.

The inner segment contains the usual cytoplasm of the cell with the usual cytoplasmic organelles. Particularly important are the mitochondria, for we shall see later that the mitochondria in this segment play an important role in providing most of the energy for function of the photoreceptors.

The synaptic body is the portion of the rod and cone that connects with the subsequent neuronal cells, the horizontal and bipolar cells, that represent the next stages in the vision chain.

Figure 17–3. Schematic drawing of the functional parts of the rods and cones. (Redrawn from R. Young: General Cell Biology.)

Figure 17–4 shows in more detail the photoreceptor discs in the outer segments of the rods and cones. Note especially their attachments to the cell membrane from which they originated.

Regeneration of Photoreceptors. The inner segments of the rods continually synthesize new rhodopsin. This in turn migrates to the base of the outer segment, where the cell membrane is continually forming new folds that become the discs of the rod and to which the rhodopsin attaches. Several new discs are formed each hour, and these migrate outward along the rod toward the tip, carrying the new rhodopsin with them. When the discs reach the top they degenerate and are dissoluted by the pigment epithelium. Thus, the light receptor portion of the rod is continually being replaced.

On the other hand, new disc formation does not seem to occur in the cones. However, new visual pigment does migrate throughout the outer segment and local repair of the disc system does seem to occur.

These processes of disc generation and repair are probably important to the provision of continually viable photoreceptor chemical mechanisms in the photoreceptors.

The Pigment Layer of the Retina. The black pigment *melanin* in the pigment layer, and still more melanin in the choroid, prevents light reflection throughout the globe of the eyeball, and this is extremely important for acute vision. This pigment performs the same function in the eye as the black paint inside the bellows of a camera. Without it, light rays would be reflected in all directions within the eyeball and would cause diffuse lighting of the retina rather than the contrasts between dark and light spots required for formation of precise images.

The importance of melanin in the pigment layer and choroid is well illustrated by its absence in *albinos,* persons hereditarily lacking in melanin pigment in all parts of their bodies. When an albino enters a bright area, light that impinges on the retina is reflected in all directions by the white surface of the unpigmented choroid so that a single discrete spot of light that would normally excite only a few rods or cones is reflected everywhere and excites many of the receptors. Also, a large amount of diffuse light enters the eye through the unpigmented iris. Thus, the lack of melanin causes the visual acuity of albinos, even with the best of optical correction, to be rarely better than 20/100 to 20/200. The pigment layer

Figure 17–4. Membranous structures of the outer segments of a rod (left) and a cone (right). (Courtesy of Dr. Richard Young.)

also stores large quantities of *vitamin A*. This vitamin A is exchanged back and forth through the membranes of the outer segments of the rods and cones which themselves are embedded in the pigment layer. We shall see later that vitamin A is an important precursor of the photosensitive pigments and that this interchange of vitamin A is very important for adjustment of the light sensitivity of the receptors.

The Blood Supply of the Retina—the Retinal Arterial System and the Choroid. The nutrient blood supply for the inner layers of the retina is derived from the central retinal artery, which enters the inside of the eye along with the optic nerve and then divides to supply the entire inner retinal surface. Thus, to a great extent, the retina has its own blood supply independent of the other structures of the eye.

However, the outer layer of the retina is adherent to the *choroid,* which is a highly vascular tissue between the retina and the sclera. The outer layers of the retina, including the outer segments of the rods and cones, depend mainly on diffusion from the choroid vessels for their nutrition, especially for their oxygen.

Retinal Detachment. The neural retina occasionally detaches from the pigment epithelium. In a few instances the cause of such detachment is injury to the eyeball that allows fluid or blood to collect between the retina and the pigment epithelium, but more often it is caused by contracture of fine collagenous fibrils in the vitreous humor, which pull the retina unevenly toward the interior of the globe.

Fortunately, partly because of diffusion across the detachment gap and partly because of the independent blood supply to the retina through the retinal artery, the retina can resist degeneration for a number of days and can become functional once

again if surgically replaced in its normal relationship with the pigment epithelium. But, if not replaced soon, the retina finally degenerates and then is unable to function even after surgical repair.

PHOTOCHEMISTRY OF VISION

Both the rods and cones contain chemicals that decompose on exposure to light and, in the process, excite the nerve fibers leading from the eye. The chemical in the *rods* is called *rhodopsin,* and the light-sensitive chemicals in the *cones* have compositions only slightly different from that of rhodopsin.

In the present section we will discuss principally the photochemistry of rhodopsin, but we may apply almost exactly the same principles to the photochemistry of the light-sensitive substances of the cones.

THE RHODOPSIN-RETINENE VISUAL CYCLE, AND EXCITATION OF THE RODS

Rhodopsin and its Decomposition by Light Energy. The outer segment of the rod that projects into the pigment layer of the retina has a concentration of about 40 per cent of the light-sensitive pigment called *rhodopsin* or *visual purple*. This substance is a combination of the protein *scotopsin* and the carotenoid pigment *retinene*. Furthermore, the retinene is a particular type called 11-*cis* retinene (also called neo-b retinine). This *cis* form of the retinene is important because only this form can combine with scotopsin to synthesize rhodopsin.

When light energy is absorbed by rhodopsin, the rhodopsin immediately begins to decompose, as shown in Figure 17–5. The cause of this is an instantaneous change of the *cis* form of retinene into an all-*trans* form, which still has the same chemical structure as the *cis* form but has a different physical structure—a straight molecule rather than a curved molecule. Because the stereoscopic orientation of the reactive sites of the all-*trans* retinene no longer fit with that of the reactive sites on the protein scotopsin, it begins to pull away from the scotopsin. The immediate product is *prelumirhodopsin,* which is a partially split combination of the all-*trans* retinene and scotopsin. However, prelumirhodopsin is an extremely unstable compound and decays in a small fraction of a second to *lumirhodopsin.* This decays in another fraction of a second to *metarhodopsin I,* then successively to *metarhodopsin II*

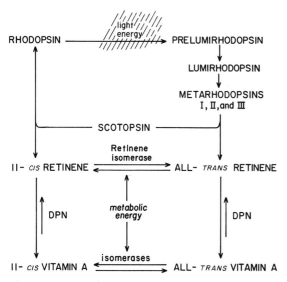

Figure 17–5. Photochemistry of the rhodopsin-retinene-vitamin A visual cycle.

and *metarhodopsin III*. All of these are loose combinations of the all-*trans* retinene and scotopsin, but the metarhodopsin III, too, is unstable, and it slowly decomposes during the next few seconds into completely split products—scotopsin and all-*trans* retinene. During the process of splitting, the rods are excited, and signals are transmitted into the central nervous system.

Reformation of Rhodopsin. The first stage in reformation of rhodopsin, as shown in Figure 17–5, is to reconvert the all-*trans* retinene into 11-*cis* retinene. This process is catalyzed by the enzyme *retinene isomerase*. However, this process also requires active metabolism and energy transfer to the 11-*cis* retinene; once the 11-*cis* retinene is formed, it automatically recombines with the scotopsin to reform rhodopsin, an exergonic process (which means that it gives off energy). The product, rhodopsin, is a stable compound until its decomposition is again triggered by absorption of light energy.

Excitation of the Rods When Rhodopsin Decomposes. Although the exact way in which rhodopsin decomposition excites the rod is still speculative, it is believed to occur in the following general way: When the all-*trans* retinene begins to split away from the scotopsin, several ionized radicals are momentarily exposed, and these are believed to excite the rod in one of several ways. One suggestion has been that the instantaneous ionic field of the radicals causes changes in the membrane of the rod that are responsible for the rod excitation. The physical construction of the outer segment of the rod is compatible with this concept because the cell membrane folds inward to form tremendous numbers of shelf-like discs lying one on top of the other, each one lined on the inside of the membrane with aggregates of rhodopsin. This extensive relationship between rhodopsin and the cell membrane could explain why the rod is so exquisitely sensitive to light, being capable of detectable excitation following absorption of only one quantum of light energy.

A second theory for excitation of the rod is that the momentarily ionized all-*trans* retinene-scotopsin complex acts as an enzyme to promote some yet unspecified chemical reaction in the outer segment of the rod. This reaction in turn supposedly leads to rod excitation.

Generation of the Receptor Potential. Regardless of the precise mechanism by which the membrane of the outer segment becomes altered in the presence of decomposing rhodopsin, it is known that this excitation process *de-creases* the conductance of this membrane for sodium ions. It has also been shown that the inner segment of the rod continually pumps sodium from inside the rod to the outside. Based on these two facts, the following theory for development of the receptor potential has been proposed:

Figure 17–6 illustrates movement of sodium ions in a complete electrical circuit through the inner and outer segments of the rod. The inner segment continually pumps sodium from inside the rod to the outside, thereby creating a negative potential on the inside of the entire cell. However, the membrane of the outer segment of the rod, in the unexcited condition, is very leaky to sodium. Therefore, sodium continually leaks back to the inside of the rod and thereby

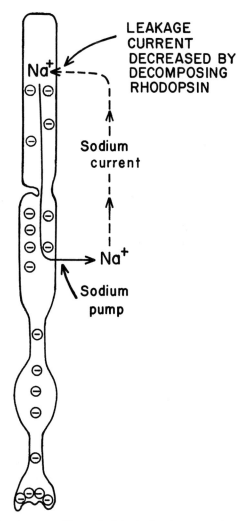

Figure 17–6. Theoretical basis for the generation of a hyperpolarization receptor potential caused by rhodopsin decomposition.

neutralizes much of the negativity on the inside of the entire cell. Thus, under normal conditions, when the rod is not excited, there is a reduced amount of electronegativity inside the membrane of the rod.

When the rhodopsin in the outer segment of the rod is exposed to light and begins to decompose, however, this *decreases* the leakage of sodium to the interior of the rod even though still more and more sodium continues to be pumped out. Thus, a net loss of sodium from the rod creates increased negativity inside the membrane, and the greater the amount of light energy striking the rod, the greater the electronegativity. This process is called *hyperpolarization*. Furthermore, it is exactly opposite to the effect that occurs in almost all other sensory receptors in which the degree of negativity is generally reduced during stimulation rather than increased, producing a state of depolarization rather than hyperpolarization.

Characteristics of the Receptor Potential. The receptor potential has two phases: an instantaneous very low voltage phase, the electrical potential of which is directly proportional to the light energy; and a secondary phase of much greater voltage, the potential of which is proportional to the logarithm of the light energy. The first potential is believed to result from the immediate interaction of light with the rhodopsin. The second is believed to result from the sodium current mechanism described above.

This transduction of light energy into a logarithmic type of receptor potential seems to be an exceedingly important one for function of the eye, because it allows the eye to discriminate light intensities through a range many thousand times as great as would otherwise be possible. In general, regardless of the original light intensity, the eye can detect an increase in light intensity when this increase is about 0.5 to 1 per cent over the intensity already existing, which again illustrates a logarithmic type of response of the retina.

Relationship Between Retinene and Vitamin A. The lower part of the scheme in Figure 17–5 illustrates that each of the two types of retinene can be converted into a corresponding type of vitamin A, and in turn the two types of vitamin A can be reconverted into the two types of retinene. Thus, the two retinenes are in equilibrium with vitamin A. Most of the vitamin A of the retina is stored in the pigment layer of the retina rather than in the rods themselves, but this vitamin A is readily available to the rods.

Retinene is formed from vitamin A by dehydrogenation in accordance with the following reaction:

$$C_{19}H_{27}CH_2OH + DPN^+ \quad \underset{\xrightarrow{\hspace{2cm}}}{\overset{\text{Alcohol dehydrogenase}}{\xleftarrow{\hspace{2cm}}}}$$

$$\underset{\text{Vitamin A}}{}$$

$$\underset{\text{Retinene}}{C_{19}H_{27}CHO} + DPNH + H^+$$

The equilibrium of this equation is strongly in favor of vitamin A. Therefore, vitamin A concentration is normally far greater than free retinene concentration in the retina.

Another important feature of the conversion of retinene into vitamin A, or the converse conversion of vitamin A into retinene, is that these processes require a much longer time to approach equilibrium than it takes for conversion of retinene and scotopsin into rhodopsin, or for conversion (under the influence of strong light energy) of rhodopsin into retinene and scotopsin. Therefore, all the reactions of the upper part of Figure 17–5 can take place relatively rapidly in comparison with the slow interconversions between retinene and vitamin A.

Yet, if the retina remains exposed to strong light for a long time, most of the stored rhodopsin will eventually be converted into retinene and then into vitamin A, thereby decreasing the concentration of all the photochemicals in the rods much more than would be true were it not for this subsequent interconversion from retinene to vitamin A.

Conversely, during total darkness, essentially all the retinene in the rods becomes converted into rhodopsin, thereby reducing the concentration of retinene almost to zero. This then allows much of the vitamin A to be converted into retinene, which also becomes rhodopsin within another few minutes. Thus, in complete darkness not only is almost all the retinene of the rods converted into rhodopsin but also much of the vitamin A stored in the pigment layer of the retina is absorbed by the rods and also converted into rhodopsin.

Night Blindness. Night blindness occurs in severe vitamin A deficiency. When the total quantity of vitamin A in the blood becomes greatly reduced, the quantities of vitamin A, retinene, and rhodopsin in the rods, as well as the color photosensitive chemicals in the cones, are all depressed, thus decreasing the sensitivities of the rods and cones. This condition is called night blindness because at night the amount of available light is far too little to permit adequate vision, though in daylight, sufficient light is available to excite the rods and cones despite their reduction in photochemical substances.

For night blindness to occur, a person often must remain on a vitamin A deficient diet for weeks or months, because large quantities of vitamin A are normally stored in the liver and are made available to the rest of the body in times of need. However, once night blindness does develop it can sometimes be completely cured in a half hour or more by intravenous injection of vitamin A. This results from the ready conversion of vitamin A into retinene and thence into rhodopsin.

PHOTOCHEMISTRY OF COLOR VISION BY THE CONES

It was pointed out at the outset of this discussion that the photochemicals in the cones have almost exactly the same chemical compositions as rhodopsin in the rods. The only difference is that the protein portions, the opsins, called *photopsins* in the cones, are different from the scotopsin of the rods. The retinene portions are exactly the same in the cones as in the rods. The color-sensitive pigments of the cones, therefore, are combinations of retinene and photopsins.

In the discussion of color vision later in the chapter, it will become evident that three different types of pigments are present in different cones, thus making these cones selectively sensitive to the different colors, blue, green, and red. The absorption characteristics of the pigments in the three types of cones show peak absorbancies at light wavelengths, respectively, of 430, 535, and 575 millimicrons. These are also the wavelengths for peak light sensitivity for each type of cone, which begins to explain how the retina differentiates the colors. The approximate absorption curves for these three pigments are shown in Figure 17–7. The peak absorption for the rhodopsin of the rods, on the other hand, occurs at 505 millimicrons.

Note that the peak absorption of the so-called "red" cone is actually in the orange color band. It is called the "red" cone because it responds to red more intensely than do any of the other cones.

AUTOMATIC REGULATION OF RETINAL SENSITIVITY—DARK AND LIGHT ADAPTATION

Relationship of Sensitivity to Pigment Concentration. The sensitivity of rods is approximately proportional to the antilogarithm of the rhodopsin concentration, and it is assumed that

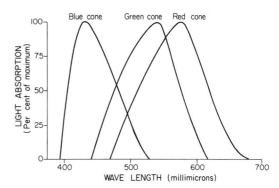

Figure 17–7. Light absorption by the respective pigments of the three color receptive cones of the human retina. (Drawn from curves recorded by Marks, Dobelle, and MacNichol, Jr.: *Science,* 143:1181, 1964, and by Brown and Wald: *Science,* 144:45, 1964.)

this relationship also holds true in the cones. This means that a minute decrease in rhodopsin reduces the sensitivity of rods tremendously. For instance, the sensitivity of a rod is reduced about 8.5 times when its concentration of rhodopsin is reduced from maximum by only 0.006 per cent, and the sensitivity decreases over 3000 times when the rhodopsin concentration is reduced 0.6 per cent. This antilog effect is postulated to result from the fact that the first rhodopsin to be decomposed on exposure to light lies near the surface of the membrane discs in the rod. After this portion has decomposed, far greater decomposition of the deeper layers of rhodopsin is required to excite the rods.

In summary, the sensitivity of the rods and cones can be altered up or down tremendously by only slight changes in concentrations of the photosensitive chemicals.

Light and Dark Adaptation. If a person has been in bright light for a long time, large proportions of the photochemicals in both the rods and cones have been reduced to retinene and opsins. Furthermore, most of the retinene of both the rods and cones has been converted into vitamin A. Because of these two effects, the concentrations of the photosensitive chemicals are considerably reduced, and the sensitivity of the eye to light is even more reduced. This is called *light adaptation.*

On the other hand, if the person remains in the darkness for a long time, essentially all the retinene and opsins in the rods and cones become converted into light-sensitive pigments. Furthermore, large amounts of vitamin A are converted into retinene, which is then changed into additional light-sensitive pigments, the final limit being determined by the amount of opsins in the rods and cones. Because of these two effects, the visual receptors gradually become so sensitive that even the minutest amount of light causes excitation. This is called *dark adaptation*.

Figure 17–8 illustrates the course of dark adaptation when a person is exposed to total darkness after having been exposed to bright light for several hours. Note that retinal sensitivity is very low when one first enters the darkness, but within 1 minute the sensitivity has increased 10-fold—that is, the retina can respond to light of one-tenth intensity. At the end of 20 minutes the sensitivity has increased about 6000-fold, and at the end of 40 minutes it has increased about 25,000-fold.

The resulting curve of Figure 17–8 is called the *dark adaptation curve*. Note, however, the inflection in the curve. The early portion of the curve is caused by adaptation of the cones, for these adapt much more rapidly than the rods because of a basic difference in the rate at which they resynthesize their photosensitive pigments. On the other hand, the cones do not achieve anywhere near the same degree of sensitivity as the rods. Therefore, despite rapid adaptation by the cones, they cease adapting after only a few minutes, while the slowly adapting rods continue to adapt for many minutes or even hours, their sensitivity increasing tremendously. However, a large share of the greater sensitivity of the rods is caused by convergence of as many as 100 rods onto a single ganglion cell in the retina; these rods summate to increase their sensitivity, as will be discussed in the following chapter.

Figure 17–9. Dark and light adaptation. (The retina is considered to have a sensitivity of 1 when maximally light-adapted.)

Figure 17–9 illustrates dark adaptation, but in this figure it is shown that the rate of dark adaptation differs depending on the previous degree of exposure of the retina to light. Curve number 1 shows the dark adaptation after a person had been in bright light for approximately 20 minutes, curve number 2 shows the rate after he had been in bright light for only a minute or so, and curve number 3 after he had been in bright light for many hours. Note that the eye exposed to bright light for a long time adapts slowly in comparison with the eye that has been in bright light for only a few minutes. The cause of this difference is probably the slowness of the interconversions between vitamin A and retinene, particularly the necessity for vitamin A to be absorbed into the rods and cones from the pigment layer of the retina. The eye that has remained in bright light for only a minute or so has not converted significant quantities of its retinene into vitamin A. Therefore, this eye can resynthesize its photosensitive pigments in a short time. Conversely, the eye that has been exposed to prolonged bright light will have had time to convert most of its retinene into vitamin A, and since the reconversion from vitamin A to retinene is very slow, dark adaptation of the eye also is slow.

To the right in Figure 17–9 is shown a typical light adaptation curve, illustrating that light adaptation occurs much more rapidly than dark adaptation. Also, the slow component caused by retinene-vitamin A interconversion does not play as prominent a role in light adaptation as in dark adaptation. Therefore, a person exposed to extremely bright light after having been in prolonged darkness becomes adjusted to the new light conditions in only a few minutes. This is in contrast to dark adaptation, which requires 10 to 20 minutes for moderate adaptation and 10 to 18 hours for maximal adaptation.

Other Mechanisms of Light and Dark Adaptation. In addition to adaptation caused by changes in concentrations of rhodopsin or color photochemicals, the eye has two other mechanisms for light and dark adaptation. The first of these is the *change in pupillary size,* which was discussed in the previous chapter. This can cause a degree of adaptation by approximately 20- to 30-fold because of changes in the light allowed through the pupillary opening.

Figure 17–8. Dark adaptation, illustrating the relationship of cone adaptation to rod adaptation.

The other mechanism is *neural adaptation,* involving the neurons in the successive stages of the visual chain in the retina itself. That is, when the light intensity first increases, the intensity of the signals transmitted by the bipolar cells, the horizontal cells, the amacrine cells, and the ganglion cells, are all very intense. However, the intensities of these signals all decrease rapidly with time. Although the degree of this adaptation is only a few-fold rather than the many thousand-fold that occurs during adaptation of the photochemical system, this neural adaptation occurs in seconds in contrast to the many minutes required for full adaptation by the photochemicals.

Value of Light and Dark Adaptation in Vision.

Between the limits of maximal dark adaptation and maximal light adaptation, the eye can change its sensitivity to light by as much as 500,000 to 1,000,000 times, the sensitivity automatically adjusting to changes in illumination.

Since the registration of images by the retina requires detection of both dark and light spots in the image, it is essential that the sensitivity of the retina always be adjusted so that the receptors respond to the lighter areas and not to the darker areas. An example of maladjustment of the retina occurs when a person leaves a movie theater and enters the bright sunlight, for even the dark spots in the images then seem exceedingly bright, and, as a consequence, the entire visual image is bleached, having little contrast between its different parts. Obviously, this is poor vision, and it remains poor until the retina has adapted sufficiently that the dark spots of the image no longer stimulate the receptors excessively.

Conversely, when a person enters darkness, the sensitivity of the retina is usually so slight that even the light spots in the image cannot excite the retina. But, after dark adaptation, the light spots begin to register. As an example of the extremes of light and dark adaptation, the light intensity of the sun is approximately 30,000 times that of the moon; yet the eye can function well both in bright sunlight and in bright moonlight.

Negative After-Images.

If one looks steadily at a scene for a while, the bright portions of the image cause light adaptation of the retina while the dark portions of the image cause dark adaptation. In other words, areas of the retina that are stimulated by light become less sensitive while areas that are exposed only to darkness gain in sensitivity. If the person then moves his eyes away from the scene and looks at a bright white surface he sees exactly the same scene that he had been viewing, but the light areas of the scene now appear dark, and the dark areas appear light. This is known as the negative after-image, and

it is a natural consequence of light and dark adaptation.

The negative after-image persists as long as any degree of light and dark adaptation remains in the respective portions of the retina. Referring back to Figure 17–9, one can see from the dark adaptation curves that a negative after-image could possibly persist as long as an hour under favorable conditions.

Photopic versus Scotopic Vision.

Photopic vision means vision capable of discriminating color, whereas *scotopic vision* means vision capable of discriminating only between shades of black and white. In bright light one finds that his vision is photopic, whereas below a critical light intensity his vision is scotopic. The reasons for this difference is the following: In very dim light, only rods are capable of becoming dark-adapted to a sensitivity level required for light detection. Therefore, in dim light the retina is capable only of scotopic vision. On the other hand, in very bright light, the rods become light-adapted to the point that they either become inoperative or overshadowed by the signals from the cones; in contrast, the cones find bright light especially suitable for optimal function. Some physiologists believe that the cones in bright light inhibit rod function by transmitting inhibiting signals through the horizontal cells to the synaptic bodies of the rods. At any rate, in bright light, function of the retina appears to be based almost entirely on cone detection of the light signals.

FUSION OF FLICKERING LIGHTS BY THE RETINA

A flickering light is one whose intensity alternately increases and decreases rapidly. An instantaneous flash of light excites the visual receptors for as long as $1/10$ to $1/5$ second, and because of the *persistence* of excitation, rapidly successive flashes of light become *fused* together to give the appearance of being continuous. This effect is well known when one observes motion pictures or television. The images on the motion picture screen are flashed at a rate of 24 frames per second, while those of the television screen are flashed at a rate of 60 frames per second. As a result, the images fuse together, and continuous motion is observed.

The frequency at which flicker fusion occurs, called the *critical frequency for fusion,* varies with the light intensity. Figure 17–10 illustrates the effect of intensity of illumination on the critical fusion frequency. At a low intensity, fusion results even when the rate of flicker is as low as 2 to 6 per second. However, in bright illumina-

Figure 17–10. Relationship of intensity of illumination to the critical frequency for fusion.

tion, the critical frequency for fusion rises to as great as 60 flashes per second. This difference results at least partly from the fact that the cones, which operate mainly at high levels of illumination, can detect much more rapid alterations in illumination than can the rods, which are the important receptors in dim light.

COLOR VISION

From the preceding sections, we know that different cones are sensitive to different colors of light. The present section is a discussion of the mechanisms by which the retina detects the different gradations of color in the visual spectrum.

THE TRI-COLOR THEORY OF COLOR PERCEPTION

Many different theories have been proposed to explain the phenomenon of color vision, but they are all based on the well-known observation that the human eye can detect almost all gradations of colors when red, green, and blue monochromatic lights are appropriately mixed in different combinations.

The first important theory of color vision was that of Young, which was later expanded and given more experimental basis by Helmholtz. Therefore, the theory is known as the *Young-Helmholtz theory*. According to this theory, there are three different types of cones, each of which responds maximally to a different color.

As time has gone by, the Young-Helmholtz theory has been expanded, and more details have been worked out. It now is generally accepted as the mechanism of color vision.

Spectral Sensitivities of the Three Types of Cones. On the basis of psychological tests, the spectral sensitivities of the three different types of cones in human beings are essentially the same as the light absorption curves for the three types of pigment found in the respective cones. These were illustrated in Figure 17–7, and they can readily explain almost all the phenomena of color vision.

Interpretation of Color in the Nervous System. Referring again to Figure 17–7, one can see that a red monochromatic light with a wavelength of 610 millimicrons stimulates the red cones to a stimulus value of approximately 0.75 (75 per cent of the peak stimulation at optimum wavelength), while it stimulates the green cones to a stimulus value of approximately 0.13 and the blue cones not at all. Thus, the ratios of stimulation of the three different types of cones in this instance are 75:13:0. The nervous system interprets this set of ratios as the sensation of red. On the other hand, a monochromatic blue light with a wavelength of 450 millimicrons stimulates the red cones to a stimulus value of 0, the green cones to a value of 0.14 and the blue cones to a value of 0.86. This set of ratios—0:14:86—is interpreted by the nervous system as blue. Likewise, ratios of 100:50:0 are interpreted as orange-yellow and 50:85:15 as green.

This scheme also shows how it is possible for a person to perceive a sensation of yellow when a red light and a green light are shone into the eye at the same time, for this stimulates the red and green cones approximately equally, which gives a sensation of yellow even though no wavelength of light corresponding to yellow is present.

Perception of White Light. Approximately equal stimulation of all the red, green, and blue cones gives one the sensation of seeing white. Yet there is no wavelength of light corresponding to white; instead, white is a combination of all the wavelengths of the spectrum. Furthermore, the sensation of white can be achieved by stimulating the retina with a proper combination of only three chosen colors that stimulate the respective types of cones.

Integration of Color Sensations by the Retina and the Brain. From psychological studies, we know that the interpretation of color

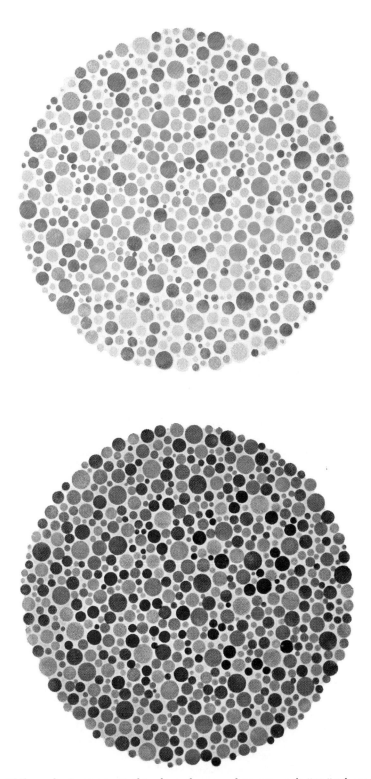

Figure 17–11. Two Ishihara charts: *Upper:* In this chart, the normal person reads "74," whereas the red-green color blind person reads "21." *Lower:* In this chart, the red-blind person (protanope) reads "2," while the green-blind person (deuteranope) reads "4." The normal person reads "42." (From Ishihara: Tests for Colour-Blindness. Tokyo, Kanehara and Co.)

is performed partly by the retina and partly by the brain. If a person places a monochromatic green filter in front of his left eye and a monochromatic red filter in front of his right eye the visual object appears mainly yellow. This integration of color sensations obviously could not be occurring in the retina because one retina is allowed to respond only to green light and the other only to red light. However, sensations perceived in this way are not as clearly mixed as those perceived when the two monochromatic lights are mixed in the same retina. Therefore, at least some degree of the interpretation of color occurs in the retina itself even before the light information is transmitted into the brain. Some of the known features of color signal processing in the neuronal cells of the retina will be presented in the following chapter.

COLOR BLINDNESS

Red-Green Color Blindness. When a single group of color receptive cones is missing from the eye, the person is unable to distinguish some colors from others. As can be observed by studying Figure 17-7, if the red cones are missing, light of 525 to 625 millimicrons wavelength can stimulate only the green-sensitive cones, so that the *ratio* of stimulation of the different cones does not change as the color changes from green all the way through the red spectrum. Therefore, within this wavelength range, all colors appear to be the same to this "color blind" person.

On the other hand, if the green-sensitive cones are missing, the colors in the range from green to red can stimulate only the red-sensitive cones, and the person also perceives only one color within these limits. Therefore, when a person lacks either the red or green types of cones, he is said to be "red-green" color blind. However, when one or more types of cones are abnormal but still function partially, a person has "color weakness," instead of color blindness.

The person with loss of red cones is called a *protanope;* his overall visual spectrum is noticeably shortened at the long wavelength end because of lack of the red cones. The color blind person who lacks green cones is called a *deuteranope;* this person has a perfectly normal visual spectral width because the absent green cones operate in the middle of the spectrum where red or blue cones also operate.

Blue Weakness. Occasionally, a person has "blue weakness," which results from diminished or absent blue receptors. If we observe Figure 17-7 once again, we can see that the blue cones are sensitive to a spectral range almost entirely different from that of both the red and green cones. Therefore, if the blue receptors are completely absent, the person has a greater preponderance of green, yellow, orange,

and red in his visual spectrum than he has of blue, thus producing this rarely observed type of color weakness or blindness.

Tests for Color Blindness. Tests for color blindness depend on the person's ability to distinguish various colors from each other and also on his ability to judge correctly the degree of contrast between colors. For instance, to determine whether or not a person is red-green color blind, he may be given many small tufts of wool whose colors encompass the entire visual spectrum. He is then asked to place those tufts that have the same colors in the same piles. If he is not color blind, he recognizes immediately that all the tufts have slightly different colors; however, if he is red-green color blind, he places the red, orange, yellow, and yellow-green colors all together as having essentially the same color.

Stilling and Ishihara Test Charts. A rapid method for determining color blindness is based on the use of spot-charts such as those illustrated in Figure 17-11. These charts are arranged with a confusion of spots of several different colors. In the top chart, the normal person reads "74," while the red-green color blind person reads "21." In the bottom chart, the normal person reads "42," while the red blind protanope reads "2," and the green blind deuteranope reads "4."

If one will study these charts while at the same time observing the spectral sensitivity curves of the different cones in Figure 17-7, he can readily understand how excessive emphasis can be placed on spots of certain colors by color blind persons in comparison with normal persons.

Genetics of Color Blindness. Color blindness is sex-linked and probably results from absence of appropriate color genes in the X chromosomes. This lack of color genes is a recessive trait; therefore, color blindness will not appear as long as another X chromosome carries the genes necessary for development of the respective color-receptive cones.

Because the male human being has only one X chromosome, all three color genes must be present in this single chromosome if he is not to be color blind. In approximately 1 out of every 50 times, the X chromosome lacks the red gene; in approximately 1 out of every 16 it lacks the green gene; and rarely it lacks the blue gene. This means, therefore, that 2 per cent of all men are red color blind (protanopes) and that 6 per cent are green color blind (deuteranopes), making a total of approximately 8 per cent who are red-green color blind. Because a female has two X chromosomes, red-green color blindness is a rare abnormality in the female, occurring in only 1 out or every 250 women.

REFERENCES

Alpern, M.: Distal mechanisms of vertebrate color vision. *Ann. Rev. Physiol.*, 30:279, 1968.
Bitensky, M. W., Miki, N., Marcus, F. R., and Keirns, J. J.: The role of cyclic nucleotides in visual excitation. *Life Sci.*, 13:1451, 1973.

Brindley, G. S.: Physiology of the Retina and Visual Pathway, 2nd Ed. Baltimore, The Williams & Wilkins Company, 1970.

Brown, J. L.: Visual sensitivity. *Ann. Rev. Psychol.*, 24:151, 1973.

Ciba Foundation: Color Vision: Physiology and Experimental Psychology. Boston, Little, Brown and Company, 1965.

Davson, H.: The Physiology of the Eye, 3rd Ed. New York, Academic Press, Inc., 1972.

Daw, N. W.: Neurophysiology of color vision. *Physiol. Rev.*, 53:571, 1973.

Duke-Elder, S. (ed.): Diseases of the Retina. *In* Systems of Ophthalmology. Vol. 10. St. Louis, The C. V. Mosby Company, 1967.

Enright, J. T.: Stereopsis, visual latency, and three-dimensional moving pictures. *Amer. Sci.*, 58:536, 1970.

Fine, B. S., and Yanoff, M.: Ocular Histology. Hagerstown, Md., Harper & Row, Publishers, 1972.

Gamow, R. I., and Harris, J. F.: The infrared receptors of snakes. *Sci. Amer.*, 228:94, 1973.

Graymore, C. N. (ed.): Biochemistry of the Eye. New York, Academic Press, Inc., 1970.

Linksz, A.: An Essay on Color Vision and Clinical Color Vision Tests. New York, Grune & Stratton, Inc., 1964.

MacNichol, E. F., Jr.: Three-pigment color vision. *Sci. Amer.*, 211:48, 1964.

Marks, W. B., Dobelle, W. H., and MacNichol, E. E., Jr.: Visual pigments of single primate cones. *Science, 143*:1181, 1964.

Maturana, H. R., Uribe, G., and Frenk, S.: A biological theory of relativistic color coding in the primate retina. *Arch. Biol. Med. Exp. (Santiago), 1*:1, 1968.

Michael, C. R.: Color vision. *New Engl. J. Med., 288*:724, 1973.

Millodot, M.: Variation of visual acuity in the central region of the retina. *Brit. J. Physiol. Opt., 27*:24, 1972.

Padgham, C. A., and Saunders, J. E.: The Perception of Light and Color. New York, Academic Press, Inc., 1975.

Ripps, H., and Weale, R. A.: The photophysiology of vertebrate color vision. *Photophysiology, 5*:127, 1970.

Stabell, B., and Stabell, U.: Chromatic rod vision. IX. A theoretical survey. *Vision Res., 13*:449, 1973.

Tomita, T., Miller, W. H., Hashimoto, Y., and Saito, T.: Electrical response of retinal cells as a sign of transport. *Exp. Eye Res., 16*:327, 1973.

Van der Tweel, L. H., and Estévez, O.: Subjective and objective evaluation of flicker. *Ophthalmologica, 169*:70, 1974.

Wald, G.: Proceedings: visual pigments and photoreceptors—review and outlook. *Exp. Eye Res., 18*:333, 1974.

Wasserman, G. S.: Invertebrate color vision and the tuned-receptor paradigm. *Science, 180*:268, 1973.

Werblin, F. S.: The control of sensitivity in the retina. *Sci. Amer., 228*:70, 1973.

Young, R. W.: Visual cells, *Sci. Amer., 223*:80, 1970.

Young, R. W.: Proceedings: Biogenesis and renewal of visual cell outer segment membranes. *Exp. Eye Res., 18*:215, 1974.

| 18 |

The Eye:
III. Neurophysiology of Vision

THE VISUAL PATHWAY

Figure 18–1 illustrates the visual pathway from the two retinae back to the *visual cortex*. After impulses leave the retinae they pass backward through the *optic nerves*. At the *optic chiasm* all the fibers from the opposite nasal halves of the retinae cross to the side where they join the fibers from the opposite temporal retinae to form the *optic tracts*. The fibers of each optic tract synapse in the *lateral geniculate body* and from here, the *geniculocalcarine fibers* pass through the *optic radiation*, or *geniculocalcarine tract*, to the *optic* or *visual cortex* in the calcarine area of the occipital lobe.

In addition, visual fibers pass to lower areas of the brain: (1) from the lateral geniculate body to the lateral thalamus, the superior colliculi, and the pretectal nuclei; (2) from the optic tracts directly to the superior colliculi; and (3) from the optic tracts directly into the pretectal nuclei of the brain stem.

NEURAL FUNCTION OF THE RETINA

NEURAL ORGANIZATION OF THE RETINA

The detailed anatomy of the retina was illustrated in Figure 17–1 of the preceding chapter, and Figure 18–2 illustrates the basic essentials of the retina's neural connections; to the left is the general organization of the neural elements in a peripheral retinal area and to the right the

organization of the foveal area. Note that in the peripheral region both rods and cones converge on *bipolar cells* which in turn converge on *ganglion cells*. In the fovea, where only cones exist, there is little or no convergence; instead, the cones are represented by approximately equal numbers of bipolar and ganglion cells.

Not emphasized in the figure is the fact that in both the outer and inner plexiform layers (where the neurons synapse with each other) there are many lateral connections between the different neural elements. Many of these lateral

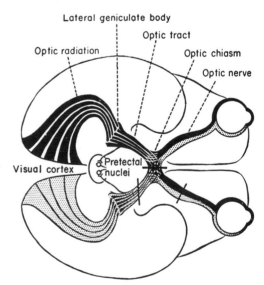

Figure 18–1. The visual pathways from the eyes to the visual cortex. (Modified from Polyak: The Retina. University of Chicago Press, 1941.)

256

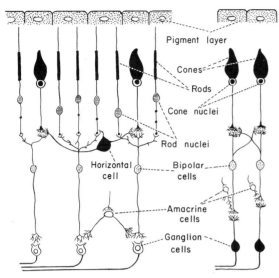

Figure 18–2. Neural organization of the retina: peripheral area to the left, foveal area to the right.

connections are collateral branches of the dendrites and axons of the bipolar and ganglion cells. But, in addition, two special types of cells are present in the inner nuclear layer that transmits signals laterally: (1) the *horizontal cells,* and (2) the *amacrine cells.*

Each retina contains about 125 million rods and 5.5 million cones; yet, as counted with the light microscope, only 900,000 optic nerve fibers lead from the retina to the brain. Thus, an average of 140 rods plus 6 cones converge on each optic nerve fiber. However, there are major differences between the peripheral retina and the central retina, for nearer the fovea, fewer and fewer rods and cones converge on each optic fiber, and the rods and cones both become slenderer. These two effects progressively increase the acuity of vision toward the central retina. In the very central portion, in the fovea, there are no rods at all. Also, the number of optic nerve fibers leading from this part of the retina is almost equal to the number of cones in the fovea, as shown to the right in Figure 18–2. This mainly explains the high degree of visual acuity in the central portion of the retina in comparison with the very poor acuity in the peripheral portions.

Another difference between the peripheral and central portions of the retina is that there is considerably greater sensitivity of the peripheral retina to weak light. This results partly from the fact that as many as 600 rods converge on the same optic nerve fiber in the most peripheral portions of the retina; the signals from these rods summate to give intense stimulation of the peripheral ganglion cells. The rods are also more sensitive to weak light than are the cones.

STIMULATION OF THE RODS AND CONES—THE RECEPTOR POTENTIAL

Stimulation of the rods and cones was discussed at length in the preceding chapter. Briefly, when light strikes either of these receptors, it decomposes a photochemical that in turn acts on the membrane of the *outer segment* of the receptor (the part that protrudes into the pigment layer) to cause a sustained *receptor potential* that lasts as long as the light continues. However, as pointed out in the previous chapter, this receptor potential is different from all other receptor potentials that have been recorded, for it is a hyperpolarization signal rather than a depolarization signal, and its intensity is proportional to the logarithm of light energy in contrast to the more linear response of many other receptors. This logarithmic response seems to be very important to vision, because it allows the eyes to detect contrasts in the image even when light intensities vary many thousand-fold, an effect that would not be possible if there were linear transduction of the signal.

Receptor potentials are transmitted unchanged through the bodies of the rods and cones. Neither the rods nor the cones generate action potentials. Instead, the receptor potentials themselves, acting at the synaptic bodies, induce signals directly in the successive neurons by *electrotonic* current flow across the synaptic gaps.

STIMULATION OF THE BIPOLAR AND HORIZONTAL CELLS

The synaptic bodies of the rods and cones make intimate contact with the dendrites of both the bipolar and horizontal cells. The hyperpolarization that occurs in the rods and cones during stimulation (the receptor potential) is transferred directly to both the bipolar and the horizontal cells. Also, the excitation signal summates in both these cells; that is, the greater the number of rods and cones exciting a single bipolar or horizontal cell, the more intense will be the signal in each of these cells. Furthermore, in both the bipolar and the horizontal cells the transmitted signals are the hyperpolarization potentials themselves—not action potentials. Indeed, action potentials have never been recorded from horizontal cells and only under rare conditions have they been recorded in bipolar cells. Therefore, it is doubtful that any part of the normal physiological visual signal is transmitted in the form of action potentials by either of these two types of cells.

Function of the Bipolar Cells. The bipolar cells are the main transmitting link for the visual signal from the rods and cones to the ganglion cells. In the foveal region of the eye, the region of greatest visual acuity, there is approximately one bipolar cell for each cone, and also approximately one ganglion cell. In the peripheral region several cones converge on a single ganglion cell, and as many as several hundred rods converge. Thus, the peripheral retina is properly organized for great retinal sensitivity to very low light intensities, whereas the central retina (the foveal region) is organized for greatest possible visual acuity and faithfulness of transmission of the signals into the brain.

The bipolar cells are entirely excitatory cells. That is, they can only excite the ganglion cells.

Function of the Horizontal Cells. The horizontal cells lie in the inner nuclear layer and spread widely in the retina, transmitting signals laterally as far as several hundred microns. They are excited directly by the synaptic bodies of the rods and cones and in turn transmit signals mainly to bipolar cells located in areas lateral to the excited rods and cones.

The horizontal cells are *inhibitory* cells, in contrast to the bipolar cells, which are of an excitatory nature. Therefore, the signals transmitted by the horizontal cells from the excited rods and cones cause inhibition of the bipolar cells lateral to the excited point in the retina. That is, excited rods and cones transmit excitatory signals in a direct line through the bipolar cells in the area of excitation but transmit inhibitory signals through the surrounding bipolar cells.

The horizontal cells are of major importance for enhancing and helping to detect contrasts in the visual scene. They are probably also of importance in helping to differentiate colors. Both of these functions will be discussed in subsequent sections of this chapter.

Stimulation and Function of the Amacrine Cells. The amacrine cells, also located in the inner nuclear layer, are excited mainly by the bipolar cells but possibly also directly by the synaptic bodies of the rods and cones. These cells in turn *inhibit* the ganglion cells. However,

their response is a *transient* one rather than the steady, continuous response of the bipolar and horizontal cells. That is, when the photoreceptors are first stimulated, the inhibitory signal transmitted by the amacrine cells is very intense; this signal dies away to almost nothing in a fraction of a second.

Two other differences between the amacrine cells and the bipolar and horizontal cells are that (1) the signal of the amacrine cells is a depolarization signal rather than a hyperpolarization signal, and (2) the amacrine cells transmit their signals to the ganglion cells in two different ways—either as a simple electrotonic depolarization or as occasional action potentials that occur at the onset of the initial depolarization.

STIMULATION OF THE GANGLION CELLS

Spontaneous, Continuous Discharge of the Ganglion Cells. The ganglion cells transmit their signals through the optic nerve fibers to the brain in the form of action potentials. These cells, even when unstimulated, transmit continuous nerve impulses at an average rate of about 5 per second. The visual signal is superimposed onto this basic level of ganglion cell stimulation. It can be either an excitatory signal, with the number of impulses increasing to greater than 5 per second, or it can be an inhibitory signal, with the number of nerve impulses decreasing to below 5 per second—often all the way to zero.

Summation of the Ganglion Cells by Signals from the Bipolar Cells, the Horizontal Cells, and the Amacrine Cells. The bipolar cells transmit the main direct *excitatory* information from the rods and the cones to the ganglion cells: the horizontal cells transmit *inhibitory* information from laterally displaced rods and cones; the amacrine cells transmit direct but short-lived transient signals that signal a *change* in the level of illumination of the retina. Thus, each of these three types of cells performs a separate function in stimulating the ganglion cells.

DIFFERENT TYPES OF SIGNALS TRANSMITTED BY THE GANGLION CELLS THROUGH THE OPTIC NERVE

Transmission of Luminosity Signals. The ganglion cells are of several different types, and they also have different patterns of stimulation by the bipolar, horizontal, and amacrine cells. Some of the ganglion cells respond to the intensity (*luminosity*) of the light falling on the photoreceptors. The rate of impulses from these cells remains at a level greater than the natural rate of firing as long as the luminosity is high. It is the signals from these cells that apprise the brain of the overall level of light intensity of the observed scene. The light and dark flat areas of the scene are also transmitted in this way, but far more information concerning the form of the scene is generally transmitted in terms of contrast borders, as will be discussed below.

Transmission of Signals Depicting Contrasts in the Visual Scene—the Process of Lateral Inhibition.   A large share of the ganglion cells barely respond to the actual level of illumination of the scene; instead they respond only to contrast borders in the scene. Since it seems that this is the major means by which the form of the scene is transmitted to the brain, let us explain how this process occurs.

When flat light is applied to the entire retina—that is, when all the photoreceptors are stimulated equally by the incident light— the contrast type of ganglion cell is neither stimulated nor inhibited. The reason for this is that the signals transmitted *directly* from the photoreceptors through the bipolar cells are excitatory, whereas the signals transmitted from *laterally displaced* photoreceptors through the horizontal cells are inhibitory. These two effects neutralize each other. Now, let us examine what happens when a contrast border occurs in the visual scene. Figure 18–3 shows a spot of light shining on the retina and exciting

Figure 18–4.   Responses of ganglion cells to light in (1) an area excited by a spot of light and (2) an area immediately adjacent to the excited spot; the ganglion cells in this area are inhibited by the mechanism of lateral inhibition. (Modified from Granit: Receptors and Sensory Perception: A Discussion of Aims, Means, and Results of Electrophysiological Research into the Process of Reception. Yale University Press, 1955.)

the photoreceptors. The signal is transmitted directly through the bipolar cells and thence to the ganglion cells in the same area to cause excitation. At the same time these same excited photoreceptors transmit *lateral inhibitory* signals through the horizontal cells to the surrounding bipolar and ganglion cells. Thus, when there is a contrast border, with stimulated photoreceptors on one side of the border and unstimulated photoreceptors on the opposite side of the border, the mutual cancellation of the excitatory signals through the bipolar cells and the inhibitory signals through the horizontal cells no longer occurs. Consequently, the ganglion cells on either side of this border become either excited or inhibited—excited on the light side of the border and inhibited on the dark side.

A linear contrast border acts in almost identically the same way as does a spot of light; all of the ganglion cells on the light side of the border are stimulated and all the dark side are inhibited. On the other hand, all of the contrast type of ganglion cells that lie in the flatly illuminated portion of the scene still remain unstimulated.

This process of contrasting an excitatory signal with an inhibitory signal is exactly the same as the process of *lateral inhibition* that occurs in most other types of sensory signal transmission. The process is a mechanism used by the nervous system for contrast enhancement.

When impulses are recorded from ganglion cells, it is possible to observe the effects of contrast borders on the signals transmitted in the optic nerve fibers. Figure 18–4 illustrates this effect. The upper recording is from a ganglion cell located in the area excited by a spot of light, whereas the lower recording is from a ganglion cell located a few hundred microns to the side of the spot. Note that when the spot of light is turned on the ganglion cell in the center of the

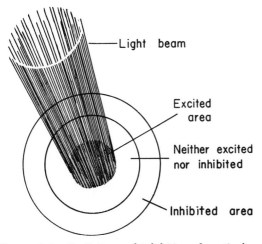

Figure 18–3.   Excitation and inhibition of a retinal area caused by a small beam of light.

light becomes excited while the ganglion cell located laterally becomes inhibited.

Detection of Instantaneous Changes in Light Intensity—the On-Off Response. Many of the ganglion cells are especially excited by *change* in light intensity; this effect most often occurs in the same ganglion cells that transmit contrast border signals. For instance, the upper tracing of Figure 18–4 shows that when the light was first turned on the ganglion cell became strongly excited for a fraction of a second, and then the level of excitation diminished. The bottom tracing shows that a second ganglion cell located in the dark area lateral to the spot of light was deeply depressed at the same time. Then when the light was turned off, exactly the opposite effects occurred. Thus, the responses of these two types of cells are called the "on-off" and the "off-on" responses.

This ability of the retina to detect and transmit signals related to *change* in light intensity is caused by a rapid phase of "adaptation" of some of the neurons in the visual chain. Since this effect is extremely marked in the amacrine cells, it is believed that the amacrine cells are peculiarly adapted to detecting light intensity change.

This capability to detect change in light intensity is especially well developed in the peripheral retina. For instance, a minute gnat flying across the peripheral field of vision is instantaneously detected. On the other hand, the same gnat sitting quietly in the peripheral field of vision remains entirely below the threshold of visual detection.

Transmission of Color Signals by the Ganglion Cells. A single ganglion cell may be stimulated by a number of cones or by only a very few. When all three types of cones—the red, blue, and green types—all stimulate the same ganglion cell, the signal transmitted through the ganglion cell is the same for any color of the spectrum. Therefore, this signal plays no role in the detection of the different colors. Instead, it is called a "luminosity" signal.

On the other hand, many of the ganglion cells are excited by only one color type of cone but are inhibited by a second type. For instance, this frequently occurs for the red and green cones, red causing excitation and green causing inhibition—or, vice versa, that is, green causing excitation and red inhibition. The same type of reciprocal effect also occurs between some blue cones and either red or green cones.

The mechanism of this opposing effect of col-

ors is the following: One color type of cones excites the ganglion cell by the direct excitatory route through a bipolar cell, while the other color type excites the ganglion cell by the indirect inhibitory route through a horizontal cell.

The importance of these color-contrast mechanisms is that they represent a mechanism by which the retina itself differentiates colors. Thus each color-contrast type of ganglion cell is excited by one color but inhibited by the opposite color. Therefore, the process of color analysis begins in the retina and is not entirely a function of the brain.

REGULATION OF RETINAL FUNCTION BY CENTRIFUGAL FIBERS FROM THE CENTRAL NERVOUS SYSTEM

The sensitivity of the retina is at least partially controlled by signals from the central nervous system. Centrifugal fibers pass in the retrograde direction in the optic nerve from the brain to the retina and synapse directly with the ganglion cells. Stimulation of specific areas in the brain can enhance in some instances and diminish in other instances the sensitivities of specific areas of the retina. It is supposed that this represents a mechanism by which the central nervous system can direct one's attention to specific portions of the visual field.

FUNCTION OF THE LATERAL GENICULATE BODY

Anatomical Organization of the Lateral Geniculate Nuclei. Each lateral geniculate body is composed of six nuclear layers. Layers 2, 3, and 5 (from the surface inward) receive signals from the temporal portion of the ipsilateral retina, while layers 1, 4, and 6 receive signals from the nasal retina of the opposite eye.

All layers of the lateral geniculate body relay visual information to the *visual cortex* through the *geniculocalcarine tract*.

The pairing of layers from the two eyes probably plays a major role in *fusion of vision*, because corresponding retinal fields in the two eyes connect with respective neurons that are approximately superimposed over each other in the successive layers. Also, with a little imagination, one can postulate that interaction between the successive layers could be part of the mechanism by which stereoscopic visual depth perception occurs, because this depends on comparing the visual images of the two eyes and determining their slight differences, as was discussed in Chapter 16.

Characteristics of the Visual Signals in the Lateral Geniculate Body

The signals recorded in the relay neurons of the lateral geniculate body are similar to those recorded in the ganglion cells of the retina. A few of the neurons transmit luminosity signals, whereas the majority transmit signals depicting only contrast borders in the visual image; also, many of the neurons are particularly responsive to movement of objects across the visual scene. However, the signals of the geniculate neurons are different from those in the ganglion cells in that a greater number of the complex interactions are found. That is, a much higher percentage of the neurons respond to contrast in the visual scene or to movement. These more complex reactions presumably result from convergence of excitatory and inhibitory signals from two or more ganglion cells on the relay neurons of the lateral geniculate body.

Color Signals in the Lateral Geniculate Body. Signals related to black and white vision are mainly found in layers 1 and 2 of the lateral geniculate body, while color signals occur mainly in layers 3 through 6. A few of the neurons in these last four layers respond to all colors and therefore transmit "white-light" information. However, about three-quarters of the neurons respond to "opponent colors;" that is, a given cell may be excited by red but be inhibited by green. Another cell will operate exactly oppositely. These are called the "red-green" cells. Still other lateral geniculate body cells respond to the opponent colors blue and yellow, with one of these exciting the cell and the other inhibiting it. The mechanism of this effect is the same as in the retina; that is, the effect is caused by convergence of signals from red and green cones onto the same neuron, one of these signals causing inhibition while the other causes excitation.

By various interactions of this type, the color information in the visual scene is gradually dissected, and the information is then transmitted to other sections of the brain as signals that express the *ratios* of different colors in the different areas of the visual scene.

FUNCTION OF THE PRIMARY VISUAL CORTEX

The ability of the visual system to detect spatial organization of the visual scene—that is, to detect the forms of objects, brightness of the individual parts of the objects, shading, and so forth—is dependent on function of the *primary visual cortex*, the anatomy of which is illustrated in Figure 18–5. This area lies mainly in the calcarine fissure located bilaterally on the medial aspect of each occipital cortex. Specific points of the retina connect with specific points of the visual cortex, the right halves of the two respective retinae connecting with the right visual cortex and the left halves connecting with the left visual cortex. The macula is represented at the occipital pole of the visual cortex and the peripheral regions of the retina are represented in concentric circles farther and farther forward from the occipital pole. The upper portion of the retina is represented superiorly in the visual cortex and the lower portion inferiorly. Note the large area of cortex receiving signals from the macular region of the retina. It is in this region that the fovea is represented, which gives the highest degree of visual acuity.

DETECTION OF LINES AND BORDERS BY THE PRIMARY VISUAL CORTEX

If a person looks at a blank wall, only a few neurons of the primary visual cortex will be stimulated, whether the illumination of the wall be bright or weak. Therefore, the question must be asked: What does the visual cortex do? To answer this question, let us now place on the wall a large black cross such as that illustrated to the left in Figure 18–6. To the right is illustrated the spatial pattern of the greater majority of the excited neurons that one finds in the visual cortex. *Note that the areas of excitation occur along the sharp borders of the visual pattern.* Thus, by the time the visual signal is recorded in the primary visual cortex, it is concerned mainly with the *contrasts* in the visual

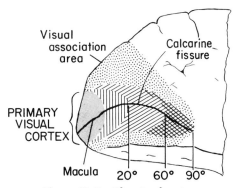

Figure 18–5. The visual cortex.

Retinal Image   Cortical Stimulation

Figure 18–6. Pattern of excitation occurring in the visual cortex in response to a retinal image of a black cross.

scene rather than with the flat areas. At each point in the visual scene where there is a change from dark to light or light to dark, the corresponding area of the primary visual cortex becomes stimulated. The intensity of stimulation is determined by the *gradient of contrast*. That is, the greater the sharpness in the contrast border and the greater the difference in intensities between the light and dark areas, the greater is the degree of stimulation.

Thus, the *pattern of contrasts* in the visual scene is impressed upon the neurons of the visual cortex, and this pattern has a spatial orientation roughly the same as that of the retinal image.

Detection of Orientation of Lines and Borders. Not only does the visual cortex detect the *existence* of lines and borders in the different areas of the retinal image, but it also detects the *orientation* of each line or border—that is, whether it is a vertical or horizontal border, or lies at some degree of inclination. The mechanism of this effect is the following:

In each small area of the visual cortex there are multiple neurons arranged in columns, each column having a diameter of about 0.5 to 1 mm. and extending downward from the surface of the cortex through its six layers. The signals arriving in the cortex from the lateral geniculate body terminate in layer 4, and from here secondary signals spread upward or downward in the column and eventually also to adjacent columns. Some columns of neurons respond to vertical lines or borders, others to lines or borders slightly angulated, still others to lines or borders even more angulated, and so forth. This process of selective stimulation of the separate columns is presumably caused by convergence of signals from two or more nerve fibers arriving from the lateral geniculate body. The effect is similar to that which occurs in the retina, one of the fibers causing inhibition and the other exci-

tation. If the orientation of the border between the dark area and the light area in the visual scene corresponds with the orientation of the neural connections of inhibitory and excitatory input fibers to a given column of the visual cortex, the column would be excited. By having many different cortical columns with slightly different synaptic connections, such interactions could lead to selective stimulation of one column for one orientation of a border, another column for another orientation, and so forth. This represents another stage in the mechanism for deciphering information in the visual scene.

Detection of Length of Lines. Still a higher order for deciphering information from the visual scene is the ability of yet other neuronal columns of cells to be stimulated by lines or borders of specific lengths. An interesting feature of this type of detection is that the lines can be displaced laterally from each other to a slight extent in the visual field and the detection process will continue to occur. This type of detection presumably results from convergence of signals within the visual cortex from the first-stimulated columns of neurons.

To perform all of these functions for deciphering visual information, the primary visual cortex has approximately 200 million neurons—200 times as great as the number of optic nerve fibers from each retina.

Analysis of Color by the Visual Cortex. One finds in the primary visual cortex specific cells that are stimulated by color intensity or by contrasts of the opponent colors, the red-green opponent colors and the blue-yellow opponent colors. These effects are almost identical to those found in the lateral geniculate body. However, the proportion of cells excited by the opponent color contrasts is vastly reduced from the proportion found in the lateral geniculate body. Since neuronal excitation by color contrasts is a means of deciphering color, it is believed that the primary visual cortex is concerned with an even higher order of detection of color than simply the deciphering of color itself, a process that seems to have been mainly completed by the time the signals have passed through the lateral geniculate body.

PERCEPTION OF LUMINOSITY

Although most of the neurons in the visual cortex are mainly responsive to contrasts caused by lines, borders, moving objects, or opponent colors in the visual scene, a few are directly responsive to the levels of luminosity in the different areas of the visual scene. Presumably, it is these cells that detect flat areas in the scene and also the overall level of luminosity.

EFFECT OF REMOVING THE PRIMARY VISUAL CORTEX

Removal of the primary visual cortex in human beings always causes complete blindness for detection of visual patterns. However, a few such persons have displayed very slight capability for detection of crude levels of light intensity. In lower level monkeys this ability to detect light intensity is strongly preserved, with even the capability to determine very crude signals of form, especially visual images related to movement.

TRANSMISSION OF VISUAL INFORMATION INTO OTHER REGIONS OF THE CEREBRAL CORTEX

The primary visual cortex is located in the *calcarine fissure area*, mainly on the medial aspect of each hemisphere but also spreading slightly over the occipital pole. It is known as *Brodmann area 17* of the cortex, and it is also called the *striate area* because of its striated appearance to the naked eye.

Signals from the striate area project laterally in the occipital cortex into area 18 and then into area 19, as illustrated in Figure 18–7. These areas are frequently called the *prestriate areas*, and they are also known as *visual association areas*. In reality, they are simply the loci for additional processing of visual information.

The visual projection images in areas 18 and 19 are organized into columns of cells in the same manner as that described earlier for the primary visual cortex. There is a topographic representation of the visual field as also found in the primary visual cortex. However, the neuronal cells respond to more complex patterns than do those in the primary visual cortex. For instance, some cells are stimulated by simple geometric patterns, such as curving borders, an-

gles, and so forth. It is presumably these progressively more complex interpretations that eventually decode the visual information, giving the person his overall impression of the visual scene that he is observing.

Projection of Visual Information into the Temporal Cortex. From areas 18 and 19 visual signals next proceed to the posterior portion of the inferior temporal gyrus and from here to the posterior portion of the medial temporal gyrus, areas 20 and 21 of the cortex. In these areas simple visual patterns such as lines, borders, angles, and so forth fail to cause excitation of specific neurons. The degree of integration of visual information at this level, such as interpretation of letters or words, is presumably much higher.

Effects of Destruction of the Visual Association Areas. Human beings who have destructive lesions of any of the visual association areas, areas 18 and 19 in the occipital cortex, or areas 20 and 21 in the temporal cortex, have difficulty with certain types of visual perception and visual learning. For instance, destruction in areas 18 and 19 generally makes it difficult to perceive form, such as shapes of objects, their sizes, and their meanings. It is believed that this type of lesion can cause the abnormality known as *dyslexia* or *word blindness*, which means that the person has difficulty understanding the meanings of words that he sees.

Destruction of the temporal projections of the visual system makes it especially difficult for animals, and presumably for human beings as well, to learn tasks that are based upon visual perceptions. For instance, the person might be able to see his plate of food perfectly well but be unable to utilize this visual information to direct his fork toward his food. Yet, when he feels the plate with his other hand, he can use stereotaxic information from the somesthetic cortex to direct the fork accurately.

Effects of Electrical Stimulation of the Visual Areas. Electrical stimulation in the primary visual cortex or in the parietal association areas, areas 18 and 19, causes a person to have simple optic auras—that is, flashes of light, simple colors, or simple forms such as lines, stars, or so forth—but he does not see complicated forms.

Stimulation of the visual association areas of the temporal cortex, areas 20 and 21, occasionally elicits complicated visual perceptions, sometimes causing the person to see a scene that he had known many years before. This is in keeping with the interpretative function of this area for visual function.

THE FIELDS OF VISION; PERIMETRY

The *field of vision* is the area seen by an eye at a given instant. The area seen to the nasal side is called the *nasal field of vision,* and the area seen to the lateral side is called the *temporal field of vision.*

To diagnose blindness in specific portions of the

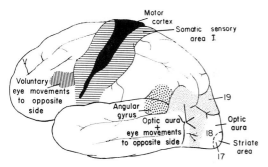

Figure 18–7. The visual association fields and the cortical areas for control of eye movements.

retinae, one charts the field of vision for each eye by a process known as *perimetry*. This is done by having the subject look with one eye toward a central spot directly in front of the eye. Then a small dot of light or a small object is moved back and forth in all areas of the field of vision, both laterally and nasally and upward and downward, and the person indicates when he can see the spot of light or object and when he cannot see it. At the same time, a chart (Fig. 18–8) is made for the eye, showing the areas in which the subject can see the spot and in which he cannot see it. Thus, the field of vision is plotted.

In all perimetry charts, a blind spot caused by lack of rods and cones in the retina over the optic disc is found approximately 15 degrees lateral to the central point of vision, as illustrated in the figure.

Abnormalities in the Fields of Vision. Occasionally blind spots are found in other portions of the field of vision besides the optic disc area. Such blind spots are called *scotomata;* they frequently result from allergic reactions in the retina or from toxic conditions, such as lead poisoning or even excessive use of tobacco.

Still another condition that can be diagnosed by perimetry is *retinitis pigmentosa*. In this disease, portions of the retina degenerate and excessive melanin pigment deposits in the degenerated areas. Retinitis pigmentosa generally causes blindness in the peripheral field of vision first and then gradually encroaches on the central areas.

Effect of Lesions in the Optic Pathway on the Fields of Vision. One of the most important uses of perimetry is for localization of lesions in the visual nervous system. Lesions in the optic nerve, in the optic chiasm, in the optic tract, and in the geniculocalcarine tract all cause blind areas in the visual fields, and the "patterns" of these blind areas indicate the location of the lesion in the optic pathway.

Destruction of an entire *optic nerve* obviously causes blindness of the respective eye. Destruction of the *optic chiasm,* as shown by the longitudinal line

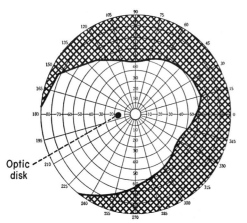

Figure 18–8. A perimetry chart, showing the field of vision for the left eye.

across the chiasm in Figure 18–1, prevents the passage of impulses from the nasal halves of the two retinae to the opposite optic tracts. Therefore, the nasal halves are both blinded, which means that the person is blind in both temporal fields of vision; this condition is called *bitemporal hemianopsia*. Such lesions frequently result from tumors of the adenohypophysis pressing upward on the optic chiasm.

Interruption of an *optic tract,* which is also shown by a line in Figure 18–1, denervates the corresponding half of each retina on the same side as the lesion, and, as a result, neither eye can see objects to the opposite side. This condition is known as *homonymous hemianopsia*. Destruction of the *optic radiation* or the *visual cortex* of one side also causes homonymous hemianopsia. A common condition that destroys the visual cortex is thrombosis of the posterior cerebral artery, which infarcts the occipital cortex except for the foveal area, thus sparing central vision.

One can differentiate a lesion in the optic tract from a lesion in the geniculocalcarine tract or visual cortex by determining whether impulses can still be transmitted into the pretectal nuclei to initiate a pupillary light reflex. To do this, light is shown onto the blinded half of one of the retinae, and, if a pupillary light reflex can still occur, it is known that the lesion is at or beyond the lateral geniculate body, that is, in the geniculocalcarine tract or visual cortex. However, if the light reflex is also lost, then the lesion is in the optic tract itself.

EYE MOVEMENTS AND THEIR CONTROL

To make use of the abilities of the eye, almost equally as important as the system for interpretation of the visual signals from the eyes is the cerebral control system for directing the eyes toward the object to be viewed.

Muscular Control of Eye Movements. The eye movements are controlled by three separate pairs of muscles shown in Figure 18–9: (1) the medial and lateral recti, (2) the superior and inferior recti, and (3) the superior and inferior obliques. The medial and lateral recti contract reciprocally to move the eyes from side to side. The superior and inferior recti contract reciprocally to move the eyes upward or downward. And the oblique muscles function mainly to rotate the eyeballs to keep the visual fields in the upright position.

Neural Pathways for Control of Eye Movements. Figure 18–9 also illustrates the nuclei of the third, fourth, and sixth cranial nerves and their innervation of the ocular muscles. Shown, too, are the interconnections among these three nuclei through the *medial longitudinal fas-*

Figure 18–9. The extraocular muscles of the eye and their innervation.

ciculus. Either by way of this fasciculus or by way of other closely associated pathways, each of the three sets of muscles to each eye is *reciprocally* innervated so that one muscle of the pair relaxes while the other contracts.

Figure 18–10 illustrates cortical control of the oculomotor apparatus, showing spread of signals from the occipital visual areas through occipitotectal and occipitocollicular tracts into the pretectal and superior colliculus areas of the brain stem. In addition, a frontotectal tract passes from the frontal cortex into the pretectal area. From both the pretectal and the superior colliculus areas, the oculomotor control signals then pass to the nuclei of the oculomotor nerves. Finally, strong signals are also transmitted into the oculomotor system from the vestibular nuclei by way of the medial longitudinal fasciculus.

CONJUGATE MOVEMENT OF THE EYES

Simultaneous movement of both eyes in the same direction is called *conjugate movement* of the eyes. The signals to the two eyes to cause precise synchronized movement of both eyes at the same time probably originate in the reticular nuclei of the mesencephalon and pons in close association with the oculomotor nuclei. However, the conjugate

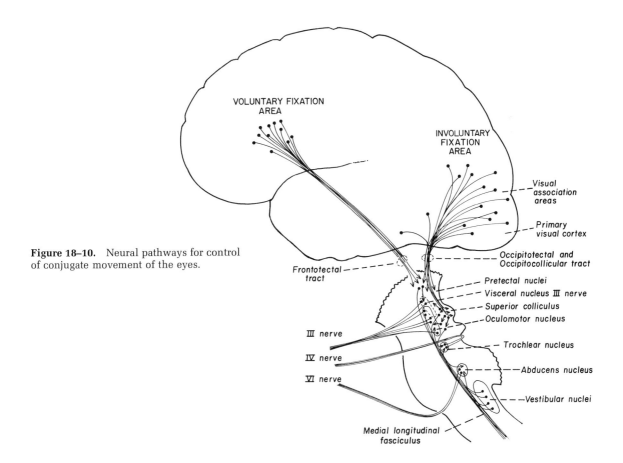

Figure 18–10. Neural pathways for control of conjugate movement of the eyes.

movements are under strong control of the cerebral cortex, which transmits signals into the reticular nuclei by way of the pretectal nuclei and the superior colliculi. Signals from the vestibular nuclei also elicit conjugate movement of the eyes, probably by sending signals through the medial longitudinal fasciculi.

FIXATION MOVEMENTS OF THE EYES

Perhaps the most important conjugate movements of the eyes are those that cause the eyes to "fix" on a discrete portion of the field of vision.

Fixation movements are controlled by two entirely different neuronal mechanisms. The first of these allows the person to move his eyes voluntarily to find the object upon which he wishes to fix his vision; this is called the *voluntary fixation mechanism*. The second is an involuntary mechanism that holds the eyes firmly on the object once it has been found; this is called the *involuntary fixation mechanism*.

The voluntary fixation movements are controlled by a small cortical field located bilaterally in the premotor cortical regions of the frontal lobes, as illustrated in Figure 18–10. Bilateral dysfunction or destruction of these areas makes it difficult or almost impossible for the person to "unlock" his eyes from one point of fixation and then move them to another point. It is usually necessary for him to blink his eyes or put his hand over his eyes for a short time, which then allows him to move the eyes.

On the other hand, the fixation mechanism that causes the eyes to "lock" on the object of attention once it is found is controlled by the *eye fields of the occipital cortex*—mainly area 19—which are also illustrated in Figure 18–10. When these areas are destroyed bilaterally, the person has difficulty or becomes completely unable to keep his eyes directed toward a given fixation point.

To summarize, the posterior eye fields automatically "lock" the eyes on a given spot of the visual field and thereby prevent movement of the image across the retina. To unlock this visual fixation, voluntary impulses must be transmitted from the "voluntary" eye fields located in the frontal areas.

Mechanism of Fixation. Visual fixation results from a negative feedback mechanism that prevents the object of attention from leaving the foveal portion of the retina. The eyes even normally have three types of continuous but almost imperceptible movements: (1) a *continuous tremor* at a rate of 30 to 80 cycles per second caused by successive contractions of the motor units in the ocular muscles, (2) a *slow drift* of the eyeballs in one direction or another, and (3) sudden *flicking movements* which are controlled by the involuntary fixation mechanism. When a spot of light has become fixed on the foveal region of the retina, the tremorous movements cause the spot to move back and forth at a rapid rate across the cones, and the drifting movements cause it to drift slowly across the cones. However, each time the spot of light drifts as far as the edge of the fovea, a sudden

flicking movement moves the spot away from this edge back toward the center, which is an automatic response to move the image back toward the central portion of the fovea. These drifting and flicking motions are illustrated in Figure 18–11, which shows by the dashed lines the slow drifting across the retina and by the solid lines the flicks that keep the image from leaving the foveal region.

Fixation of the Eyes on Important Visual Highlights—Role of the Superior Colliculi. The eyes have an automatic capability for instantaneously *fixing* on an important highlight in the visual field. However, this capability is mostly lost when the superior colliculi are destroyed even though most other conjugate movements of the eyes occur normally in the absence of the superior colliculi. The signals for fixation on the visual scene originate in the visual areas of the occipital cortex, primarily in the visual association areas, then pass to the superior colliculi, from there to reticular areas around the oculomotor nuclei, and thence into the motor nuclei themselves.

The superior colliculi are also important in causing sudden turning of the eyes to the side when a flash of light or some other sudden visual disturbance occurs on that side. In addition, signals are transmitted through the superior colliculi into the medial longitudinal fasciculus and other areas of the brain stem to cause turning of the whole head and perhaps even of the whole body toward the direction of the light. Other types of disturbances besides visual disturbances, such as strong sounds or even stroking the side of the body, will cause similar turning of the eyes, head, and body if the superior colliculi are intact. This effect, however, is absent or severely disturbed when the superior colliculi are destroyed. Therefore, it is frequently said that the superior

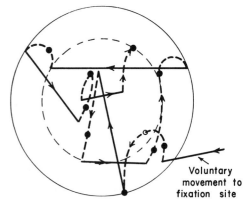

Voluntary
movement to
fixation site

Figure 18–11. Movements of a spot of light on the fovea, showing sudden "flicking" movements to move the spot back toward the center of the fovea whenever it drifts to the foveal edge. (The dashed lines represent slow drifting movements, and the solid lines represent sudden flicking movements.) (Modified from Whitteridge: Handbook of Physiology, Vol. 2, Sec. 1. Baltimore, The Williams & Wilkins Co., 1960, p. 1089.)

colliculi play an important role in orienting the eyes, the head, and the body with respect to external signals—visual signals, auditory signals, somatic signals, and perhaps even others.

Saccadic Conjugate Movement of the Eyes. When the visual scene is moving continually before the eyes, such as when a person is riding in a car or when he is turning around, the eyes fix on one highlight after another in the visual field, jumping from one to the next at a rate of two to three jumps per second. These jumps are called *saccades*. The saccades occur so rapidly that not more than 10 per cent of the total time is spent in moving the eyes, 90 per cent of the time being allocated to the fixation sites. Also, the brain suppresses the visual image during the saccades so that one is completely unconscious of the movements from point to point.

Saccadic Movements During Reading. During the process of reading, a person usually makes several saccadic movements of the eyes for each line. In this case the visual scene is not moving past the eyes, but the eyes are trained to scan across the visual scene to extract the important information. Similar saccades occur when a person observes a painting, except that the saccades occur in one direction after another from one highlight of the painting to another, then another, and so forth.

Fixation on Moving Objects—"Pursuit Movements." The eyes can also remain fixed on a moving object, which is called *pursuit movement*. A highly developed cortical mechanism automatically detects the course of movement of an object and then gradually develops a similar course of movement of the eyes. For instance, if an object is moving up and down in a wavelike form at a rate of several times per second, the eyes at first may be completely unable to fixate on it. However, after a second or so the eyes begin to jump coarsely in approximately the same pattern of movement as that of the object. Then after a few more seconds, the eyes develop progressively smoother and smoother movements and finally follow the course of movement almost exactly. This represents a high degree of automatic, subconscious computational ability by the cerebral cortex.

Opticokinetic Nystagmus. A particularly important type of pursuit movement is that called *nystagmus,* which allows the eyes to fixate on successive points in a continuously moving scene. For instance, if a person is looking out the window of a train, his eyes fix on successive points in the visual scene. To do this, the eyes fixate on some object and move slowly backward as the object also moves backward. When the eyes have moved far to the side, they automatically jump forward to fix on a new object, which is followed again by slow movement in the backward direction. This type of movement in one direction is called *opticokinetic nystagmus.* The slow movement in one direction is called the *slow component* of the nystagmus, while the rapid movement in the other direction is called the *fast component.*

Opticokinetic nystagmus obviously is a type of pursuit movement. That is, after an initial second or so of orientation, the visual system automatically calculates the course and rate of movement of the visual scene, then follows this exactly until the eyes reach a lateral limit, at which time they jump to a new point in the scene.

Vestibular Control of Eye Movements. Another type of eye movement is elicited by stimulation of the vestibular apparatus. The vestibular nuclei are connected directly with the brain stem nuclei that control ocular movements, and, any time the head is accelerated in a vertical, longitudinal, lateral or angular direction, an immediate compensatory motion of the eyes occurs in the opposite direction. This allows the eyes to remain fixed on an object of attention despite rapid movements of the body or head.

Vestibular control of the eyes is especially valuable when a person is subjected to jerky motions of his body. For instance, when a person with bilateral destruction of his vestibular apparatuses rides over rough roads, he has extreme difficulty fixing his eyes on the road or on any horizontal scene. The optikokinetic type of pursuit movement is not capable of keeping the eyes fixed under such conditions because it has a latent period of about one-fifth second before the direction of movement can be detected and followed by the eyes. On the other hand, the vestibular type of eye movement has a short latent period, measured in hundredths of a second rather than one-fifth second.

Also when a person begins to rotate, his vestibular apparatuses cause a vestibular type of nystagmus. That is, the eyes lag behind the rotating head, then jump forward, then lag behind again, jump again, and so forth. This type of nystagmus is discussed in Chapter 10 in relation to vestibular function.

Pathologic Types of Nystagmus. Occasionally, abnormalities occur in the control system for eye movements that cause continuous nystagmus despite the fact that neither the visual scene nor the body is moving. This is likely to occur when one of the vestibular apparatuses is damaged or when severe damage is sustained in the deep nuclei of the cerebellum. This is discussed further in Chapter 11.

Another pathologic type of eye movement that is sometimes called nystagmus occurs when the foveal regions of the two eyes have been destroyed or when the vision in these areas is greatly weakened. In such a condition the eyes attempt to fix the object of attention on the foveae but always overshoot the mark because of foveal insensitivity. Therefore, they oscillate back and forth but never achieve foveal fixation. Even though this condition is known clinically as a type of nystagmus, physiologically it is completely different from the nystagmus that keeps the eyes fixed on a moving scene.

FUSION OF THE VISUAL IMAGES

To make the visual perceptions more meaningful and also to aid in depth perception by the mechanism of stereopsis, which was discussed in Chapter 16, the visual images in the two eyes normally *fuse* with each other on "corresponding points" of the two retinae. Furthermore, three different types of fusion are required: lateral fusion, vertical fusion, and torsional fusion (same rotation of the two eyes about their optical axes.)

Fusion of the images of the two eyes probably results from two mechanisms in the visual system. First, crude fusion is inherent in the newborn baby because of inherited conjugate movements of the eyes. Second, as the visual system becomes more and more developed, the ability of the two eyes to fixate on the same object of attention causes even greater accuracy of fusion. Then, as the visual system develops its pursuit abilities, the pathways for controlling the conjugate movements of the two eyes normally develop equally. And the more the two eyes are moved in unison with each other the more "set" become the patterns of movement for the eyes, and, consequently, the more exact becomes the degree of fusion that can be maintained regardless of the position or rapidity of movement of the eyes.

Both the lateral geniculate body and the visual cortex play very important roles in this process of fusion. It was pointed out earlier in the chapter that corresponding points of the two retinae transmit visual signals, respectively, to successive nuclear layers of the lateral geniculate body. Interactions occur between the layers of the lateral geniculate body where the signals from the retinal images of the two eyes overlap each other; these cause *interference patterns of stimulation* in specific cells of the visual cortex. That is, when the two corresponding points of the retinae are not precisely in fusion, specific cells in the visual cortex become excited; this excitation presumably provides the signal that is transmitted to the oculomotor apparatus to cause convergence or divergence of the eyes so that fusion can be reestablished. Once the corresponding points of the retinae are precisely *in register* with each other, the excitation of the specific cells in the visual cortex disappears.

The Neural Mechanism for Stereopsis. The visual images that appear on the retina during the process of stereopsis were discussed in Chapter 16. It was pointed out that because the two eyes are a little more than 2 inches apart the images on the two retinae are not exactly the same. The closer the object is to the eye the greater is the disparity between the two images. Consequently, it is impossible for all corresponding points in the visual image to be in complete register at the same time. Furthermore, the nearer the object is to the eye the less is the degree of register. Here again, specific cells in the primary visual cortex become excited in the areas of the visual field where highlights are out of register. Presumably, this excitation is the source of the signals for detection of the distance of the object in front of the eyes; this mechanism is called *stereopsis*.

Strabismus. Strabismus, which is also called *squint* or *cross-eyedness*, means lack of fusion of the eyes in one or more of the coordinates described above. Three basic types of strabismus are illustrated in Figure 8–12: *horizontal strabismus, vertical strabismus,* and *torsional strabismus.* However, combinations of two or even of all three of the different types of strabismus often occur.

Strabismus is believed to be caused by an abnormal "set" of the fusion mechanism of the visual system. That is, in the early efforts of the child to fixate the two eyes on the same object, one of the eyes fixates satisfactorily while the other fails to fixate, or they both fixate satisfactorily but never simultaneously. Soon, the patterns of conjugate movements of the eyes become abnormally "set" so that the eyes never fuse.

Frequently, some abnormality of the eyes contributes to the failure of the two eyes to fixate on the same point. For instance, if at birth one eye has poor vision in comparison with the other, the good eye tends to fixate on the object of attention while the poor eye might never do so. Also, in hypermetropic infants, intense impulses must be transmitted to the ciliary muscles to focus the eyes, and some of these impulses overflow into the oculomotor nuclei to cause simultaneous convergence of the eyes, as will be discussed below. As a result, the child's fusion mechanism becomes "set" for continual inward deviation of the eyes.

Suppression of Visual Image from a Repressed Eye. In most patients with strabismus the eyes alternate in fixing on the object of attention. However, in some patients, one eye alone is used all the time while the other eye becomes repressed and is never used for vision. The vision in the repressed eye develops only slightly, usually remaining 20/400 or less. If the dominant eye then becomes blinded, vision in the repressed eye can develop to only a slight extent in the adult but far more rapidly in young children. This illustrates that visual acuity is highly dependent on the proper development of the central synaptic connections from the eyes.

AUTONOMIC CONTROL OF ACCOMMODATION AND PUPILLARY APERTURE

The Autonomic Nerves to the Eyes. The eye is innervated by both parasympathetic and sympathetic fibers, as illustrated in Figure 18–13. The parasym-

Horizontal   Torsional   Vertical
strabismus   strabismus   strabismus

Figure 18–12.   The three basic types of strabismus.

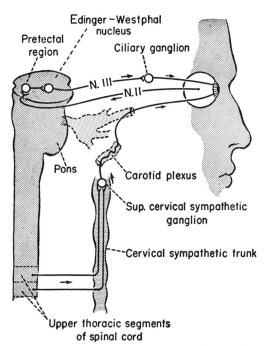

Figure 18–13. Autonomic innervation of the eye, showing also the reflex arc of the light reflex. (Modified from Ranson and Clark: Anatomy of the Nervous System, 1959.)

pathetic fibers arise in the *Edinger-Westphal nucleus* (the visceral nucleus of the third nerve) and then pass in the *third nerve* to the *ciliary ganglion*, which lies about 1 cm. behind the eye. Here the fibers synapse with postganglionic parasympathetic neurons that pass through the *ciliary nerves* into the eyeball. These nerves excite the ciliary muscle and the sphincter of the iris.

The sympathetic innervation of the eye originates in the *intermediolateral horn cells* of the first thoracic segment of the spinal cord. From here, sympathetic fibers enter the sympathetic chain and pass upward to the *superior cervical ganglion* where they synapse with postganglionic neurons. Fibers from these spread along the carotid artery and along successively smaller arteries until they reach the eyeball. There the sympathetic fibers innervate the radial fibers of the iris as well as several extraocular structures around the eye, which are discussed shortly in relation to Horner's syndrome. Also, they supply very weak innervation to the ciliary muscle.

CONTROL OF ACCOMMODATION

The accommodation mechanism—that is, the mechanism which focuses the lens system of the eye—is essential to a high degree of visual acuity. Accommodation results from contrac-

tion or relaxation of the ciliary muscle, contraction causing increased strength of the lens system, as explained in Chapter 16, and relaxation causing decreased strength. The question that must be answered now is: How does one adjust his accommodation to keep his eyes in focus all the time?

Accommodation of the lens is regulated by a negative feedback mechanism that automatically adjusts the focal power of the lens for the highest degree of visual acuity. When the eyes have been fixed on some far object and then suddenly fix on a near object, the lens accommodates for maximum acuity of vision usually within one second; the precise control mechanism that causes this rapid and accurate focusing of the eye is still unclear. Some of the known features of the mechanism are the following:

First, when the eyes suddenly change the distance of their fixation point, the lens changes its strength almost invariably in the proper direction to achieve a new state of focus. In other words, the lens usually *does not hunt* back and forth on the two sides of focus in an attempt to find the focus.

Second, different types of cues that can help the lens change its strength in the proper direction include the following: (1) *Chromatic aberration* appears to be important. That is, the red light rays focus slightly posteriorly to the blue light rays. The eyes appear to be able to detect which of these two types of rays is in better focus, and this cue relays the information to the accommodating mechanism as to whether to make the lens stronger or weaker. (2) When the eyes fixate on a near object they also converge toward each other. The neural mechanisms for *convergence causes a simultaneous signal to strengthen the lens of the eye.* (3) *Since the fovea is a depressed area, the clarity of focus in the depth of the fovea versus the clarity of focus on the edges will be different.* It has been suggested that this also gives clues as to which way the strength of the lens needs to be changed. (4) It has been found that *the degree of accommodation of the lens oscillates slightly* all of the time at a frequency of approximately one-half to two times per second. It has been suggested that the visual image becomes clearer when the oscillation of the lens strength is in the appropriate direction and poorer when the lens strength is in the wrong direction. This could give a rapid cue as to which way the strength of the lens needs to change to provide appropriate focus.

It is presumed that the cortical areas that control accommodation closely parallel those that control fixation movements of the eyes, with integration of visual signals in areas 18 and 19 and transmission of motor signals to the ciliary muscle through the pretectal area and Edinger-Westphal nucleus.

CONTROL OF THE PUPILLARY APERTURE

Stimulation of the parasympathetic nerves excites the pupillary sphincter, thereby decreasing the pupillary aperture; this is called *miosis*. On the other hand, stimulation of the sympathetic nerves excites the radial fibers of the iris and causes pupillary dilatation, which is called *mydriasis*.

The Pupillary Light Reflex. When light is shone into the eyes the pupils constrict, a reaction that is called the pupillary light reflex. The neuronal pathway for this reflex is illustrated in Figure 18–13. When light impinges on the retina, the resulting impulses pass through the optic nerves and optic tracts to the pretectal nuclei. From here, impulses pass to the *Edinger-Westphal nucleus* and finally back through the *parasympathetic nerves* to constrict the sphincter of the iris. In darkness, the Edinger-Westphal nucleus becomes inhibited, which results in dilatation of the pupil.

The function of the light reflex is to help the eye adapt extremely rapidly to changing light conditions, the importance of which was explained in relation to retinal adaptation in the previous chapter. The limits of pupillary diameter are about 1.5 mm. on the small side and 8 mm. on the large side. Therefore, the range of light adaptation that can be effected by the pupillary reflex is about 30 to 1.

Pupillary Reflexes in Syphilis. Central nervous system syphilis almost always eventually blocks the light reflex pathway between the retina and the Edinger-Westphal nucleus. It is believed that this block most likely occurs in the pretectal region of the brain stem, though it could result from destruction of small afferent fibers in the optic nerves. One of the distinguishing features of the loss of the light reflex in syphilis is that pupillary constriction, which also occurs with lens accommodation, is not lost at the same time because the parasympathetic pathways to the eyes are not involved in syphilis.

When the impulses to the Edinger-Westphal nuclei are blocked by syphilis, these nuclei are also released from inhibitory impulses arriving from some outside source. As a result, the nuclei become tonically active, causing the pupils thereafter to remain constricted in addition to their failure to respond to light. Such a pupil that fails to respond to light and also is very small (an *Argyll Robertson pupil*) is an important diagnostic sign of central nervous system syphilis. However, a few other conditions, including central nervous system damage from alcoholism, encephalitis, and so forth, can occasionally also cause an Argyll Robertson pupil.

Horner's Syndrome. The sympathetic nerves to the eye are occasionally interrupted, and this interruption frequently occurs in the cervical chain. This results in Horner's syndrome, which consists of the following effects: First, because of interruption of fibers to the pupillary dilator muscle, the pupil remains persistently constricted to a smaller diameter than that of the pupil of the opposite eye. Second, the superior eyelid droops because this eyelid is normally maintained in an open position during the waking hours partly by contraction of a smooth muscle, the *superior palpebral muscle*, which is innervated by the sympathetics. Therefore, destruction of the sympathetics makes it impossible to open the superior eyelid nearly as widely as normally. Third, the blood vessels on the corresponding side of the face and head become persistently dilated. And, fourth, sweating cannot occur on the side of the face and head affected by Horner's syndrome.

REFERENCES

Armington, J. C.: The Electroretinogram. New York, Academic Press, Inc., 1974.

Ashworth, B.: Clinical Neuro-Ophthalmology. Philadelphia, J. B. Lippincott Company, 1973.

Bach-y-Rita, P., and Collins, C. C. (eds.): The Control of Eye Movements. New York, Academic Press, Inc., 1971.

Becker, W.: The control of eye movements in the saccadic system. Bibl. Ophthalmol., 82:233, 1972.

Bouman, M. A., and Koenderink, J. J.: Psychophysical basis of coincidence mechanisms in the human visual system. Ergeb. Physiol., 65:126, 1972.

Brindley, G. S.: Central pathways of vision. Ann. Rev. Physiol., 32:259, 1970.

Cooper, I. S., Riklan, M., and Rakic, P. T.: The Pulvinar–LP Complex. Springfield, Ill., Charles C Thomas, Publisher, 1974.

Crone, R. A.: Diplopia. New York, American Elsevier Publishing Co., Inc., 1974.

Gerrits, H. J., and Vendrik, A. J.: Eye movements necessary for continuous perception during stabilization of retinal images. Bibl. Ophthalmol., 82:339, 1972.

Glezer, V. D., Leushina, L. I., Nevskaya, A. A., and Prazdnikova, N. V.: Studies on visual pattern recognition in man and animals. Vision Res., 14:555, 1974.

Gombrich, E. H.: The visual image. Sci. Amer., 227:82, 1972.

Gordon, B.: The superior colliculus of the brain. Sci. Amer., 227:72, 1972.

Gordon, B.: Superior colliculus: structure, physiology, and possible functions. In Guyton, A. C. (ed.): MTP International Review of Science: Physiology. Vol. 3. Baltimore, University Park Press, 1974, p. 185.

Guyton, J. S., and Kirkman, N.: Ocular movement: I. Mechanics, pathogenesis, and surgical treatment of alternating hypertropia (dissociated vertical divergence, double hypertropia) and some related phenomena. Amer. J. Ophthalmol., 41:438, 1956.

Hagen, M. A.: Picture perception: toward a theoretical model. Psychol. Bull., 81:471, 1974.

Hassler, R.: Supranuclear structures regulating binocular eye and head movements. *Bibl. Ophthalmol., 82*:207, 1972.

Hubel, D. H.: Eleventh Bowditch Lecture. *Physiologist, 10*:17, 1967.

Hubel, D. H., and Wiesel, T. N.: Receptive fields of cells in striate cortex of very young, visually inexperienced kittens. *J. Neurophysiol., 26*:994, 1963.

Hubel, D. H., and Wiesel, T. N.: Cortical and callosal connections concerned with the vertical meridian of visual fields in the cat. *J. Neurophysiol., 30*:1561, 1967.

Janisse, M. P. (ed.): Pupillary Dynamics and Behavior. New York, Plenum Publishing Corporation, 1974.

Jung, R.: How do we see with moving eyes? *Bibl. Ophthalmol., 82*:377, 1972.

Kommerell, G., and Täumer, R.: Investigations of the eye tracking system through stabilized retinal images. *Bibl. Ophthalmol., 82*:288, 1972.

Kuffler, S. W.: The single-cell approach in the visual system and the study of receptive fields. *Invest. Ophthalmol., 12*:794, 1973.

Lindenberg, R., Walsh, F. B., and Sacks, J. G.: Neuropathology of Vision. Philadelphia, Lea & Febiger, 1973.

McIlwain, J. T.: Central vision: visual cortex and superior colliculus. *Ann. Rev. Physiol., 34*:291, 1972.

Mansourian, P. G.: System analysis of the vestibulo-ocular control mechanism. *Adv. Ophthalmol., 28*:175, 1974.

Matin, E.: Saccadic suppression: a review and a analysis. *Psychol. Bull., 81*:899, 1974.

Matin, L., and Matin, E.: Visual perception of direction and voluntary saccadic eye movements. *Bibl. Ophthalmol., 82*:358, 1972.

Michael, C. R.: Retinal processing of visual images. *Sci. Amer., 220*:104, 1969.

Noton, D., and Stark, L.: Eye Movements and visual perception. *Sci. Amer., 224*:34, 1971.

Oster, G.: Phosphenes. *Sci. Amer., 222*:82, 1970.

Pettigrew, J. D.: The neurophysiology on binocular vision. *Sci. Amer., 227*:84, 1972.

Polyak, S.: The Retina. Chicago, University of Chicago Press, 1941.

Rock, I.: The perception of disoriented figures. *Sci. Amer., 230*:78, 1974.

Straschill, M., and Rieger, P.: Optomotor integration in the colliculus superior of the cat. *Bibl. Ophthalmol., 82*:130, 1972.

Szentágothai, J.: Lateral geniculate body structure and eye movement. *Bibl. Ophthalmol., 82*:178, 1972.

Toates, F. M.: Accommodation function of the human eye. *Physiol. Rev., 52*:828, 1972.

Tomita, T., Miller, W. H., Hashimoto, Y., and Saito, T.: Electrical response of retinal cells as a sign of transport. *Exp. Eye Res., 16*:327, 1973.

Westheimer, G., and Blair, S. M.: Concerning the supranuclear organization of eye movements. *Bibl. Ophthalmol., 82*:28, 1972.

Whitteridge, D.: Binocular vision and cortical function. *Proc. Roy. Soc. Med., 65*:947, 1972.

Wist, E. R.: Eye movements and space perception. *Bibl. Ophthalmol., 82*:348, 1972.

Wurtz, R. H., and Goldberg, M. E.: The role of the superior colliculus in visually-evoked eye movements. *Bibl. Ophthalmol., 82*:149, 1972.

19

The Sense of Hearing

Hearing, like many somatic senses, is a mechanoreceptive sense, for the ear responds to mechanical vibration of the sound waves in the air. The purpose of the present chapter is to describe and explain the mechanism by which the ear receives sound waves, discriminates their frequencies, and finally transmits auditory information into the central nervous system.

THE TYMPANIC MEMBRANE AND THE OSSICULAR SYSTEM

TRANSMISSION OF SOUND FROM THE TYMPANIC MEMBRANE TO THE COCHLEA

Figure 19–1 illustrates the *tympanic membrane* (commonly called the *eardrum*) and the *ossicular system,* which transmits sound through the middle ear. The tympanic membrane is cone shaped, with its concavity facing downward toward the auditory canal. Attached to the very center of the tympanic membrane is the *handle* of the *malleus.* At its other end the malleus is tightly bound to the *incus* by ligaments so that whenever the malleus moves the incus generally moves in unison with it. The opposite end of the incus in turn articulates with the stem of the *stapes,* and the *faceplate* of the stapes lies against the membranous labyrinth in the opening of the oval window where sound waves are transmitted into the inner ear, the *cochlea.*

The ossicles of the middle ear are suspended by ligaments in such a way that the combined malleus and incus act as a single lever having its fulcrum approximately at the border of the tympanic membrane. The large *head* of the malleus, which is on the opposite side of the fulcrum from the handle, almost exactly balances the other end of the lever so that changes in position of the body will not increase or decrease the tension on the tympanic membrane.

The articulation of the incus with the stapes causes the stapes to push forward on the cochlea fluid every time the handle of the malleus moves inward and to pull backward on the fluid every time the malleus moves outward, which promotes inward and outward motion of the faceplate at the oval window.

The handle of the malleus is constantly pulled inward by ligaments and by the tensor tympani muscle, which keeps the tympanic membrane tensed. This allows sound vibrations on *any* portion of the tympanic membrane to be transmitted to the malleus, which would not be true if the membrane were lax.

Impedance Matching by the Ossicular System. The amplitude of movement of the stapes faceplate with each sound vibration is only three-fourths as much as the amplitude of the

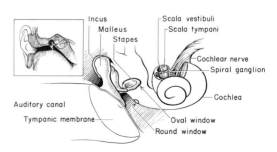

Figure 19–1. The tympanic membrane, the ossicular system of the middle ear, and the inner ear.

handle of the malleus. Therefore, the ossicular lever system does not amplify the movement distance of the stapes, as is commonly believed, but instead the system increases the *force* of movement about 1.3 times. However, the surface area of the tympanic membrane is approximately 55 sq. mm., whereas the surface area of the stapes averages 3.2 sq. mm. This 17-fold difference times the 1.3-fold ratio of the lever system, allows all the energy of a sound wave impinging on the tympanic membrane to be applied to the small faceplate of the stapes, causing approximately 22 times as much *pressure* on the fluid of the cochlea as is exerted by the sound wave against the tympanic membrane. Since fluid has far greater inertia than air, it is easily understood that increased amounts of pressure are needed to cause vibration in the fluid. Therefore, the tympanic membrane and ossicular system provide *impedance matching* between the sound waves in air and the sound vibrations in the fluid of the cochlea. Indeed, the impedance matching is probably 50 to 75 per cent of perfect for sound frequencies between 300 to 3000 cycles per second, which allows almost full utilization of the energy in the incoming sound waves.

In the absence of the ossicular system and tympanum, sound waves can travel directly through the air of the middle ear and can enter the cochlea at the oval window. However, the sensitivity for hearing is then 30 decibels less than for ossicular transmission—equivalent to a decrease from a very loud shouting voice to a barely audible voice level.

Transmission Characteristics of the Ossicular System. Every vibrating system that has inertia and that has an elastic component also has a natural frequency at which it can vibrate back and forth most easily. This is called its *resonant frequency*. Since the ossicular system does have inertia and since it is suspended by elastic ligaments, it has a broadly tuned natural resonating frequency between 700 and 1400 cycles per second. However, the ligaments and other structures attached to the ossicles are also viscous, which prevents excessive resonance; this is called *damping of the vibrations*. Because of the slight amount of resonance that does occur, sound waves of approximately 1200 cycles per second can be transmitted through the ossicular system with slightly greater ease than can sound waves of other frequencies.

The external auditory canal, because of its dimensions, acts as an air column resonator and has a natural resonating frequency of about 3000 cycles per second. But here again, the degree of resonance is slight and potentiates the 3000 cycle sound only a minute amount.

Combining the resonant effects of the ossicular system and of the auditory canal, transmission of sound from the air to the cochlea is excellent between the limits of 600 and 6000 cycles per second and fades both above and below these limits.

Attenuation of Sound by Contraction of the Stapedius and Tensor Tympani Muscles. When loud sounds are transmitted through the ossicular system into the central nervous system, a reflex occurs after a latent period of only 40 milliseconds to cause contraction of both the stapedius and tensor tympani muscles. The tensor tympani muscle pulls the handle of the malleus inward while the stapedius muscle pulls the stapes outward. These two forces oppose each other and thereby cause the entire ossicular system to develop a high degree of rigidity, thus greatly reducing the transmission of low frequency sound, frequencies below 1000 cycles per second, to the cochlea.

This *attenuation reflex* can reduce the intensity of sound transmission by as much as 30 to 40 decibels, which is about the same difference as that between a whisper and the sound emitted by a loud speaker. The function of this mechanism is probably two-fold:

1. To *protect* the cochlea from damaging vibrations caused by excessively loud sound. It is mainly low-frequency sounds (the ones that are attenuated) that are frequently loud enough to damage the basilar membrane of the cochlea. Unfortunately, because of the 40 or more millisecond latency for reaction of the reflex, the sudden loud thunderous sounds that result from explosions can still cause extensive cochlear damage.

2. To *mask* low-frequency sounds in loud environments. This usually removes a major share of the background noise and allows a person to concentrate on sounds above 1000 cycles per second frequency. It is in this upper-frequency range that most voice communication is achieved.

Another function of the tensor tympani and stapedius muscles is to decrease the person's hearing sensitivity to his own speech. This effect is activated by collateral signals transmitted to these muscles at the same time that his brain activates his voice mechanism.

TRANSMISSION OF SOUND THROUGH THE BONE

Because the inner ear, the *cochlea,* is embedded in a bony cavity in the temporal bone, vibrations of the entire skull can cause fluid vibrations in the cochlea itself. Therefore, under appropriate conditions, a tuning fork or an electronic vibrator placed on any bony protuberance of the skull causes the person to hear the sound if it is intense enough. Unfortunately, the energy available even in very loud sound in the air is not sufficient to cause hearing through the bone except when a special electromechanical sound-transmitting device is applied directly to the bone, usually to the mastoid process.

THE COCHLEA

FUNCTIONAL ANATOMY OF THE COCHLEA

The cochlea is a system of coiled tubes, shown in Figure 19–1 and in cross-section in Figure 19–2, with three different tubes coiled side by side: the *scala vestibuli,* the *scala media,* and the *scala tympani.* The scala vestibuli and scala media are separated from each other by the *vestibular membrane,* and the scala tympani and scala media are separated from each other by the *basilar membrane.* On the surface of the basilar membrane lies a structure, the *organ of Corti,* which contains a series of mechanically sensitive cells, the *hair cells.* These are the receptive end-organs that generate nerve impulses in response to sound vibrations.

Figure 19–3 illustrates schematically the functional parts of the uncoiled cochlea for transmission of sound vibrations. First, note that the

Figure 19–3. Movement of fluid in the cochlea following forward thrust of the stapes.

vestibular membrane is missing from this figure. This membrane is so thin and so easily moved that it does not obstruct the passage of sound vibrations from the scala vestibuli into the scala media at all. Therefore, so far as the transmission of sound is concerned, the scala vestibuli and scala media are considered to be a single chamber. The importance of the vestibular membrane is to maintain a special fluid in the scala media that is required for normal function of the sound receptive hair cells, as discussed later in the chapter.

Sound vibrations enter the scala vestibuli from the faceplate of the stapes at the oval window. The faceplate covers this window and is connected with the window's edges by a relatively loose annular ligament so that it can move inward and outward with the sound vibrations. Inward movement causes the fluid to move into the scala vestibuli and scala media, which immediately increases the pressure in the entire cochlea and causes the round window to bulge outward.

Note from Figure 19–3 that the distal end of the scala vestibuli and scala tympani are continuous with each other by way of the *helicotrema.* If the stapes moves inward *very slowly,* fluid from the scala vestibuli is pushed through the helicotrema into the scala tympani, and this causes the round window to bulge outward. However, if the stapes vibrates inward and outward rapidly, the fluid simply does not have time to pass all the way to the helicotrema, then to the round window, and back again to the oval window between each two successive vibrations. Instead, the fluid wave takes a shortcut through the basilar membrane, causing it to bulge back and forth with each sound vibration. We shall see later that each frequency of sound causes a different "pattern" of vibration in the basilar membrane and that this is one of

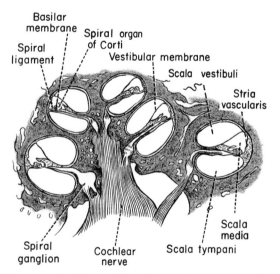

Figure 19–2. The cochlea. (From Goss, C. M. (ed.): Gray's Anatomy of the Human Body. Lea & Febiger.)

the important means by which the sound frequencies are discriminated from each other.

The Basilar Membrane and Resonance in the Cochlea. The basilar membrane contains about 20,000 or more *basilar fibers* that project from the bony center of the cochlea, the *modiolus*, toward the outer wall. These fibers are stiff, elastic, reedlike structures that are not fixed at their distal ends except that they are embedded in the basilar membrane. Because they are stiff and free at one end, they can vibrate like reeds of a harmonica.

The lengths of the basilar fibers increase progressively from the base of the cochlea to the helicotrema, from approximately 0.04 mm. at the base to 0.5 mm. at the helicotrema, a 12-fold increase in length.

The diameters of the fibers, on the other hand, decrease from the base to the helicotrema, so that their overall stiffness decreases more than 100-fold. As a result, the stiff, short fibers near the base of the cochlea have a tendency to vibrate at a high frequency, whereas the long, limber fibers near the helicotrema have a tendency to vibrate at a low frequency.

In addition to the differences in stiffness of the basilar fibers, they are also differently "loaded" by the fluid mass of the cochlea. That is, when a fiber vibrates back and forth, all the fluid between the vibrating fiber and the oval and round windows must also move back and forth at the same time. For a fiber vibrating near the base of the cochlea, the total mass of moving fluid is slight in comparison with that for a fiber vibrating near the helicotrema. This difference, too, favors high frequency vibration near the windows and low frequency vibration near the tip of the cochlea.

Thus, high frequency resonance of the basilar membrane occurs near the base, and low frequency resonance occurs near the apex because of (1) difference in stiffness of the fibers and (2) difference in "loading."

TRANSMISSION OF SOUND WAVES IN THE COCHLEA— THE "TRAVELING WAVE"

If the foot of the stapes moves inward instantaneously, the round window must also bulge outward instantaneously because the cochlea is bounded on all sides by bony walls. Since the fluid wave will not have time to move all the way from the oval window to the helicotrema and back to the round window, the initial effect is to cause the basilar membrane at the very base of the cochlea to bulge in the direction of the round window. However, the elastic tension that is built up in the basilar fibers as they bend toward the round window initiates a wave that "travels" along the basilar membrane toward the helicotrema, as illustrated in Figure 19–4. Figure 19–4A shows movement of a high frequency wave down the basilar membrane, Figure 19–4B a medium frequency wave, and Figure 19–4C a very low frequency wave. Movement of the wave along the basilar membrane is comparable to the movement of a pressure wave along the arterial walls, causing pulsation in the peripheral arteries, or it is also comparable to the wave that travels along the surface of a pond.

Pattern of Vibration of the Basilar Membrane for Different Sound Frequencies. Note in Figure 19–4 the different patterns of transmission for sound waves of different frequencies. Each wave is relatively weak at the outset but becomes strong when it reaches that portion of the basilar membrane that has a natural resonant frequency equal to the respective sound frequency. At this point the basilar membrane can vibrate back and forth with such great ease that the energy in the wave is completely dissipated. Consequently, the wave ceases at this point and fails to travel the remaining distance along the basilar membrane. Thus, a high frequency sound wave travels only a short distance along the basilar membrane be-

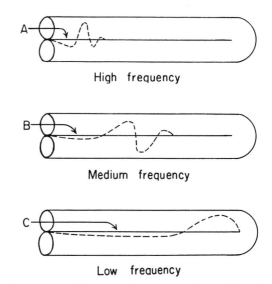

Figure 19–4. Diagrammatic representation of "traveling waves" along the basilar membrane for high, medium, and low frequency sounds.

fore it reaches its resonant point and dies out; a medium frequency sound wave travels about halfway and then dies out; and, finally, a very low frequency sound wave travels the entire distance along the membrane.

Another feature of the traveling wave is that it travels fast along the initial portion of the basilar membrane but progressively more slowly as it goes farther and farther into the cochlea. The cause of this is the high coefficient of elasticity of the basilar fibers near the stapes but a progressively decreasing coefficient farther along the membrane. This rapid initial transmission of the wave allows the high frequency sounds to travel far enough into the cochlea to spread out and separate from each other on the basilar membrane. Without this spread, all the high frequency waves would be bunched together within the first millimeter or so of the basilar membrane, and their frequencies could not be discriminated one from the other.

Amplitude Pattern of Vibration of the Basilar Membrane. The dashed curves of Figure 19–5A show the position of a sound wave on the basilar membrane when the stapes *(a)* is all the way inward, *(b)* has moved back to the neutral point, *(c)* is all the way outward, and *(d)* has moved back again to the neutral point but is moving inward. The shaded area around these different waves shows the maximum extent of vibration of the basilar membrane during a

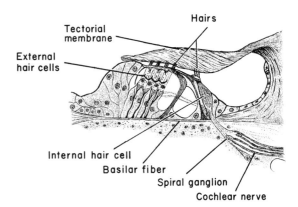

Figure 19–6. The organ of Corti, showing especially the hair cells and the tectorial membrane against the projecting hairs.

complete vibratory cycle. This is the amplitude pattern of vibration of the basilar membrane for this particular sound frequency.

Figure 19–5B shows the amplitude patterns of vibration for different frequencies, showing that the maximum amplitude for 8000 cycles occurs near the base of the cochlea, while that for frequencies of 50 to 100 cycles per second occurs near the helicotrema.

Note in Figure 19–5B that the basal end of the basilar membrane vibrates at least weakly for all frequencies. However, beyond the resonant area for each given frequency, the vibration of the basilar membrane cuts off sharply. The principal method by which sound frequencies are discriminated from each other is based on the "place" of maximum stimulation of the nerve fibers from the basilar membrane, as will be explained in the following section.

FUNCTION OF THE ORGAN OF CORTI

The organ of Corti, illustrated in Figures 19–2 and 19–6, is the receptor organ that generates nerve impulses in response to vibration of the basilar membrane. Note that the organ of Corti lies on the surface of the basilar fibers and basilar membrane. The actual sensory receptors in the organ of Corti are two types of *hair cells,* a single row of *internal hair cells,* numbering about 3500 and measuring about 12 microns in diameter, and three to four rows of *external hair cells,* numbering about 20,000 and having diameters of only about 8 microns. The bases and sides of the hair cells are enmeshed by a network of cochlear nerve endings. These lead to the *spiral ganglion of Corti,* which lies in the modiolus of the cochlea. The spiral ganglion in

Figure 19–5. (A) Amplitude pattern of vibration of the basilar membrane for a medium frequency sound. (B) Amplitude patterns for sounds of all frequencies between 50 and 8000 per second, showing the points of maximum amplitude (the resonance points) on the basilar membrane for the different frequencies.

turn sends axons into the *cochlear nerve* and thence into the central nervous system at the level of the upper medulla. The relationship of the organ of Corti to the spiral ganglion and to the cochlear nerve is illustrated in Figure 19–2.

Excitation of the Hair Cells. Note in Figure 19–6 that minute hairs, or cilia, project upward from the hair cells and either touch or are embedded in the surface gel coating of the *tectorial membrane,* which lies above the cilia in the scala media. These hair cells are similar to the hair cells found in the macula and cristae ampullaris of the vestibular apparatus which were discussed in Chapter 10. Bending of the hairs excites the hair cells, and this in turn excites the nerve fibers enmeshing their bases.

Figure 19–7 illustrates the mechanism by which vibration of the basilar membrane excites the hair endings. This shows that the upper ends of the hair cells are fixed tightly in a structure called the *reticular lamina.* Furthermore, the reticular lamina is very rigid and is continuous with a rigid triangular structure called the *rods of Corti* that rests on the basilar fibers. Therefore, the basilar fiber, the rods of Corti, and the reticular lamina all move as a unit.

Upward movement of the basilar fiber rocks the reticular lamina upward and *inward.* Then, when the basilar membrane moves downward, the reticular lamina rocks downward and *outward.* The inward and outward motion causes the hairs to sheer back and forth in the tectorial membrane, thus exciting the cochlear nerve fibers whenever the basilar membrane vibrates.

Mechanism by which the Hair Cells Excite the Nerve Fibers—Receptor Potentials. Back-and-forth bending of the hairs causes alternate changes in the electrical potential across the hair cell membrane. This alternating potential is the *receptor potential* of the hair cell; and

it in turn stimulates the cochlear nerve endings that terminate on the hair cells. Most physiologists believe that the receptor potential stimulates the endings by direct electrical excitation.

When the basilar fiber bends toward the scala vestibuli (in the upward direction in Figure 19–7), the hair cell becomes depolarized, and it is this depolarization that excites an increased number of action potentials in the nerve fiber. When the basilar fiber moves in the opposite direction, the hair cell becomes hyperpolarized, and the number of action potentials decreases.

The Endocochlear Potential. To explain even more fully the electrical potentials generated by the hair cells, we need to explain still another electrical phenomenon called the endocochlear potential: The scala media is filled with a fluid called *endolymph* in contradistinction to the *perilymph* present in the scala vestibuli and scala tympani. The scala vestibuli and scala tympani in most young children and in some adults communicate directly with the subarachnoid space around the brain, and the perilymph is almost identical with cerebrospinal fluid. On the other hand, the endolymph that fills the scala media is an entirely different fluid probably secreted by the *stria vascularis,* a highly vascular area on the outer wall of the scala media. Endolymph contains a very high concentration of potassium and a very low concentration of sodium, which is exactly opposite to the perilymph.

An electrical potential of approximately 80 mv. exists all the time between the endolymph and the perilymph, with positivity inside the scala media and negativity outside. This is called the *endocochlear potential,* and it is believed to be generated by continual secretion of positive potassium ions into the scala media by the stria vascularis.

The importance of the endocochlear potential is that the tops of the hair cells project through the reticular lamina into the endolymph of the scala media while perilymph bathes the lower bodies of the hair cells. Furthermore, the hair cells have a negative intracellular potential −70 millivolts with respect to the perilymph, but −150 millivolts with respect to the endolymph—that is, at the upper surfaces of the hair cells where the hairs project into the endolymph. It is believed that this high electrical potential at the hair border of the cell greatly sensitizes the cell, thereby increasing its ability to respond to slight movement of the hairs.

DETERMINATION OF PITCH—THE "PLACE" PRINCIPLE

In the minds of most persons, sound pitch and sound frequency are the same thing. However, the two are slightly different in the following way: Pitch is the conscious perception of the sound frequency and may not be the same as

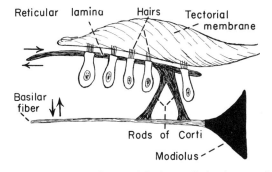

Figure 19–7. Stimulation of the hair cells by the to-and-fro movement of the hairs in the tectorial membrane.

the true sound frequency. The pitch is especially likely to deviate from the true sound frequency at both very high and very low frequencies; also, the pitch usually changes slightly as the intensity of the sound changes even though the frequency remains constant. Yet, from the point of view of the following discussion, we can still consider the two to be essentially the same.

From earlier discussions in this chapter it is already apparent that low pitch (or low frequency) sounds cause maximal activation of the basilar membrane near the apex of the cochlea, sounds of high pitch (or high frequency) activate the basilar membrane near the base of the cochlea, and intermediate frequencies activate the membrane at intermediate distances between these two extremes. Furthermore, there is spatial organization of the cochlear nerve fibers from the cochlea to the cochlear nuclei in the brain stem, the fibers from each respective area of the basilar membrane terminating in a corresponding area in the cochlear nuclei. We shall see later that this spatial organization continues all the way up the brain stem to the cerebral cortex. The recording of signals from the auditory tracts in the brain stem and from the auditory receptive fields in the cerebral cortex shows that specific neurons are activated by specific pitches. Therefore, the primary method used by the nervous system to detect different pitches is to determine the position along the basilar membrane that is most stimulated. This is called the *place principle* for determination of pitch.

Yet, low frequency sounds probably can be discriminated much less accurately in other ways as well. For instance, destruction of the apical half of the cochlea destroys the basilar membrane where low frequency sounds are normally detected, but low frequency sounds can still be discriminated from high frequency sounds to a slight degree. It is believed that the low frequency sounds cause synchronized low frequency volleys of impulses that can be distinguished from the high frequency signals.

DETERMINATION OF LOUDNESS

Loudness is determined by the auditory system in at least three different ways: First, as the sound becomes louder, the amplitude of vibration of the basilar membrane and hair cells also increases so that the hair cells excite the nerve endings at more rapid rates. Second, as the amplitude of vibration increases, it causes more and more of the hair cells on the fringes of the vibrating portion of the basilar membrane to be-

come stimulated, thus causing *spatial summation* of impulses—that is, transmission through many nerve fibers rather than through a few. Third, certain hair cells do not become stimulated until the vibration of the basilar membrane reaches a relatively high intensity, and it is believed that stimulation of these cells in some way apprises the nervous system that the sound is then very loud.

Detection of Changes in Loudness—The Power Law. It was pointed out in Chapter 48 that a person interprets changes in intensity of sensory stimuli approximately in proportion to a power function of the actual intensity. In the case of sound, the interpreted sensation changes approximately in proportion to the cube root of the actual sound intensity. To express this another way, the ear can discriminate changes in sound intensity from the softest whisper to the loudest possible noise of *approximately one trillion times* as much sound energy. Yet the ear interprets this much difference in sound level as approximately a 10,000-fold change. Thus, the scale of intensity is greatly "compressed" by the sound perception mechanisms of the auditory system. This obviously allows a person to interpret differences in sound intensities over an extremely wide range, a far broader range than would be possible were it not for compression of the scale.

The Decibel Unit. Because of the extreme changes in sound intensities that the ear can detect and discriminate, sound intensities are usually expressed in terms of the logarithm of their actual intensities. A 10-fold increase in sound energy (or a $\sqrt{10}$-fold increase in sound pressure, because energy is proportional to the square of pressure) is called 1 *bel,* and one-tenth bel is called 1 *decibel.* One decibel represents an actual increase in intensity of 1.26 times.

Another reason for using the decibel system in expressing changes in loudness is that, in the usual sound intensity range for communication, the ears can detect approximately a 1 decibel change in sound intensity.

The "Zero" Decibel Reference Level. The usual method for expressing the intensity of sound is to state the pressure difference between the peak of the sound compression wave and the trough of the wave. A pressure difference of *1 dyne per square centimeter* is considered to have unit intensity, and this is expressed as zero decibels when converted to the decibel scale because the logarithm of one is zero. However, it should be remembered that the decibel scale is an *energy scale*—not a pressure scale. Furthermore, energy changes are proportional to the square of the pressure changes. Therefore, if the pressure of the sound increases to 10 dynes per square centimeter, this will be equivalent to a 100-fold increase in sound energy above zero reference level. Consequently, the sound intensity will be +20 decibels. A 100-fold increase in pressure will change the sound intensity to +40 decibels.

Threshold for Hearing Sound at Different Frequencies. Figure 19–8 shows the energy threshold at which sounds of different frequencies can barely be heard by the ear. This figure illustrates that a 2000 cycle per second sound can be heard even when its intensity is as low as −70 decibels, which is one ten-millionth microwatt/cm.^{2}. On the other hand, a 100 cycle per second sound can be detected only if its intensity is 10,000 times as great as this—that is, at an intensity of −30 decibels.

Frequency Range of Hearing. The frequencies of sound that a young person can hear, before aging has occurred in the ears, is generally stated to be between 30 and 20,000 cycles per second. However, referring again to Figure 19–8, we see that the sound range depends to a great extent on intensity. If the intensity is only −60 decibels, the sound range is 500 to 5000 cycles per second, but, if the sound intensity is −20 decibels, the frequency range is about 70 to 15,000 cycles per second, and only with intense sounds can the complete range of 30 to 20,000 cycles be achieved. In old age, the frequency range falls to 50 to 8,000 cycles per second or less, as is discussed later in the chapter.

CENTRAL AUDITORY MECHANISMS

THE AUDITORY PATHWAY

Figure 19–9 illustrates the major auditory pathways. It shows that nerve fibers from the *spiral ganglion of the organ of Corti* enter the *cochlear nuclei* located in the upper part of the medulla. At this point, all the fibers synapse, and second order

Figure 19–8. Relationship of the threshold of hearing and the threshold of somesthetic perception to the sound energy level at each sound frequency. (Modified from Stevens and Davis: Hearing. John Wiley & Sons.)

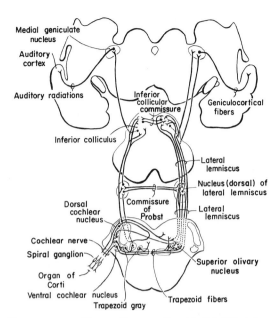

Figure 19–9. The auditory pathway. (Modified from Crosby, Humphrey, and Lauer: Correlative Anatomy of the Nervous System. The Macmillan Co., 1962.)

neurons pass mainly to the opposite side of the brain stem through the *trapezoid body* to the *superior olivary nucleus*. However, some of the second order fibers pass ipsilaterally to the superior olivary nucleus on the same side. Most of the fibers entering the superior olivary nucleus on either side terminate here, but some pass on through this nucleus. From the superior olivary nucleus the auditory pathway then passes upward through the *lateral lemniscus*, and many of the fibers terminate in the *nucleus of the lateral lemniscus*, but many also bypass this nucleus and pass on to the inferior colliculus where most terminate; a few pass on without terminating to higher levels. A few fibers cross from the nucleus of the lateral lemniscus through the *commissure of Probst* to the contralateral nucleus, and still other fibers cross through the *inferior collicular commissure* from one inferior colliculus to the other. From the inferior colliculus, the pathway passes through the *peduncle of the inferior colliculus* to the *medial geniculate nucleus,* where all the fibers synapse. From here, the auditory tract spreads by way of the *auditory radiation* to the *auditory cortex* located mainly in the superior temporal gyrus.

Several points of importance in relation to the auditory pathway should be noted. First, impulses from either ear are transmitted through the auditory pathways of both sides of the brain stem with only slight preponderance of transmission in the contralateral pathway. In at least three different places in the brain stem crossing-over occurs between the two pathways: (a) in the trapezoid body, (b) in the commissure of Probst, and (c) in the commissure connecting the two inferior colliculi.

Second, many collateral fibers from the auditory tracts pass directly into the reticular activating system of the brain stem. This system projects diffusely upward into the cerebral cortex and downward into the spinal cord.

Third, the pathway for transmission of sound impulses from the cochlea to the cortex consists of at least four neurons and sometimes as many as six. Neurons *may* or *may not* synapse in the superior olivary nuclei, in the nuclei of the lateral lemniscus, and in the inferior colliculi. Therefore, some of the tracts are more direct than others, which means that some impulses arrive at the cortex well ahead of others even though they might have originated at exactly the same time.

Fourth, several important pathways also exist from the auditory system into the cerebellum: (a) directly from the cochlear nuclei, (b) from the inferior colliculi, (c) from the reticular substance of the brain stem, and (d) from the cerebral auditory areas. These activate the *cerebellar vermis* instantaneously in the event of a sudden noise.

Fifth, a high degree of spatial orientation is maintained in the fiber tracts from the cochlea all the way to the cortex. In fact, there are three different spatial representations of sound frequencies in the cochlear nuclei, two representations in the inferior colliculi, one very precise representation for discrete sound frequencies in the auditory cortex, and several less precise representations in the auditory association areas.

Firing Rates at Different Levels of the Auditory Tract. Single nerve fibers entering the cochlear nuclei from the eighth nerve can fire at rates up to 1000 per second, the rate being determined mainly by the loudness of the sound. At low sound frequencies, the nerve impulses are usually synchronized with the sound waves but they do not necessarily occur with every wave.

In the auditory tracts of the brain stem, the firing is usually no longer synchronized with the sound frequency except at sound frequencies below 200 cycles per second. Furthermore, the firing rates are often considerably different from those in the eighth nerve. These findings demonstrate that the sound signals are not transmitted unchanged directly from the ear to the higher levels of the brain; instead, information from the sound signals begins to be dissected from the impulse traffic at levels as low as the cochlear nuclei. We will have more to say about this later, especially in relation to perception of direction from which sound comes.

Another significant feature of the auditory pathways is that low rates of impulse firing continue even in the absence of sound all the way from the cochlear nerve fibers to the auditory cortex. When the basilar membrane moves toward the scala vestibuli, the impulse traffic increases; and when the basilar membrane moves toward the scala tympani, the impulse traffic decreases. Thus, the presence of this background signal allows information to be transmitted from the basilar membrane when the membrane moves in either direction: positive information in one direction and negative information in the opposite direction. Were it not for the background signal, only the positive half of the information could be transmitted. This type of so-called "carrier wave" method for transmitting information is utilized in many parts of the brain, as has been discussed in several of the preceding chapters.

Function of the Auditory Relay Nuclei. Very little is known about the function of the different nuclei in the auditory pathway. However, cats and even monkeys can still detect barely threshold sounds when the cerebral cortex is removed bilaterally, which indicates that the nuclei in the brain stem and thalamus can perform many auditory functions even without the cerebral cortex. However, discrimination of pitch and tonal patterns is considerably impaired. In man, *bilateral* destruction of the cortical auditory centers probably gives a different picture: it is said to cause almost total deafness; unfortunately, this has not been studied adequately. This indicates that in man, however, the elements of the lower centers might be greatly suppressed.

One of the important features of auditory transmission through the relay nuclei is the spatial orientation of the pathways for sounds of different frequencies. For instance, in the dorsal cochlear nucleus, high frequencies are represented along the medial edge while low frequencies are represented along the lateral edge, and a similar type of spatial orientation occurs throughout the auditory pathway as it travels upward to the cortex.

FUNCTION OF THE CEREBRAL CORTEX IN HEARING

The projection of the auditory pathway to the cerebral cortex is illustrated in Figure 19–10, which shows that the auditory cortex lies principally on the *supratemporal plane of the superior temporal gyrus* but also extends over the *lateral border of the temporal lobe,* over much of the *insular cortex,* and even into the most lateral portion of the *parietal operculum.*

Two separate areas are shown in Figure 19–10; the *primary auditory cortex* and the *au-*

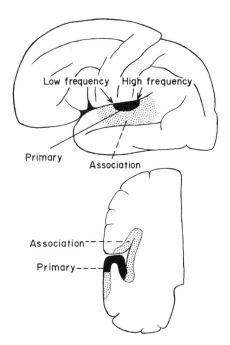

Figure 19–10. The auditory cortex.

ditory association cortex. The primary auditory cortex is directly excited by projections from the medial geniculate body, while the auditory association areas are usually excited secondarily by impulses from the primary auditory cortex and by projections from thalamic association areas adjacent to the medial geniculate body.

Locus of Sound Frequency Perception in the Primary Auditory Cortex. Certain parts of the primary auditory cortex are known to respond to high frequencies and other parts to low frequencies. In monkeys, the posterior part of the supratemporal plane responds to high frequencies, while the anterior part responds to low frequencies. Presumably, the same frequency localization occurs in the human cortex but this is yet unproven.

The frequency range to which each individual neuron in the auditory cortex responds is much narrower than that in the cochlear and brain stem relay nuclei. Referring back to Figure 19–5B, we note that the basilar membrane near the base of the cochlea is stimulated by all frequency sounds, and in the cochlear nuclei this same breadth of sound representation is found. Yet by the time the excitation has reached the cerebral cortex, each sound-responsive neuron responds to only a narrow range of frequencies rather than to a broad range. Therefore, some-

where along the pathway processing mechanisms in some way "sharpen" the frequency response. It is believed that this sharpening effect is caused mainly by the phenomenon of lateral inhibition, which was discussed in Chapter 5 in relation to mechanisms for transmitting information in nerves. That is, stimulation of the cochlea at one frequency causes inhibition of signals caused by sound frequencies on either side of the stimulated frequency, this effect resulting from collateral fibers angling off the primary signal pathway and exerting inhibitory influences on adjacent pathways. The same effect has also been demonstrated to be important in sharpening patterns of somesthetic images, visual images, and other types of sensations.

Some of the neurons in the auditory cortex, especially in the auditory association cortex, do not respond at all to sounds in the ear. It is believed that these neurons "associate" different sound frequencies with each other or associate sound information with information from other sensory areas of the cortex. Indeed, the parietal portion of the auditory association cortex partly overlaps somatic sensory area II, which could provide easy opportunity for association of auditory information with somatic sensory information.

Discrimination of Sound "Patterns" by the Auditory Cortex. Complete bilateral removal of the auditory cortex does not prevent an animal from detecting sounds or reacting in a crude manner to the sounds. However, it does greatly reduce or sometimes even abolish his ability to discriminate different sound pitches and especially *patterns of sound.* For instance, an animal that has been trained to recognize a combination or sequence of tones, one following the other in a particular pattern, loses this ability when the auditory cortex is destroyed, and, furthermore, he cannot relearn this type of response. Therefore, the auditory cortex is important in the discrimination of *tonal patterns.*

In the human being, lesions affecting the auditory association areas but not affecting the primary auditory cortex will allow the person full capability to hear and differentiate sound tones as well as to interpret at least a few simple patterns of sound. However, he will often be completely unable to interpret the *meaning* of the sound that he hears. For instance, lesions in the posterior portion of the superior temporal gyrus often make it impossible for the person to interpret the meanings of words even though he hears them perfectly well and can often even repeat them; all the time, however, he does not know the meaning of the words. These functions of the auditory association areas and their relationship to the overall intellectual functions of the brain were discussed in detail in Chapter 13.

DISCRIMINATION OF DIRECTION FROM WHICH SOUND EMANATES

A person determines the direction from which sound emanates by at least two different mechanisms: (1) by the time lag between the entry of sound into one ear and into the opposite ear and (2) by the difference between the intensities of the sounds in the two ears. The first mechanism functions best for frequencies below 3000 cycles per second, and the intensity mechanism operates best at higher frequencies because the head acts as a sound barrier at these frequencies. The time lag mechanism discriminates direction much more exactly than the intensity mechanism, for the time lag mechanism does not depend on extraneous factors but only on an exact interval of time between two acoustical signals. If a person is looking straight toward the sound, the sound reaches both ears at exactly the same instant, while, if the right ear is closer to the sound than the left ear, the sound signals from the right ear are perceived ahead of those from the left ear.

If a sound emanates from the right side 45 degrees from the frontal direction and if still a second sound emanates also from the right but 45 degrees from behind, the difference in time of arrival of the two sounds at the two ears will be exactly the same. For this reason, it is difficult to distinguish whether the sound is originating from the frontal or the posterior quadrant. The principal method by which a person determines this is to rotate his head quickly. If he turns his head toward the right when the sound is coming from the frontal quadrant, the time lag between the two ears becomes smaller. If the sound is originating from the posterior quadrant, the time lag becomes greater. A sudden sound that occurs so rapidly that the person does not have time to move his head often cannot be properly localized to the frontal or posterior quadrant.

Neural Mechanisms for Detecting Sound Direction. Destruction of the auditory cortex on both sides of the brain, in either man or lower mammals, causes loss of almost all ability to detect the direction from which sound comes. Yet, the mechanism for this detection process begins in the superior olivary nuclei,

even though it requires the neural pathways all the way from these nuclei to the cortex for interpretation of the signals. The mechanism is believed to be the following:

When the sound enters one ear slightly before it enters the other ear, it *excites* the neurons in the medial portion of the contralateral superior olivary nucleus but, at the same time, it *inhibits* the neurons in the ipsilateral superior olivary nucleus, and this inhibition lasts for a fraction of a millisecond. Therefore, for a short period of time after the sound reaches the first ear, the pathway for sound coming from the second ear is in an inhibited state. Furthermore, certain neurons of the medial superior olivary nuclei have longer time lags of inhibition than do other portions. Therefore, when the sound signal from the second ear enters the inhibited superior olivary nucleus, the signal will pass up the auditory pathway through some of the neurons but not through others. And the specific neurons through which the signal passes are determined by the time-interval of the sound between the two ears. Thus, a spatial pattern of neuronal stimulation develops, with the short lagging sounds stimulating one set of neurons maximally and the long lagging sounds stimulating another set of neurons maximally. This spatial orientation of signals is then transmitted all the way to the auditory cortex where sound direction is determined by the locus in the cortex that is stimulated maximally. It is believed that the signals for determining sound direction are transmitted through a slightly different pathway and that this pathway terminates in the cerebral cortex in a slightly different locus from the transmission pathway and the termination locus of the tonal patterns of sound.

This mechanism for detection of sound direction indicates again how the information in sensory signals is dissected out as the signals pass through different levels of neuronal activity. In this case, the "quality" of sound direction is separated from the "quality" of sound tones at the level of the superior olivary nuclei.

CENTRIFUGAL CONDUCTION OF IMPULSES FROM THE CENTRAL NERVOUS SYSTEM

Retrograde pathways have been demonstrated at each level of the central nervous system all the way from the auditory cortex to the cochlea. The final pathway is mainly from the superior olivary nucleus to the organ of Corti.

These retrograde fibers are inhibitory. Indeed, direct stimulation of discrete points in the olivary nucleus have been shown to inhibit specific areas of the organ of Corti, reducing their sound sensitivities as much as 15 to 20 decibels. One can readily understand how this could allow a person to direct his attention to sounds of particular qualities while rejecting sounds of other qualities. This is readily demonstrated when one listens to a single instrument in a symphony orchestra.

HEARING ABNORMALITIES

TYPES OF DEAFNESS

Deafness is usually divided into two types; first, that caused by impairment of the cochlea or auditory nerve, which is usually classed under the heading "nerve deafness," and, second, that caused by impairment of the middle ear mechanisms for transmitting sound into the cochlea, which is usually called "conduction deafness." Obviously, if either the cochlea or the auditory nerve is completely destroyed the person is permanently deaf. However, if the cochlea and nerve are still intact but the ossicular system has been destroyed or ankylosed ("frozen" in place by fibrosis or calcification), sound waves can still be conducted into the cochlea by means of bone conduction.

Tuning Fork Test for Differentiation Between Nerve Deafness and Conduction Deafness. To test an ear for bone conduction with a tuning fork, one places a vibrating fork in front of the ear and the subject listens to the tone of the fork until he can no longer hear it. Then the butt of the still weakly vibrating fork is immediately placed against the mastoid process. If his bone conduction is better than his air conduction, he will again hear the sound of the tuning fork. If this occurs, his deafness may be considered to be conduction deafness. However, if on placing the butt of the fork against the mastoid process he cannot hear the sound of the tuning fork, his bone

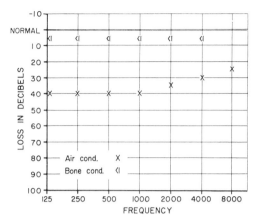

Figure 19–12. Audiogram of deafness resulting from middle ear sclerosis.

conduction is probably decreased as much as his air conduction, and the deafness is presumably due to damage in the cochlea or in the nervous system rather than in the ossicular system—that is, it is nerve deafness.

The Audiometer. To determine the nature of hearing disabilities more exactly than can be accomplished by the above method, the "audiometer" is used. This is simply an earphone connected to an electronic oscillator capable of emitting pure tones ranging from low frequencies to high frequencies. Based on previous studies of normal persons, the instrument is calibrated so that the zero intensity level of sound at each frequency is the loudness that can barely be heard by the normal person. However, a calibrated volume control can be changed to increase or decrease the loudness of each tone above or below the zero level. If the loudness of a tone must be increased to 30 decibels above normal before the subject can hear it, he is said to have a *hearing loss* of 30 decibels for that particular tone.

In performing a hearing test using an audiometer, one tests approximately 8 to 10 tones one at a time covering the auditory spectrum, and the hearing loss is determined for each of these tones. Then the so-called "audiogram" is plotted as shown in Figures 19–11 and 19–12, depicting the hearing loss for each of the tones in the auditory spectrum.

The audiometer, in addition to being equipped with an earphone for testing air conduction by the ear, is also equipped with an electronic vibrator for testing bone conduction from the mastoid process into the cochlea.

The Audiogram in Nerve Deafness. If a person has nerve deafness—this term including damage to the cochlea, to the auditory nerve, or to the central nervous system circuits from the ear—he has lost the ability to hear sound as tested by both the air conduction apparatus and the bone conduction apparatus. An audiogram depicting nerve deafness is illustrated in Figure 19–11. In this figure the deafness is mainly for

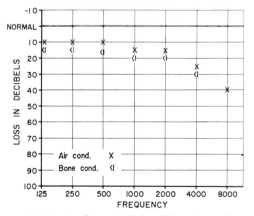

Figure 19–11. Audiogram of the old-age type of nerve deafness.

high frequency sound. Such deafness could be caused by damage to the base of the cochlea. This type of deafness occurs to some extent in almost all older persons.

The Audiogram in Conduction Deafness. A second and frequent type of deafness is that caused by fibrosis of the middle ear following repeated infection in the middle ear or in the hereditary disease called *otosclerosis*. In this instance the sound waves cannot be transmitted easily to the oval window. Figure 19–12 illustrates an audiogram from a person with "middle ear deafness" of this type. In this case the bone conduction is essentially normal, but air conduction is greatly depressed at all frequencies, more so at the low frequencies. In this type of deafness, the faceplate of the stapes frequently becomes "ankylosed" by bony overgrowth to the edges of the oval window. In this case, the person becomes totally deaf for air conduction; but he can be made to hear again almost normally by removing the stapes and replacing it with a minute teflon or metal prosthesis that transmits the sound from the incus to the oval window.

REFERENCES

Ainsworth, W. A.: The perception of speech signals. *Sci. Prog.,* 62:33, 1975.

Dallos, P.: The Auditory Periphery. New York, Academic Press, Inc., 1973.

Davis, H.: Biophysics and physiology of the inner ear. *Physiol. Rev., 37*:1, 1957.

Eldredge, D. H., and Miller, J. D.: Physiology of hearing. *Ann. Rev. Physiol., 33*:281, 1971.

Erulkar, S. D.: Comparative aspects of spatial localization of sound. *Physiol. Rev., 52*:237, 1972.

Friedmann, I.: Pathology of the Ear. Philadelphia, J. B. Lippincott Company, 1973.

Gerber, S. E.: Introductory Hearing Science. Philadelphia, W. B. Saunders Company, 1975.

Grinnell, A. D.: Comparative physiology of hearing. *Ann. Rev. Physiol, 31*:545, 1969.

Gulick, W. L.: Hearing: Physiology and Psychophysics. New York, Oxford University Press, 1971.

Harris, J. D.: The Electrophysiology and Layout of the Auditory Nervous System. Indianapolis, The Bobbs-Merrill Co., Inc., 1974.

Harrison, J. M.: The auditory system of the medulla and localization. *Fed. Proc., 33*:1901, 1974.

Moushegian, G., and Rupert, A. L.: Relations between the psychophysics and the neurophysiology of sound localization. *Fed. Proc., 33*:1924, 1974.

Oster, G.: Auditory beats in the brain. *Sci. Amer., 229*:94, 1973.

Small, A. M., Nordmark, J. O., Jeffress, L. A., Elliott, D. N., et al.: In Tobias, J. V. (ed.): Foundations of Modern Auditory Theory. Vol. 1. New York, Academic Press, Inc., 1973.

Starr, A.: Neurophysiological mechanisms of sound localization. *Fed. Proc., 33*:1911, 1974.

Stevens, K. N., House, A. S., Tanner, W. P., Sorkin, R. D. et al.: In Tobias, J. V. (ed.): Foundations of Modern Auditory Theory. Vol. 2. New York, Academic Press, Inc., 1973.

Taylor, W. (ed.): Disorders of Auditory Function. New York, Academic Press, Inc., 1973.

Tobias, J. V. (ed.): Foundations of Modern Auditory Theory. Vols. 1 and 2. New York, Academic Press, Inc., 1973.

Warren, R. M., and Warren, R. P.: Auditory illusions and confusions. *Sci. Amer., 223*:30, 1970.

Wever, E. G.: Electrical potentials of the cochlea. *Physiol. Rev., 46*:102, 1966.

Wever, E. G., and Lawrence, M.: Physiological Acoustics. Princeton, Princeton University Press, 1954.

Whitfield, I. C.: Auditory Pathway. Baltimore, The Williams & Wilkins Company, 1968.

20

The Chemical Senses—
Taste and Smell

THE SENSE OF TASTE

Taste is a function of the *taste buds* in the mouth, and its importance lies in the fact it allows the person to select his food in accord with his desires and perhaps also in accord with the needs of the tissues for specific nutritive substances.

On the basis of psychologic studies, there are generally believed to be at least four *primary* sensations of taste: *sour, salty, sweet, and bitter*. Yet we know that a person can perceive literally hundreds of different tastes. These are all supposed to be combinations of the four primary sensations in the same manner that all the colors of the spectrum are combinations of three primary color sensations, as described in Chapter 17. However, there might be other less conspicuous classes or subclasses of primary sensations. Nevertheless, the following discussion is based on the usual classification of only four primary tastes.

THE PRIMARY SENSATIONS OF TASTE

The Sour Taste. The sour taste is caused by acids, and the intensity of the taste sensation is approximately proportional to the logarithm of the *hydrogen ion concentration*. That is, the more acidic the acid, the stronger becomes the sensation.

The Salty Taste. The salty taste is elicited by ionized salts. The quality of the taste varies somewhat from one salt to another because the salts also elicit other taste sensations besides saltiness. The cations of the salts are mainly reponsible for the salty taste, but the anions also contribute at least to some extent.

The Sweet Taste. The sweet taste is not caused by any single class of chemicals. A list of some of the types of chemicals that cause this taste includes: sugars, glycols, alcohols, aldehydes, ketones, amides, esters, amino acids, sulfonic acids, halogenated acids, and inorganic salts of lead and beryllium. Note specifically that almost all the substances that cause a sweet taste are organic chemicals; the only inorganic substances that elicit the sweet taste at all are certain salts of lead and beryllium.

Table 20–1 shows the relative intensities of taste of certain substances that cause the sweet taste. *Sucrose*, which is common table sugar, is considered to have an index of 1. Note that one of the substances has a sweet index 5000 times as great as that of sucrose. However, this extremely sweet substance, known as *P-4000*, is unfortunately extremely toxic and therefore cannot be used as a sweetening agent. *Saccharin*, on the other hand, is also more than 600 times as sweet as common table sugar, and since it is not toxic it can be used with impunity as a sweetening agent.

The Bitter Taste. The bitter taste, like the sweet taste, is not caused by any single type of chemical agent, but, here again, the substances that give the bitter taste are almost entirely organic substances. Two particular classes of substances are especially likely to cause bitter taste sensations, (1) long chain organic substances and (2) alkaloids. The alkaloids include many of the drugs used in medicines such as quinine, caffeine, strychnine, and nicotine.

285

TABLE 20–1. Relative Taste Indices of Different Substances

Sour Substances	Index	Bitter Substances	Index	Sweet Substances	Index	Salty Substances	Index
Hydrochloric acid	1	Quinine	1	Sucrose	1	NaCl	1
Formic acid	1.1	Brucine	11	1-propoxy-2-amino-		NaF	2
Chloracetic acid	0.9	Strychnine	3.1	4-nitrobenzene	5000	CaCl$_2$	1
Acetyllactic acid	0.85	Nicotine	1.3	Saccharin	675	NaBr	0.4
Lactic acid	0.85	Phenylthiourea	0.9	Chloroform	40	NaI	0.35
Tartaric acid	0.7	Caffeine	0.4	Fructose	1.7	LiCl	0.4
Malic acid	0.6	Veratrine	0.2	Alanine	1.3	NH$_4$Cl	2.5
Potassium H tartrate	0.58	Pilocarpine	0.16	Glucose	0.8	KCl	0.6
Acetic acid	0.55	Atropine	0.13	Maltose	0.45		
Citric acid	0.46	Cocaine	0.02	Galactose	0.32		
Carbonic acid	0.06	Morphine	0.02	Lactose	0.3		

From Derma: *Proc. Oklahoma Acad. Sc.*, 27:9, 1947; and Pfaffman: Handbook of Physiology, Sec. I, Vol. I, p. 507, 1959. Baltimore, The Williams & Wilkins Co.

Some substances that at first taste sweet have a bitter after-taste. This is true of saccharin, which makes this substance objectionable to some people. Some substances have a sweet taste on the front of the tongue, where taste buds with special sensitivity to the sweet taste are principally located, and a bitter taste on the back of the tongue, where taste buds more sensitive to the bitter taste are located.

The bitter taste, when it occurs in high intensity, usually causes the person or animal to reject the food. This is undoubtedly an important purposive function of the bitter taste sensation because many of the deadly toxins found in poisonous plants are alkaloids, and these all cause an intensely bitter taste.

Threshold for Taste

The threshold for stimulation of the sour taste by hydrochloric acid averages 0.0009 N; for stimulation of the salty taste by sodium chloride: 0.01 M; for the sweet taste by sucrose: 0.01 M; and for the bitter taste by quinine: 0.000008 M. Note especially how much more sensitive is the bitter taste sense to stimuli than all the others, which would be expected since this sensation provides an important protective function.

Table 20–1 gives the relative taste indices (the reciprocals of the taste thresholds) of different substances. In this table, the intensities of the four different primary sensations of taste are referred, repectively, to the intensities of taste of hydrochloric acid, quinine, sucrose, and sodium chloride, each of which is considered to have a taste index of 1.

Taste Blindness. Many persons are taste blind for certain substances, especially for different types of thiourea compounds. A substance used frequently by psychologists for demonstrating taste blindness is *phenylthiocarbamide*, for which approximately 15 to 30 per cent of all people exhibit taste blindness, the exact percentage depending on the method of testing.

THE TASTE BUD AND ITS FUNCTION

Figure 20–1 illustrates a taste bud, which has a diameter of about $\frac{1}{30}$ millimeter and a length of about $\frac{1}{16}$ millimeter. The taste bud is composed of about 40 modified epithelial cells called *taste cells*. These cells are continually being replaced by mitotic division from the surrounding epithelial cells so that some are young cells and others mature cells that lie toward the center of the bud and soon dissolute. The life span of each taste cell is about ten days.

The outer tips of the taste cells are arranged around a minute *taste pore*, shown in Figure

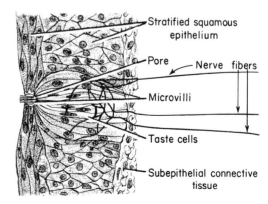

Figure 20–1. The taste bud.

20–1. From the tip of each cell, several *microvilli*, or *taste hairs*, about 2 to 3 microns in length and 0.2 micron in width, protrude outward through the taste pore to approach the cavity of the mouth. These microvilli are believed to provide the receptor surface for taste.

Interwoven among the taste cells is a branching terminal network of several *taste nerve fibers* that are stimulated by the taste cells. These fibers invaginate deeply into folds of the taste cell membranes, so that there is extremely intimate contact between the taste cells and the nerves. Several taste buds can be innervated by the same taste fiber.

An interesting feature of the taste buds is that they completely degenerate when the taste nerve fibers are destroyed. Then, if the taste fibers regrow to the epithelial surface of the mouth, the local epithelial cells regroup themselves to form new taste buds. This illustrates the important principle of "trophic" function of nerve fibers in certain parts of the body. The cause of the tropism is unknown, but it has been postulated to be a protein trophic factor secreted by the nerve endings.

Location of the Taste Buds. The taste buds are found on three out of four different types of papillae of the tongue, as follows: (1) A large number of taste buds are on the walls of the troughs that surround the circumvallate papillae, which form a V line toward the posterior of the tongue. (2) Moderate numbers of taste buds are on the fungiform papillae over the front surface of the tongue. (3) Moderate numbers are on the foliate papillae located in the folds along the posterolateral surfaces of the tongue. Additional taste buds are located on the palate and a few on the tonsillar pillars and at other points around the nasopharynx. Adults have approximately 10,000 taste buds, and children a few more. Beyond the age of 45 many taste buds rapidly degenerate causing the taste sensation to become progressively less critical.

Especially important in relation to taste is the tendency for taste buds subserving particular primary sensations of taste to be localized in special areas. The sweet taste is localized *principally* on the anterior surface and tip of the tongue, the salty and sour tastes on the two lateral sides of the tongue, and the bitter taste on the circumvallate papillae on the posterior of the tongue.

Specificity of Taste Buds for the Primary Taste Stimuli. In the foregoing paragraphs we have discussed taste buds as if each responded to a particular type of taste stimulus and not to other taste stimuli. In a statistical sense this is true, but so far as any single taste bud is concerned, it is not true, for most taste buds respond to varying extents to at least three and usually to all four of the primary taste stimuli.

Figure 20–2 illustrates the responsiveness of four different taste buds to the different primary tastes. Figure 20–2A illustrates a bud responsive to all four types of taste stimuli, but especially to saltiness. Figure 20–2B illustrates a taste bud strongly responsive to sourness and saltiness but also responsive to a moderate degree to both bitterness and sweetness. Likewise, Figures 20–2C and 20–2D illustrate responsive characteristics of two other taste buds.

Detection of Different Sensations of Taste by the Taste Buds. Since each taste bud responds to multiple primary taste stimuli, it is difficult to understand how a person perceives the different primary taste sensations independently of each other. However, a theory attempting to explain this is the following: Some area in the nervous system presumably is capable of detecting the *ratios* of stimulation of the different types of taste buds. For the sweet taste, a taste bud that responds strongly to sweet stimuli will transmit a stronger signal than will a taste bud that responds only weakly to the sweet taste. Thus, the ratio of the signal strength from the first bud to the signal strength from the second is high, and it is this *ratio* that elicits the sweet taste. Likewise, other ratios from other taste buds will theoretically be perceived as salty, sour, and bitter tastes.

Tastes besides the four primary tastes obviously would be detected as still other ratios of stimulation of the different taste buds, thus giv-

Figure 20–2. Specific responsiveness of four different types of taste buds, showing multiple stimulation by the different primary sensations of taste in the case of each of the taste buds.

ing all the different gradations of taste sensations that are known to occur.

Mechanism of Stimulation of Taste Buds. *The Receptor Potential.* The membrane of the taste cell, like that of other sensory receptor cells, normally is negatively charged on the inside with respect to the outside. Application of a taste substance to the taste hairs causes partial loss of this negative potential. The decrease in potential, within a wide range, is approximately proportional to the logarithm of concentration of the stimulating substance. This change in potential in the taste cell is the *receptor potential* for taste.

The mechanism by which the stimulating substance reacts with the taste hairs to initiate the receptor potential is unknown. It is believed by some physiologists that the substance is simply adsorbed to receptors on the surface of the taste hair and that this adsorption changes the physical characteristics of the hair membrane. This in turn makes the taste cell more permeable to ions and thus depolarizes the cell. The substance is gradually washed away from the taste hair by the saliva, thus removing the taste stimulus. Supposedly, the type of receptor substance or substances in each taste hair determine the types of taste substances that will elicit responses.

Generation of Nerve Impulses by the Taste Bud. The taste nerve fiber endings are encased by folds of the taste cell membranes. In some way not understood the receptor potentials of the taste cells generate impulses in the taste fibers. On first application of the taste stimulus, the rate of discharge of the nerve fibers rises to a peak in a small fraction of a second, but then it adapts within the next 2 seconds back to a much lower steady level. Thus, a strong immediate signal is transmitted by the taste nerve, and a much weaker continuous signal is transmitted as long as the taste bud is exposed to the taste stimulus.

TRANSMISSION OF TASTE SIGNALS INTO THE CENTRAL NERVOUS SYSTEM

Figure 20–3 illustrates the neuronal pathways for transmission of taste sensations from the tongue and pharyngeal region into the central nervous system. Taste impulses from the anterior two thirds of the tongue pass first into the *fifth nerve* and then through the *chorda tympani* into the *seventh nerve*, thence into the *tractus solitarius* in the brain stem. Taste sensations

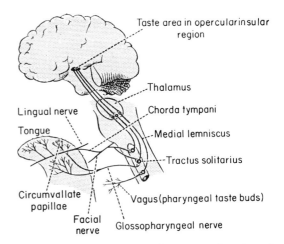

Figure 20–3. Transmission of taste impulses into the central nervous system.

from the circumvallate papillae on the back of the tongue and from other posterior regions of the mouth are transmitted through the *ninth nerve* also into the *tractus solitarius* but at a slightly lower level. Finally, a few taste impulses are transmitted into the *tractus solitarius* from the base of the tongue and other parts of the pharynegeal region by way of the *vagus nerve*. All taste fibers synapse in the *nuclei of the tractus solitarius* and send second order neurons to a small area of the *thalamus* located slightly medial to the thalamic terminations of the facial regions of the dorsal column-medial lemniscal system. From the thalamus, third order neurons are believed to be transmitted to the *parietal opercular-insular area* of the cerebral cortex. This lies at the very lateral margin of the postcentral gyrus in the sylvian fissure in close association with, or even superimposed on, the tongue area of somatic area I.

From this description of the taste pathways, it immediately becomes evident that they parallel closely the somatic pathways from the tongue.

Taste Reflexes. From the tractus solitarius a large number of impulses are transmitted directly into the *superior* and *inferior salivatory nuclei*, and these in turn transmit impulses to the submaxillary and parotid glands to help control the secretion of saliva during the ingestion of food.

Adaptation of Taste. Everyone is familiar with the fact that taste sensations adapt rapidly. Yet, from electrophysiological studies of taste nerve fibers, it seems that the taste buds themselves do not adapt enough by themselves to account for all or most of the taste adaptation. They have a rapid period of adaptation during the first 2 to 3 seconds after contact with the taste stimulus. The first burst of impulses from the taste bud allows one to detect extremely minute concentrations of taste substances, but normal concentrations of taste substances cause prolonged discharge of the taste fibers. Therefore, the progressive adaptation that occurs in the sensation of taste has been postulated to occur in the central nervous system itself, though the mechanism and site of this is not known. If this is true—and it is still questionable—it is a mechanism that is different from that of other sensory systems, which adapt almost entirely in the receptors.

SPECIAL ATTRIBUTES OF THE TASTE SENSE

Affective Nature of Taste. *Pleasantness* and *unpleasantness* are called the "affective" attributes of a sensation. Figure 20–4 illustrates the affective effects of different types of taste at different concentrations of the stimulating substances, showing, strangely enough, that the sweet taste is likely to be unpleasant at a very low concentration but very pleasant at high concentrations. The other types of taste, on the other hand, are likely to be pleasant at low concentrations but exceedingly unpleasant at high concentrations. This is particularly true of the bitter taste.

Importance of the Sense of Smell in Taste. Persons with severe colds frequently state that they have lost their sense of taste. However, on testing the

Figure 20–4. The affective nature of the different primary sensations of taste at progressively increasing degrees of taste stimulus. (From Engel in Woodworth and Schlosberg: Experimental Psychology. Holt, Rinehart & Winston, Inc., 1954.)

taste sensations, these are found to be completely normal. This illustrates that much of what we call taste is actually smell. Odors from the food can pass upward into the nasopharynx, often stimulating the olfactory system thousands of times as strongly as the taste system. For instance, if the olfactory system is intact, alcohol can be "tasted" in $1/_{50,000}$ the concentration required when the olfactory system is not intact.

Taste Preference and Control of the Diet. Taste preferences mean simply that an animal will choose certain types of food in preference to others, and he automatically uses this to help control the type of diet he eats. Furthermore, to a great extent his taste preferences change in accord with the needs of the body for certain specific substances. The following experimental studies will illustrate this ability of an animal to choose food in accord with the need of his body: First, adrenalectomized animals automatically select drinking water with a high concentration of sodium chloride in preference to pure water, and this in many instances is sufficient to supply the needs of the body and prevent death as a result of salt depletion. Second, an animal injected with excessive amounts of insulin develops a depleted blood sugar, and he automatically chooses the sweetest food from among many samples. Third, parathyroidectomized animals automatically choose drinking water with high concentration of calcium chloride.

These same phenomena are also observed in many instances of everyday life. For instance, the salt licks of the desert region are known to attract animals from far and wide, and even the human being rejects any food that has an unpleasant affective sensation, which certainly in many instances protects our bodies from undesirable substances.

The phenomenon of taste preference almost certainly results from some mechanism located in the central nervous system and not from a mechanism in the taste buds themselves, because many experiments have demonstrated that taste preference can occur in animals even in the absence of changes in stimulus threshold of the taste buds for the substances involved. Another reason for believing this to be a central phenomenon is that previous experience with unpleasant or pleasant tastes plays a major role in determining one's different taste preferences. For instance, if a person becomes sick immediately after eating a particular type of food, he generally develops a negative taste preference, or taste aversion, for that particular food thereafter; the same effect can be demonstrated in animals.

THE SENSE OF SMELL

Smell is the least well understood sense. This results partly from the location of the olfactory membrane high in the nose where it is difficult to study and partly from the fact that the sense of smell is a subjective phenomenon that cannot be studied with ease in lower animals. Still another complicating problem is the fact that the sense of smell is almost rudimentary in the human being in comparison with that of some lower animals.

THE OLFACTORY MEMBRANE

The olfactory membrane lies in the superior part of each nostril, as illustrated in Figure 20–6. Medially it folds downward over the surface of the septum, and laterally it folds over the superior turbinate and even over a small portion of the upper surface of the middle turbinate. In each nostril the olfactory membrane has a surface area of approximately 2.4 square centimeters.

The Olfactory Cells. The receptor cells for the smell sensation are the *olfactory cells*, which are actually bipolar nerve cells derived originally from the central nervous system itself. There are about 100 million of these cells in the olfactory epithelium interspersed among *sustentacular cells,* as shown in Figure 20–5. The mucosal end of the olfactory cell forms a knob called the *olfactory vesicle* from which large numbers of *olfactory hairs*, or *cilia*, 0.3 micron in diameter and 50 to 150 microns in length, project into the mucus that coats the inner surface of the nasal cavity. These projecting olfactory hairs are believed to react to odors in the air and then to stimulate the olfactory cells, as is discussed below. Spaced among the olfactory cells in the olfactory membrane are many small *glands of Bowman* that secrete mucus onto the surface of the olfactory membrane.

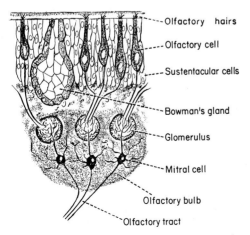

Figure 20–5. Organization of the olfactory membrane. (After Maximow and Bloom: A Textbook of Histology.)

STIMULATION OF THE OLFACTORY CELLS

The Necessary Stimulus for Smell. We do not know what it takes chemically to stimulate the olfactory cells. Yet we do know the physical characteristics of the substances that cause olfactory stimulation: First, the substance must be volatile so that it can be sniffed into the nostrils. Second, it must be at least slightly water soluble so that it can pass through the mucus to the olfactory cells. And, third, it must also be lipid soluble, presumably because the olfactory hairs and outer tips of the olfactory cells are composed principally of lipid materials.

Regardless of the basic mechanism by which the olfactory cells are stimulated, it is known that they become stimulated only when air blasts upward into the superior region of the nose. Therefore, smell occurs in cycles along with the inspirations, which indicates that the olfactory receptors respond in milliseconds to the volatile agents. Because smell intensity is exacerbated by blasting air through the upper reaches of the nose, a person can greatly increase his sensitivity of smell by the well known sniffing technique.

Receptor Potentials in Olfactory Cells. The olfactory cells are believed to react to olfactory stimuli in the same manner that most other sensory receptors react to their specific stimuli; that is, by generating a receptor potential, which in turn initiates nerve impulses in the olfactory nerve fibers. An experiment that demonstrates this property of the olfactory receptors is the following: An electrode is placed on the surface of the olfactory membrane, and its electrical potential with respect to the remainder of the body is recorded. When an odorous substance is insufflated into the nostril, the potential becomes negative and remains negative as long as the odorous air continues to pass through the nostril. This electrical recording is called the *electro-olfactogram*, and it is believed to result from summation of receptor potentials developed in the receptor olfactory cells.

Over a wide range, both the amplitude of the electro-olfactogram and the rate of olfactory nerve impulses are approximately proportional to the logarithm of the stimulus strength, which illustrates that the olfactory receptors tend to obey principles of transduction similar to those of other sensory receptors.

Adaptation. The olfactory receptors adapt approximately 50 per cent in the first second or so after stimulation. Thereafter, they adapt further very slowly. Yet we all know from our own experience that smell sensations adapt almost to extinction within a minute or more after one enters a strongly odorous atmosphere. Since the psychological adaptation seems to be more rapid than the adaptation of the receptors, it has been suggested that at least part of this adaptation occurs in the central nervous system, as has also been postulated for adaptation of taste sensations.

Search for the Primary Sensations of Smell. Most physiologists are convinced that the many smell sensations are subserved by a few rather discrete primary sensations in the same way that taste is subserved by sour, sweet, bitter, and salty sensations. Thus far, only minor success has been achieved in classifying the primary sensations of smell. Yet, on the basis of psychological tests and action potential studies from various points in the olfactory nerve pathways, it has been postulated that about seven different primary classes of olfactory stimulants preferentially excite separate olfactory cells. These classes of olfactory stimulants may be characterized as follows:

1. Camphoraceous
2. Musky
3. Floral
4. Pepperminty
5. Ethereal
6. Pungent
7. Putrid

However, it is unlikely that this list actually represents the true primary sensations of smell even though it does illustrate the results of one of the many attempts to classify them. Indeed, several clues in recent years have indicated that there may be as many as *50* or more primary sensations of smell—a marked contrast to there being only *three* primary sensations of color detected by the eyes and only *four* primary sensations of taste detected by the tongue. For instance, individual persons have been found who are specifically *odor-blind* for more than 50 different substances. Since it is presumed that odor-blindness for each substance represents a lack of the appropriate receptor for that substance, it is postulated that the sense of smell might be subserved by 50 or more primary smell sensations.

Two basic theories have been postulated to explain the abilities of different receptors to respond selectively to different types of olfactory stimulants, the *chemical theory* and the *physical theory*. The chemical theory assumes that *receptor chemicals* in the membranes of the olfactory hairs react specifically with the different types of olfactory stimulants. The type of receptor chemical determines the type of stimulant that will elicit a response in the olfactory cell. The reaction between the stimulant and the re-ceptor substance supposedly increases the permeability of the olfactory hair membrane, and this in turn creates the receptor potential in the olfactory cell that generates impulses in the olfactory nerve fibers.

The physical theory assumes that differences in *physical receptor sites* on the olfactory hair membranes of separate olfactory cells allow specific olfactory stimulants to adsorb to the membranes of different olfactory cells. A fact that supports this theory is that many substances that have very different chemical properties but that have almost identical molecular shapes have the same odor. This indicates that a physical property of the stimulant might determine the odor.

Affective Nature of Smell. Smell, equally as much as taste, has the affective qualities of either pleasantness or unpleasantness. Because of this, smell is as important as, if not more important than, taste in the selection of food. Indeed, a person who has previously eaten food that has disagreed with him is often nauseated by the smell of that same type of food on a second occasion. Other types of odors that have proved to be unpleasant in the past may also provoke a disagreeable feeling; on the other hand, perfume of the right quality can wreak havoc with the masculine emotions. In addition, in some lower animals odors are the primary excitant of sexual drive.

Threshold for Smell. One of the principal characteristics of smell is the minute quantity of the stimulating agent in the air required to effect a smell sensation. For instance, the substance *methyl mercaptan* can be smelled when only 1/25,000,000,000 milligram is present in each milliliter of air. Because of this low threshold, this substance is mixed with natural gas to give it an odor that can be detected when it leaks from a gas pipe.

Measurement of Smell Threshold. One of the problems in studying smell has been difficulty in obtaining accurate measurements of the threshold stimulus required to induce smell. The simplest technique is simply to allow a person to sniff different substances in his usual manner of smelling. Indeed, some investigators feel that this is equally as satisfactory as almost any other procedure. However, to eliminate variations from person to person, more objective methods have been developed: One of these has been to place the subject's head into a box containing the volatilized agent. Appropriate precautions are taken to exclude odors from the person's own body. The person is allowed to breathe naturally, but the volatilized agent is distributed evenly in the air that is breathed.

Gradations of Smell Intensities. Though the threshold concentrations of substances that evoke smell are extremely slight, concentrations only 10 to 50 times above the threshold values evoke maximum intensity of smell. This is in contrast to most other sensory systems of the body, in which the ranges of detection are tremendous–for instance 500,000 to 1 in the case of the eyes and 1,000,000,000,000 to 1 in the case of the ears. This perhaps can be explained by the fact that smell is concerned more with detecting the presence or absence of odors than with quantitative detection of their intensities.

TRANSMISSION OF SMELL SENSATIONS INTO THE CENTRAL NERVOUS SYSTEM

The function of the central nervous system in olfaction is almost as vague as the function of the peripheral receptors. However, Figures 20–5 and 20–6 illustrate the general plan for transmission of olfactory sensations into the central nervous system. Figure 20–5 shows a number of separate *olfactory cells* sending axons into the *olfactory bulb* to end on *dendrites from mitral cells* in a structure called the *glomerulus*. Approximately 25,000 axons enter each glomerulus and synapse with about 25 mitral cells that in turn send signals into the brain.

Figure 20–6 shows the major pathways for transmission of olfactory signals from the mitral cells into the brain. The fibers from the mitral cells travel through the olfactory tract and terminate either primarily or through relay neurons in two principal areas of the brain called the *medial olfactory area* and the *lateral olfactory area*, respectively. The medial olfactory

area is composed of a large group of nuclei located in the midportion of the brain superiorly and anteriorly to the hypothalamus. This group includes the *septum pellucidum*, the *gyrus subcallosus*, the *paraolfactory area*, the *olfactory trigone*, and the *medial part of the anterior perforated substance*.

The lateral olfactory area is composed of the *prepyriform area*, the *uncus*, the *lateral part of the anterior perforated substance*, and part of the *amygdaloid nuclei*.

Secondary olfactory tracts pass from the nuclei of both the medial olfactory area and the lateral olfactory area into the *hypothalamus*, *thalamus*, *hippicampus*, and *brain stem nuclei*. These secondary areas control the automatic responses of the body to olfactory stimuli, including automatic feeding activities and also emotional responses, such as fear, excitement, pleasure and sexual drives.

Secondary olfactory tracts also spread from the lateral olfactory area into the temporal cortex and prefrontal cortex. It is probably in this lateral olfactory area, especially in the amygdala and its associated cortical regions, that the more complex aspects of olfaction are integrated, such as association of olfactory sensations with somatic, visual, tactile, and other types of sensation. However, complete removal of the lateral olfactory area hardly affects the primitive responses to olfaction, such as licking the lips, salivation, and other feeding responses caused by the smell of food or such as the various emotions associated with smell. On the other hand, its removal does abolish the more complicated conditioned reflexes depending on olfactory stimuli. Therefore, this region is often considered to be the *primary olfactory cortex* for smell. In human beings, tumors in the region of the uncus and amygdala frequently cause the person to perceive abnormal smells.

Centrifugal Control of the Olfactory Bulb by the Central Nervous System. The central nervous system also transmits impulses in a backward direction to the olfactory bulb. These originate mainly from undetermined areas in the brain stem and olfactory portion of the cerebrum and terminate in the small *granule* cells in the center of the bulb, which in turn send axons to the mitral cells to inhibit these cells.

Mechanism of Function of the Olfactory Tracts. Electrophysiological studies of the olfactory system show that the mitral cells are continually active, and superimposed on this background are increases or decreases in impulse traffic caused by different odors. Thus, the olfactory stimuli presumably *modulate* the rate of impulses in the olfactory system and in this way transmit the olfactory information.

Figure 20–6. Neural connections of the olfactory system.

REFERENCES

Alberts, J. R.: Producing and interpreting experimental olfactory deficits. *Physiol. Behav., 12*:657, 1974.

Bradley, R. M. and Mistretta, C. M.: Investigations of taste function and swallowing in fetal sheep. *Symp. Oral Sens. Percept., 4*:185, 1973.

Dastoli, F. R.: Taste receptor proteins. *Life Sci., 14*:1417, 1974.

Denton, D. A.: Salt appetite. *In* Code, C. F., and Heidel, W. (eds.): Handbook of Physiology. Sec. 6, Vol. 1. Baltimore, The Williams & Wilkins Company, 1967, p. 433.

Douek, E.: The Sense of Smell and Its Abnormalities. New York, Churchill Livingstone, Div. of Longman, Inc., 1974.

Forss, D. A.: Odor and flavor compounds from lipids. *Prog. Chem. Fats Other Lipids., 13*:177, 1972.

Hodgson, E. S.: Taste receptors. *Sci. Amer., 204*:135, 1961.

Kare, M. R., and Maller, O.: The Chemical Sense and Nutrition. Baltimore, The Johns Hopkins Press, 1967.

Lat, J.: Self-selection of dietary components. *In* Code, C. F., and Heidel, W. (eds.): Handbook of Physiology. Sec. 6, Vol. 1. Baltimore, The Williams & Wilkins Company, 1967, p. 367.

Moulton, D. G., and Beidler, L. M.: Structure and function in the peripheral olfactory system. *Physiol. Rev., 47*:1, 1967.

Norsiek, F. W.: The sweet tooth. *Amer. Sci., 60*:41, 1972.

Oakley, B., and Benjamin, R. M.: Neural mechanisms of taste. *Physiol. Rev., 46*:173, 1966.

Ohloff, G., and Thomas, A. F. (eds.): Gustation and Olfaction. New York, Academic Press, Inc., 1971.

Schultz, E. F., and Tapp, J. T.: Olfactory control of behavior in rodents. *Psychol. Bull., 79*:21, 1973.

Shepherd, G. M.: Synaptic organization of the mammalian olfactory bulb. *Physiol. Rev., 52*:864, 1972.

Todd, J. H.: The chemical languages of fishes. *Sci. Amer., 224*:98, 1971.

Wenzel, B. M., and Sieck, M. H.: Olfaction. *Ann. Rev. Physiol., 28*:381, 1966.

Zotterman, Y.: Olfaction and Taste. New York, The Macmillan Company, 1963.

INDEX

Illustrations are indicated by page numbers in *italic* type. Tables are indicated by *(t)* following page numbers.